# MISTAKE-BASED LEARNING IN CARDIOLOGY

## AVOIDING MEDICAL ERRORS

# MISTAKE-BASED LEARNING IN CARDIOLOGY

## AVOIDING MEDICAL ERRORS

## Bliss J. Chang, MD

**Resident**
Department of Medicine
Columbia University
New York, New York

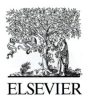

ELSEVIER

Elsevier
1600 John F. Kennedy Blvd.
Ste 1800
Philadelphia, PA 19103-2899

MISTAKE-BASED LEARNING IN CARDIOLOGY:
AVOIDING MEDICAL ERRORS

978-0-323-93157-1

---

**Notice**

Practitioners and researchers must always rely on their own experience and knowledge in evaluating and using any information, methods, compounds, or experiments described herein. Because of rapid advances in the medical sciences, in particular, independent verification of diagnoses and drug dosages should be made. To the fullest extent of the law, no responsibility is assumed by Elsevier, authors, editors, or contributors for any injury and/or damage to persons or property as a matter of product liability, negligence or otherwise, or from any use or operation of any methods, products, instructions, or ideas contained in the material herein.

---

*Senior Content Strategist:* Marybeth Thiel
*Senior Content Development Specialist:* Vaishali Singh
*Publishing Services Manager:* Shereen Jameel
*Senior Project Manager:* Beula Christopher
*Senior Book Designer:* Patrick Ferguson

Working together
to grow libraries in
developing countries

www.elsevier.com • www.bookaid.org

Printed in India
Last digit is the print number: 9 8 7 6 5 4 3 2 1

**To my dad Moon,**
*The kindest person to ever walk the planet.*
*You will always be in my heart.*

**To all the Mentors in my life,**
*I would not be me without you.*
*I hope to become as great a mentor as you.*

# CONTRIBUTORS

**Paul Yong Kyu Lee, MD**
Resident Physician
Department of Medicine
Rutgers New Jersey Medical School
Newark, New Jersey
CHAPTER 13 – VASCULAR CARDIOLOGY

**Yonatan Mehlman, MD**
Resident Physician
Department of Internal Medicine
Columbia University Medical Center
New York, New York
CHAPTER 6 – CORONARY ARTERY DISEASE

**Chinelo Lynette Onyilofor, MD, MPH**
Resident Physician
Department of Internal Medicine
Columbia University Medical Center
New York, New York
CHAPTER 15 – HYPERTENSION

**Balakrishnan Pillai, MD**
Resident Physician
Department of Internal Medicine
Stanford University, Stanford Hospital
Palo Alto, California
CHAPTER 7 – ACUTE CORONARY SYNDROMES

**Ashkon Alexander Rahbari, MD**
Resident Physician
Department of Internal Medicine
Columbia University Medical Center
New York, New York
CHAPTER 14 – VENOUS THROMBOEMBOLISM

**Richard John Sekerak III, MD**
Resident Physician
Department of Internal Medicine
Columbia University Medical Center
New York, New York
CHAPTER 10 – VALVULAR DISEASE

# FACULTY REVIEWERS

**Timothy Crimmins, MD, RPVI**
**Chief Medical Information Officer**
Columbia University
**Director**
Division of Cardiology, Vascular Laboratory
**Associate Professor of Medicine**
Columbia University Medical Center
New York, New York
CHAPTER 6 – CORONARY ARTERY DISEASE

**Jose Dizon, MD**
**Director**
Columbia Electrocardiography Laboratory
**Director**
Columbia Pacemaker and Defibrillator Clinic
**Associate Professor of Medicine**
Columbia University Medical Center
New York, New York
CHAPTER 9 – ARRHYTHMIAS

**Timothy Fernandez, MD**
**Fellow in Cardiovascular Medicine**
PGY-5, Emory University
Atlanta, Georgia
CHAPTER 5 – DEVICES
CHAPTER 12 – PERICARDIAL DISEASE

**Ian Kronish, MD, MPH**
**Co-Director**
Columbia Doctors Hypertension Center
**Associate Director**
NYP/Columbia Center for Behavioral
    Cardiovascular Health
**Associate Professor of Medicine**
Columbia University Medical Center
New York, New York
CHAPTER 15 – HYPERTENSION

**Leonard Lilly, MD**
**Chief of Cardiology**
Brigham and Women's Faulkner Hospital
**Professor of Medicine**
Harvard Medical School
Boston, Massachusetts
CHAPTER 8 – HEART FAILURE

**Nino Mihatov, MD**
**Structural Interventional Fellow**
Columbia University Medical Center, New York
Presbyterian Hospital
New York, New York
CHAPTER 10 – VALVULAR DISEASE

**Sahil Parikh, MD**
**Director**
Columbia Endovascular Services
**Associate Professor of Medicine**
Columbia University Medical Center
New York, New York
CHAPTER 13 – VASCULAR CARDIOLOGY

**Todd Pulerwitz, MD**
**Assistant Professor of Medicine**
Columbia University Medical Center
New York, New York
CHAPTER 4 – CARDIAC IMAGING

**Risheen Reejhsinghani, MD**
**Assistant Professor of Medicine**
Stanford University
**Associate Program Director**
Stanford Cardiovascular Medicine Fellowship
**Associate Director**
Stanford Consultative Cardiology
Stanford, California
CHAPTER 7 – ACUTE CORONARY SYNDROMES

**Keri Shafer, MD**
**Assistant Professor of Pediatrics**
Harvard Medical School
Boston Children's Hospital
Brigham and Women's Hospital
Boston, Massachusetts
CHAPTER 11 – PULMONARY HYPERTENSION

**Natalie Tapaskar, MD**
**Fellow in Cardiovascular Medicine**
PGY-6, Stanford University
Stanford, California
CHAPTER 7 – ACUTE CORONARY SYNDROMES

**Layla Van Doren, MD**
**Assistant Professor of Medicine**
Columbia University Medical Center
New York, New York
CHAPTER 14 – VENOUS THROMBOEMBOLISM

**Hirad Yarmohammadi, MD, MPH, FACC, FAHA, FHRS**
**Assistant Professor of Medicine**
Columbia University Medical Center
New York, New York
CHAPTER 3 – ELECTROCARDIOGRAM INTERPRETATION

# PREFACE

Toward the end of medical school, I became fascinated by how some "master" clinicians would almost always make the optimal clinical decisions, even in uncommon and tricky scenarios. Naturally, I asked a master clinician how to become as such and was surprised to hear "decades of screwing up." As I kept thinking about that humble response, it resonated with me more and more. Since our existence as a species, we have made tremendous strides because of trial and error, understanding what works and what should be avoided.

However, our current medical education system fails to adequately protect us from making mistakes. We are almost exclusively taught what to do rather than what not to do, which is equally as important. The result is that medical errors are the third leading cause of mortality in the United States, a statistic that continues to startle me today. Given the enormous morbidity and mortality associated with medical errors, and their immense learning potential, I thought it would be essential to create this work to educate on easy-to-commit errors.

Much of our most significant growth results from errors given their unique, striking emotional and psychological effects. Since recognizing the immense power of learning from mistakes, I have embraced learning from each mistake in a rigorous fashion, which I term "mistake-based learning." I hope that this term will destigmatize mistakes in medicine and open up the medical education field to new learning strategies and opportunities. I firmly believe that we can significantly reduce our collective burden of clinical mistakes by carefully analyzing each mistake in terms of why it occurred, what we can do to reverse the mistake, and how to prevent the same mistake in the future. The mere awareness of what mistakes can occur with each clinical decision we make is half the battle—it is much easier to avoid falling when you know where the edge of a cliff is!

Last but most importantly, I am lucky to have known Marybeth Thiel at Elsevier for a number of years, dating back to a prior collaboration on another textbook. Thank you for believing in this unique idea, your willingness to work with trainees, and all the invaluable guidance along the way. Without you, this work would not exist today. Thank you also to my mother, Ahn Hyee, and father, Moon, as well as my dear friends Iyas Daghlas, Alex Bonilla, and Timothy Fernandez for always allowing me to bounce off ideas. Finally, a heartfelt thank you to all the patients that have facilitated our profession to learn every day.

*Bliss J. Chang*

Bliss J. Chang is a passionate educator who reimagines medical education for the modern learner by capturing and infusing the fleeting yet essential trainee perspective into contemporary education. He is currently focused on creating novel pedagogical approaches to education, such as mistake-based learning, that he hopes will redefine how medicine is taught and practiced, ultimately leading to improved clinical outcomes. Uniquely, Bliss has reached an international audience with his work while still a trainee, including as lead editor and author of *Introduction to Evidence-Based Medicine* by Elsevier and *The Ultimate Medical School Rotation Guide* by Springer Nature. He has also created educational videos for the First Aid Step 1 book series. Bliss received his MD from Harvard Medical School, completed an Internal Medicine residency at Columbia University, and is now a cardiology fellow at the Cleveland Clinic.

# CONTENTS

# Mistake-Based Learning

Bliss J. Chang

Take a moment to think about how medicine is taught. We are almost entirely educated in terms of what to do rather than what not to do. In the few cases where we are taught what to avoid, such as through morbidity and mortality conferences or surgical checklists, we actively and frequently think about avoiding the potential mistakes and, by doing so, significantly decrease the rate of medical errors. Yet, despite considerable work from educators to decrease medical errors, there is yet to be a systematic method of discovering and learning from all the possible mistakes across all diseases and clinical actions within healthcare. It is the hope of this work to introduce such a method and begin the herculean task of identifying as many clinical errors as possible, eventually bringing to light all the ways in which a clinician may go astray. Learning what to do by understanding what to preemptively avoid not only harnesses a powerful side of human psychology but also adds a unique dimension to a clinician's skillset and bolsters mastery, akin to recognizing a road regardless of driving forward or backward, day or night. It is time to systematically teach all medical topics by including what not to do.

Mistakes have been and are still very taboo in healthcare. We are held to the highest standards; when we fail to meet them—even once—the pervasive response is often one of disappointment and blame. It is no wonder that many of our mistakes and the associated learning are kept to ourselves. A dear hope of this work is to not only teach medicine in a memorable manner that tangibly improves patient outcomes but also destigmatize well-intentioned errors within medicine. You would be surprised at how easy it is to commit certain errors or even recognize that an error occurred (many do not visibly affect clinical outcomes—we "get away" with them). Indeed, medical errors quietly lurk as the third leading cause of mortality in the United States, and this does not even begin to account for the morbidity that stems from medical errors. By supporting each other in these vulnerable moments, we can reframe mistakes as learning opportunities and harness their true power to maximize long-term healthcare outcomes. I hope that mistake-based learning becomes a way to articulate and learn from what may previously have been uncomfortable, discouraging, and even humiliating.

## What Is Mistake-Based Learning?

"Mistake-based learning" is a novel strategy presented with the advent of this book that represents an incredibly exciting and untapped area of learning. While the barebones concept of learning from mistakes is as ancient as our species, there are, somewhat surprisingly, no educational materials within any subject area (medicine or otherwise) that formally and systemically identify common potential mistakes and scrutinize them to forge powerful learning opportunities. Specifically, this book dissects each mistake into a brief case example, reasoning error(s), recommendations on how to avoid the mistake, immediate "antidote" for a mistake, common similar scenarios, high-yield notes, and suggestions for further reading.

The aim of the case example is to help readers "experience" committing each mistake. In fact, many mistakes are easier to commit than you might imagine, and the cases try to illustrate the human fallibility that surrounds these common clinical scenarios. Each case is carefully curated so as to maximize the memorability that is inherent to committing mistakes. Notably, for any unscrupulous lawyers reading this text, this work does not condone the making of medical errors, and the mistakes and case examples set forth are not based on real-world cases.

The phrase "reasoning error" traditionally refers to categories of cognitive errors and fallacies that are used to explain why a mistake occurred. While I respect the amazing breadth and depth of work on traditional reasoning errors, I have always thought that these are more conceptual than useful. For example, labeling an error as facilitated by premature closure does not get at the true "why"—why was there premature closure in the first place? Is it because there is a lack of a systematic approach to considering differentials, a high-pressure and time-sensitive situation, a lack of appropriately broad and relevant clinical knowledge, or something else specific to that particular clinical scenario? I believe it is far more effective and useful to provide the most likely *specific* explanations as to why an error occurred rather than a general label as done by traditional reasoning errors. As you will see in the upcoming chapters, the majority of "reasoning errors" provided are very specific to each clinical scenario and therefore very easy to take actionable steps to counter.

Each mistake is paired with a section on how to avoid the error. Every suggestion is tailored to the individual scenario and may include optimal clinical habits, high-yield clinical knowledge, or even novel approaches to thinking about a disease. The commonality is that each of these suggestions is readily actionable—there is no need to scratch one's head about how to best implement reasoning and behavioral changes to prevent future such mistakes.

In many cases, medical errors can be negated with various actions if caught early enough. As such, each mistake entry is supplied with the "antidote" when applicable. We hope that this provides a useful quick reference for when even the best clinicians occasionally falter. However, as with all references, there is no substitute for critical appraisal of the individual scenario at hand and one's own clinical judgment.

Many entries have a list of common scenarios for which similar principles apply. For example, hemodynamic collapse in the setting of aggressive diuresis may occur due to a myriad of preload-dependent conditions ranging from pulmonary hypertension to aortic stenosis and constrictive pericarditis. This will help clinicians understand rather than memorize fundamental pathophysiology and empower them to apply the valuable lessons in this book to even more scenarios.

High-yield notes for each entry provide carefully curated content knowledge that is deemed essential to high-quality and high-value care. Many of these facts may be little known pearls or interesting facts that help the content stick better. We also occasionally provide other tips such as mnemonics.

Last, many entries are associated with further readings that span primary literature to classic textbooks. Because this book is meant to be a fairly quick read and reference of common mistakes and how to avoid them, a low to moderate level of content knowledge is assumed for most entries; however, we believe that this resource is excellent for any level of training, and references are made to excellent reading materials whenever possible to help refresh and augment your content knowledge and understanding of pathophysiology.

## What Is the Best Way to Use This Book?

This book may be used as both a reference handbook and a more traditional textbook. For instance, a quick glance at potential mistakes to avoid when crafting a medication regimen for a patient with heart failure can instantly reap benefits for patient care. The mere awareness of what mistakes can occur with each clinical decision is key—it is much easier to avoid traps when you know what they are! Likewise, the book could be used as an adjunct while studying to help synergize and augment your overall understanding of a topic (which is taught in the traditional approach of what to do, without focusing on what should not be done). Lastly, the book is an excellent method of reviewing and debriefing on mistakes, whether individually or in group settings.

## Keeping Your Own Mistake Diary

After familiarizing yourself with this book, I highly recommend keeping a mistake diary of your own. Given the vast number of diseases and infinite permutations of clinical judgment, it is impossible for any resource to fully cover every possible mistake. By keeping track of mistakes, you can be better prepared for the mistakes that you are uniquely prone to and encounter more often in your own clinical practice. Entries need not be mistakes that you personally commit, but rather anyone's mistakes; furthermore, the mistakes need not actually occur (for example, they may be caught in the process of critical thinking and rounding). Moreover, the practice of dissecting clinical actions and mistakes will bolster your clinical acumen. The end of this book provides a few pages of templates to help jumpstart your journaling habits.

## A Final Word on Clinical Errors

As briefly aforementioned, the historical and present culture of healthcare is to label errors as a taboo subject, largely due to the implications for human life and its sanctity. However, to err is human, and we must strike a fine balance between discouraging mistakes and punishing clinicians (whether emotionally, psychologically, financially, and so forth) for mistakes that can and do happen to the best of us. Most important is embracing the educational value of mistakes and using them to enhance future patient care rather than merely viewing errors as negatives. I ask all professionals reading this text to commit to transforming your workplace culture into one that does not stigmatize errors. I sincerely thank you for your help.

## CHAPTER 2

# Fundamentals of Clinical Decision-Making

Bliss J. Chang

## General

### MISTAKE: FAILING TO ADMIT AND LEARN FROM MISTAKES

**Case Example**     An intern is taking care of a patient hospitalized with decompensated heart failure. During morning prerounds, the intern checks the patient's legs for edema by pressing her finger against the patient's calf for half a second. Seeing no indentations, she reports the patient to have no leg edema. Later during bedside rounds, the senior resident points out 2+ pitting edema observed when pressing firmly against the patient's shin for several seconds. The intern is unimpressed and says, "Well, it wasn't there this morning!"

**Reasoning Error(s)**
- Lack of understanding the mutual goal for optimal patient outcomes
- Excessive ego and/or pride
- Fixed mindset
- Environment that does not foster learning from genuine mistakes

| | |
|---|---|
| **How to Avoid the Mistake** | ■ Understand that the mission of a health care system is to provide the best possible care for patients. This involves putting aside one's ego and/or pride and being open to suggestions and teachings from colleagues, regardless of rank. |
| | ■ Help promote a safe practicing environment by supporting colleagues who make mistakes. The most important step is to move forward and learn from our mistakes while contributing to quality and safety improvement efforts to minimize future similar errors. You may be surprised at how easy it is to make mistakes; refrain from judging. |
| | ■ Make the most of shortcomings by reflecting on them with purpose. |
| **Antidote** | ■ Apologize and learn from the mistake! |
| **Common Scenarios** | ■ Not applicable |
| **Note(s)** | ■ You may be surprised to know that medical errors are the third leading cause (excluding the COVID-19 pandemic) of mortality in the United States, only behind cardiovascular disease and cancer. |

## MISTAKE: WELL-INTENTIONED THINKING NOT BASED ON EVIDENCE

| | |
|---|---|
| **Case Example** | The overnight intern is paged for a stable monomorphic ventricular tachycardia in a patient admitted 1 day earlier with a large anterior ST-segment elevation myocardial infarction (STEMI), now reperfused with a stent to the proximal left anterior descending coronary artery (LAD). The intern remembers that ventricular tachycardia can be treated with antiarrhythmics and suggests to the senior resident that amiodarone be started. |
| **Reasoning Error(s)** | ■ Underestimating the complexity of medicine |
| | ■ Relying on reasoning over empiric data |
| | ■ Not being up to date with evidence for clinical practices |
| | ■ Thinking "it should be okay" |
| | ■ Not thinking about each patient as your own family |
| **How to Avoid the Mistake** | ■ Understand that medicine and human physiology are immensely complex. Our understanding of physiology is often limited and may not adequately provide the optimal answers. Hence, we rely on data from studies that provide empiric results, which not uncommonly surprise medical experts. In this example, it is difficult or impossible to logically reason that suppression of stable arrhythmias postreperfusion actually increases mortality (e.g., Cardiac Arrhythmia Suppression Trial [CAST] trial). |
| | ■ Remember that clinical practices are always changing, as is their evidence base. Practices that may be deemed optimal today may be suboptimal or even incorrect years later. Always keep up to date with the latest evidence and clinical practice guidelines. |
| | ■ It is easy to think that something may be okay without actually knowing that it will indeed be okay. Furthermore, place yourself in the shoes of a close family member to the patient—would you be comfortable with your well-intentioned thinking, or would you want solid evidence? |

| | |
|---|---|
| **Antidote** | ■ When in doubt (and often when you are sure!), double check your understanding and knowledge. |
| **Common Scenarios** | ■ Not applicable |
| **Note(s)** | ■ Mistakes do not necessarily need to lead to harm. Mistakes that result in no bad outcomes are also important to identify and eliminate. In other words, getting away with a mistake is not cause for continuing an erroneous practice. |

## MISTAKE: TRUSTING WITHOUT VERIFYING

| | |
|---|---|
| **Case Example** | A 70-year-old Hungarian-speaking female with unknown medical history presents for evaluation of new shortness of breath. The medical student on the team speaks with the daughter, who speaks English, at bedside and reports back that the patient is taking ticagrelor. The intern astutely mentions ticagrelor as a potential cause of dyspnea, citing that approximately 15% of patients in the Platelet Inhibition and Patient Outcomes (PLATO) study experienced dyspnea with ticagrelor. However, when the senior resident calls the pharmacy, the team learns that the ticagrelor was discontinued several months ago. The senior resident gently advises the medical student to verify medications with the patient and pharmacy whenever possible. |
| **Reasoning Error(s)** | ■ Not thinking of redundancy and safety mechanisms<br>■ Overly trusting those in positions of power or high rank<br>■ Rushing due to time pressure |
| **How to Avoid the Mistake** | ■ Understand that the more redundancy in a system, the smaller the chances of overlooking preventable errors. Whenever possible, personally verify patient history, medications, data, and so forth.<br>■ Errors can be made by anyone and often involve factors that are unrelated to a provider's competency. For example, an extremely busy service increases the risk of errors due to rushing (which may also decrease the likelihood of providers using systematic approaches). Hence, always verify data yourself, even if the world's most preeminent cardiologist read the electrocardiogram (ECG). This is also how you learn and reconcile important points that may not have been considered before. |
| **Antidote** | ■ Not applicable |
| **Common Scenarios** | ■ Not applicable |
| **Note(s)** | ■ A commonly trusted interpretation is the machine's read of an ECG. These are very often wrong, particularly in the setting of arrhythmias. |

## MISTAKE: LACK OF DAILY GOALS FOR ADVANCING PATIENT CARE

| | |
|---|---|
| **Case Example** | A 44-year-old male with alcoholic cardiomyopathy is admitted to your service for alcohol withdrawal. After the patient improves and is no longer in withdrawal, several days pass with no active medical issues as insurance authorization to an alcohol detoxification facility is pending. |

| Reasoning Error(s) | ■ Developing excess comfort with the current plan |
| | ■ Not constantly thinking of how to advance patient care |
| | ■ Lack of experience thinking about when to optimize chronic issues |

**How to Avoid the Mistake**

■ Realize that many chronic medical conditions (e.g., heart failure guideline-directed medical therapy [GDMT] optimization) may be optimized when patients are stable and not medically active (e.g., awaiting disposition). In fact, it may be easier to carry out optimization in monitored settings such as an inpatient unit. Burnout can also lead to mental fatigue that creates complacency with existing plans. Always be on the lookout!

■ Understand that medical problems should always be reviewed daily for updates to the plan. Avoid becoming so comfortable with the plan that you only think about the major problem at hand each day. Avoid the temptation to think that there can be nothing done today—very often there is something that can be done!

■ As a patient approaches disposition, begin thinking more about any chronic issues that may be addressed while in the hospital.

**Antidote**

■ Plan daily goals for patients, including optimizing issues that may be addressed on either an inpatient or outpatient basis.

**Common Scenarios**

■ Nursing homes
■ Long-term care facilities
■ Inpatient services
■ Patients who have been on one service for an extended period
■ Patients awaiting disposition

**Note(s)**

■ Common tasks that may be easier to do while an inpatient include heart failure medication optimization, 24-hour urine collection, early morning labs (e.g., a.m. cortisol), expedited imaging, and education (more time to counsel).

## MISTAKE: NON–PATIENT-CENTERED DECISION-MAKING

**Case Example**

A patient is admitted to your service with massive pulmonary embolism. Under your excellent care, the patient improves on heparin and mechanical thrombectomy. Nearing discharge, you transition the patient to apixaban 5 mg twice daily. On the day of discharge, the patient nods in agreement as always as you explain the hospital course and medication plan on discharge. Two weeks later, the patient presents again with a recurrent pulmonary embolism. It turns out that the patient really dislikes taking medications.

**Reasoning Error(s)**

■ Thinking there are too many decisions to make in too little time
■ Assuming that the patient will speak up (voice her/his concerns)
■ Assuming that the patient will be amenable (especially an inpatient)
■ Language barriers (including time for translation)

**How to Avoid the Mistake**

- Understand that all medical treatments work only if the patient understands and is on board with the plan. Spending that little extra time to ask the patient regarding their preferences (e.g., once- versus twice-daily dosing). Have a low threshold to involve an interpreter as necessary.
- Realize that many patients are very deferential to their physicians and/or shy about questioning decisions. Thus patient preferences are best elicited by actively engaging with patients. Constant nodding and lack of questions may signal that a patient does not truly understand what is going on. Take the initiative and ask them questions to verify understanding.
- Refrain from assuming that a patient will be agreeable to your plan. Many patients want to feel involved and have some agency over their medical course. A particularly common place for assuming that patients are amenable are on the inpatient services where new medications may be ordered without explicitly informing the patient (when able).

**Antidote**

- Not applicable

**Common Scenarios**

- Inpatient hospital services
- Language barriers

**Note(s)**

- In-person interpreters are often much more efficient and better able to translate given additional information they receive from the patient's expressions and body language.

# Diagnosis

## MISTAKE: NOT COMPARING TO BASELINE

**Case Example**

A 70-year-old male is admitted with a high-risk non-STEMI (NSTEMI) and receives a stent to the mid-LAD. His hemoglobin is 8.1 and the decision is made for shorter-duration dual antiplatelet therapy (DAPT) with aspirin and clopidogrel given his anemia and fear of frequent bleeding events. At a follow-up visit, chart records show anemia of chronic disease with a baseline hemoglobin around 8.

**Reasoning Error(s)**

- Lack of experience or habit referencing baselines
- Fast thinking
- Not understanding how to find baselines

**How to Avoid the Mistake**

- Develop a habit of using baselines. They are an extremely powerful tool for providing context.
- Baselines can sometimes be difficult to obtain, especially if care is split between multiple hospital systems. If necessary, do not be shy about obtaining medical records.

**Antidote**

- Not applicable

**Common Scenarios**

- Troponins
- N-terminal prohormone of brain natriuretic peptide (NTproBNP)
- Creatinine

**Note(s)**

- Document baselines whenever possible. For example, a discharge dry weight and NTproBNP can be very helpful for the next provider.

## MISTAKE: NOT ANALYZING THE PRIMARY DATA

| | |
|---|---|
| **Case Example** | A 40-year-old female presents with typical chest pain. She has no family history of coronary artery disease (CAD) or any CAD risk factors such as smoking, diabetes, and hypertension. The patient undergoes a pharmacologic stress test and is deemed to have an inferior perfusion defect concerning for ischemia. When you show the images, your attending notes that the inferior perfusion defect is likely artifact due to the diaphragm. |
| **Reasoning Error(s)** | ■ Assuming that interpreted data are always correct<br>■ Assuming data interpreted by more senior people are always correct<br>■ Not trusting but verifying<br>■ Lack of confidence in one's own skills to interpret data |
| **How to Avoid the Mistake** | ■ Understand that self-analysis of primary data is critical for high-level patient care. Rather than a matter of right or wrong, it is the mere presence of an additional eye that can uncover important details and significantly help with learning to interpret studies/data.<br>■ Always trust but verify interpretations of data with the primary source, regardless of seniority. Every member of the health care team is valuable. Refer to the "Trust but Verify" mistake entry for further details.<br>■ Do not be afraid to interpret data. You will learn and improve, and experts are always there to guide you. Develop a habit of interpreting as much of study results as you can. |
| **Antidote** | ■ Not applicable |
| **Common Scenarios** | ■ Chest radiograph<br>■ Computed tomography (CT) scans<br>■ Transthoracic echocardiogram (TTE) |
| **Note(s)** | ■ In a similar vein, review articles are an excellent starting point for learning, but do not negate the necessity of reading and understanding the primary scientific literature. |

## MISTAKE: OVERLOOKING INAPPROPRIATELY NORMAL VALUES

| | |
|---|---|
| **Case Example** | A patient presents with hypercalcemia and is found to have a normal parathyroid hormone level. As you continue to review the lab data, wondering how to explain the hypercalcemia, your colleague astutely notes that the parathyroid hormone should be low in hypercalcemia. |
| **Reasoning Error(s)** | ■ Relying on the electronic medical record (EMR) to flag abnormal values<br>■ Habit of assuming all normal values are actually normal<br>■ Not thinking of the physiology for physiology-related lab values<br>■ Not comparing to baselines |
| **How to Avoid the Mistake** | ■ Understand the danger of trusting the EMR for flagging abnormal values. In other words, not all abnormal values (in context) are abnormal in absolute terms, raising flags. Always think through whether each value is reasonable based on a patient's physiology.<br>■ Think through the physiology related to each lab value to help with finding abnormal values that are hidden as normal.<br>■ Understand that values that are abnormal may also be "normal" for patients whose baselines were abnormal to begin with. |

| | |
|---|---|
| **Antidote** | ■ Not applicable |
| **Common Scenarios** | ■ Hormone levels (e.g., thyroid-stimulating hormone [TSH], parathyroid hormone [PTH])<br>■ Reticulocytes<br>■ Adjunct lipid particles [e.g., lipoprotein (a)]—may be accompanied by low or normal low-density lipoprotein (LDL)<br>■ Afebrile state (masked by acetaminophen)<br>■ Afebrile state (insufficient immune system to mount a fever)<br>■ Normal heart or respiratory rate in pulmonary embolism (e.g., masked by β-blockers or opioids) |
| **Note(s)** | ■ Remember that normal means "expected," which varies for each patient, yet laboratories use a single reference range to fit the majority of patient values. |

## MISTAKE: EXHIBITING RIGIDITY WITH REGARD TO CUTOFFS AND CRITERIA

| | |
|---|---|
| **Case Example** | A 40-year-old male presents to your outpatient clinic for CAD risk factor management. You check a lipid profile, which demonstrates an LDL of 189. You note that his atherosclerotic cardiovascular disease (ASCVD) risk based on the pooled-cohort equation is not significant yet for a statin and that he barely missed the cutoff for starting a statin. Your attending favors starting a statin, noting that a difference in LDL of 1 is within the margin of error for the laboratory test. |
| **Reasoning Error(s)** | ■ Familiarity with rigid cutoffs and criteria during medical training (e.g., standardized exams)<br>■ Not considering the wide range of normal<br>■ Not understanding the evidence basis from which cutoffs and criteria are derived<br>■ Inflexible mindset<br>■ Lack of patient-centered decision-making |
| **How to Avoid the Mistake** | ■ Realize that cutoffs are derived using a population basis and do not apply to all patients, unlike on standardized exams. Clinical judgment should be used to determine whether cutoffs are applicable and, if so, the extent to which they apply. For example, a patient who misses qualifying for a positive troponin (>99th percentile reference range) by 0.01 in the appropriate context may actually rule in for acute coronary syndromes (ACS) if the test were run again, due to laboratory error or small differences in timing of the blood draw.<br>■ Understand that it is rare for patients to present with the classic triads and pentads of symptoms. More often, unless the disease is very progressed, patients present with only some of the symptoms.<br>■ Maintain a flexible mind and evaluate the patients holistically in context to avoid overlooking atypical presentations.<br>■ When borderline, discuss the risks/benefits of proposed approaches with the patient. |
| **Antidote** | ■ Not applicable |

| Common Scenarios | ■ Not applicable |
|---|---|
| Note(s) | ■ Reference ranges vary even between laboratories and institutions given many variables ranging from different reagents and instruments to varying patient populations. |

## Treatment

### MISTAKE: FORGETTING COMMON RENAL DOSING OF MEDICATIONS

| Case Example | A 70-year-old male with CAD status post (s/p) multiple stents, heart failure with reduced ejection fraction (HFrEF) (EF 25%), and chronic kidney disease (CKD) stage IV is admitted to your service for acute decompensated heart failure. His creatinine is 2.2 up from a baseline of 1.6. Medications include metoprolol succinate 50 mg daily, sacubitril-valsartan 24–26 mg BID, epleronone 25 mg daily, dapagliflozin 10 mg daily, aspirin 81 daily, and rosuvastatin 40 mg daily. Home medications with the exception of sacubitril-valsartan and epleronone are continued. Three days later, the patient complains of sore arms and dark urine. Results of a urinalysis and creatine kinase confirmed rhabdomyolysis. |
|---|---|
| Reasoning Error(s) | ■ Lack of awareness of renally dosed medications<br>■ Lack of ownership over medications one prescribes |
| How to Avoid the Mistake | ■ Remember that prescribers should always be aware of key medication characteristics such as method of clearance, need for dosage adjustments (for organ function, age, body mass index [BMI], and so forth), bioavailability by route of administration. While you certainly do not need to know every detail about a medication, you should know its fundamentals, especially for very commonly prescribed medications. For example, rosuvastatin dosages should not exceed 10 mg daily for glomerular filtration rate under 30.<br>■ Learn about each medication and intervention you prescribe as if affecting your own health. While many institutions have pharmacists who are invaluable, learn to be self-sufficient on the most commonly prescribed medications such as heart failure GDMT, diuretics, statins, antiplatelets, and anticoagulants. |
| Antidote | ■ Not applicable |
| Common Scenarios | ■ Heart failure GDMT<br>■ Diuretics<br>■ Statins<br>■ Antiplatelets<br>■ Anticoagulants |
| Note(s) | ■ EMRs have many built-in flags, such as for renally dosed medications, but these are almost always not specialty specific and may miss many medications. For example, rosuvastatin is very commonly overlooked in terms of its renal dosing. |

## MISTAKE: OVERLOOKING COMMON MEDICATION INTERACTIONS

**Case Example**

A 75-year-old male with HFrEF (EF 40%) and atrial fibrillation is admitted for decompensated heart failure. Home medications include aspirin, atorvastatin, digoxin, metoprolol succinate, valsartan, and empagliflozin. The patient goes into sustained and hemodynamically stable rapid ventricular response (RVR) to the 160s. Two pushes of metoprolol tartrate IV are attempted carefully, but the rates do not improve. Amiodarone 150 mg is administered as a bolus, and then a loading dose of 1 mg/min is started. Two days later, the patient complains of nausea, blurry vision, and abdominal pain.

**Reasoning Error(s)**

- Not knowing common medications that are prone to interactions
- EMR alert fatigue

**How to Avoid the Mistake**

- Learn common medications that interact with other medications. If unsure, check with the pharmacist or a trusted reference.
- Though EMR alert fatigue is difficult to avoid, at least try to review alerts when dealing with medications you rarely use (e.g., digoxin).

**Antidote**

- Not applicable

**Common Scenarios**

- Warfarin
- Digoxin
- Amiodarone
- HIV medications
- Proton pump inhibitors

**Note(s)**

- Generally, digoxin dosing should be reduced by half when starting amiodarone.

## MISTAKE: ALWAYS TREATING WITH STANDARD OF CARE

**Case Example**

A 65-year-old female with recent STEMI presents to your office to establish care with a cardiologist. The patient notes that she has not been taking her statin. Despite repeated attempts to inform and convince her of the benefits, she refuses, stating that the statin dose is too high. When presenting the case to your attending, you frustratedly note that the patient is unwilling to take the statin due to the high dosage. Your attending suggests trialing a smaller dosage and seeing the lipid-lowering response, as every patient is different and a moderate-intensity statin is still better than none.

**Reasoning Error(s)**

- Not assessing for the patient's rationale
- Thinking in binary extremes (e.g., statin or no statin)

**How to Avoid the Mistake**

- Understand that patients often have specific reasons for their clinical actions. While it may not make sense to you, there is very likely an important reason causing them to act the way they do. It is your job to inquire about the rationale for a decision. Knowing the rationale may help achieve better medical care.
- Think about medical options on a spectrum rather than in a yes-no binary manner. If a patient does not want the full recommended treatment, is it better to be on some treatment than on nothing at all?

| | |
|---|---|
| **Antidote** | ■ Compromise |
| **Common Scenarios** | ■ Culture |
| | ■ Religion |
| | ■ Socioeconomics |
| | ■ Individual preferences/personalities |
| **Note(s)** | ■ End-of-life discussions and management are particularly prone to this mistake where medical futility is apparent to the treating team. Patients with certain religious beliefs may be unable to withdraw care or decline escalation of care, and this should be respected rather than fought. |

## CHAPTER 3

# Electrocardiogram Interpretation

Bliss J. Chang

# General Principles

## MISTAKE: TRUSTING THE ECG MACHINE READ

| | |
|---|---|
| **Case Example** | A 40-year-old male with a prior double lung transplant presents with altered mental status. An electrocardiogram (ECG) is obtained as part of the workup and the machine reads it as a sinus tachycardia to 148 beats per minute (bpm). The patient's sinus tachycardia is left alone for several days, but an astute resident recognizes that the heart rate appears fixed at 148 bpm. Adenosine challenge reveals a 2:1 atrial flutter. An echocardiogram is obtained and demonstrates a newly reduced ejection fraction to 20%. |
| **Reasoning Error(s)** | ■ Overreliance on technology without verification<br>■ Lack of awareness regarding the poor diagnostic accuracy of ECG machines reads<br>■ Lack of confidence in one's ECG-reading abilities<br>■ Laziness leading to reliance on the machine read |
| **How to Avoid the Mistake** | ■ Understand that ECG machine reads are often incorrect, particularly for determining arrhythmias. In fact, some studies demonstrate that up to 50% of nonsinus rhythms are interpreted incorrectly by the machine. Similarly, the false positivity of machine-read myocardial infarcts may be as high as 42%. That leaves a lot of room for error, often for situations in which the correct ECG reading is critical!<br>■ Develop a habit of using the ECG machine read as an aid rather than as the answer. Start by reading the ECG yourself and then compare to the machine read to sort out discrepancies. |
| **Antidote** | ■ Not applicable |
| **Common Scenarios** | ■ Not applicable |
| **Note(s)** | ■ In addition to clinical errors when based on incorrect ECG machine interpretations, providers' ECG interpretation skills deteriorate over time with exclusive reliance on machine reads. |

## MISTAKE: INTERPRETING ECGS WITHOUT A SYSTEMATIC APPROACH

| | |
|---|---|
| **Case Example** | A 78-year-old male presents with crushing substernal chest pressure that lasts for 20 minutes. Your team obtains an ECG, and you eagerly peer at the ST segments, looking to be the first to call out "STEMI!" |
| **Reasoning Error(s)** | ■ Bias toward prioritization of more "exciting" ECG findings<br>■ Applying clinical context to the ECG prior to discovery of all ECG abnormalities, which biases the interpretation toward what is being actively sought<br>■ Not possessing a systematic approach to dissecting ECGs |

| How to Avoid the Mistake | ■ Contain the excitement of jumping to search for personally appealing ECG findings and always interpret ECGs in a systematic fashion. Understand that important findings may be missed when jumping around in the interpretation of a complex data piece. |
| --- | --- |
| | ■ Learn a systematic approach that works for you in analyzing ECGs. One approach that is effective is to walk through alphabetically from the P wave through the U wave, thinking through every abnormality possible for each letter. |
| | ■ Approach every ECG as an unbiased piece of data to which clinical context may be applied after all ECG abnormalities are discovered. This will facilitate the discovery of any incidental yet important abnormalities! |
| Antidote | ■ Re-read the ECG with a systematic approach. |
| Common Scenarios | ■ Suspected acute coronary syndromes (ACS) <br> ■ Arrhythmias |
| Note(s) | ■ Whenever possible, compare ECGs to one or more prior baselines. |

## MISTAKE: NOT HOLDING A DIFFERENTIAL DIAGNOSIS FOR ALL ECG FINDINGS

| Case Example | A 70-year-old womale presents with atypical chest pain. An ECG is obtained and you peer through systematically, observing no significant abnormalities of the ST segments and T waves. You note "No ischemic changes." The pain persists, and the next team members read your interpretation and are unsure of what exactly you meant. |
| --- | --- |
| Reasoning Error(s) | ■ Lack of awareness regarding how vague descriptions may be less informative to team members (i.e., thinking that everyone interprets abnormalities on the ECG in the same manner that you do) |
| | ■ Mixing identification of findings with clinical interpretation |
| | ■ Lack of knowledge that each ECG abnormality may represent a myriad of clinical etiologies |
| How to Avoid the Mistake | ■ Understand that the first step in a successful interpretation of the ECG is to identify what is normal and what is abnormal. Applying clinical diagnoses afterward allows all team members to have a chance to think through the possibilities for each ECG finding. |
| | ■ Describe exactly what you see rather than intertwining them with a clinical diagnosis. Be specific about the exact changes you see. For example, "No ST elevations or depressions" is more informative than "No ischemic changes." |
| | ■ Understand that most ECG findings have an extensive list of possibilities. For example, an ST elevation does not always suggest ischemia; rather, it may represent benign early repolarization or pericarditis. |
| Antidote | ■ Not applicable |
| Common Scenarios | ■ Not applicable |

**Note(s)**

- Key differentials for common ECG findings:
  - ST elevation: ST-segment elevation myocardial infarction (STEMI), pericarditis/myocarditis, early repolarization, repolarization abnormalities (left ventricular [LV] hypertrophy [LVH], bundle-branch block), ventricular pacing, type 1 Brugada
  - ST depression: non-STEMI (NSTEMI), reciprocal changes for STEMI, strain, repolarization abnormalities (common in lateral leads)
  - T-wave inversions: strain, bundle-branch blocks, LVH, ventricular pacing, hypertrophic cardiomyopathy, Wellen syndrome, elevated intracranial pressure
  - U waves: bradycardia, hypokalemia, hypothermia

## MISTAKE: FORGETTING TO INCREASE THE PAPER SPEED TO REVEAL SUBTLE ECG FINDINGS

**Case Example**

A 50-year-old female presents with palpitations and is discovered with a heart rate of 170. You obtain an ECG as shown in Fig. 3.1 but are unable to discern clear P waves due to the tachycardia. Given an inability to distinguish the rhythm, you administer 6 mg followed by 12 mg of adenosine to slow the rhythm. The rhythm does not break or slow, and the patient moans of feeling severe nausea and "doom."

**Reasoning Error(s)**

- Lack of understanding regarding ECG paper speed and its effect on ECG interpretation
- Focusing only on data interpretation rather than optimizing data quality

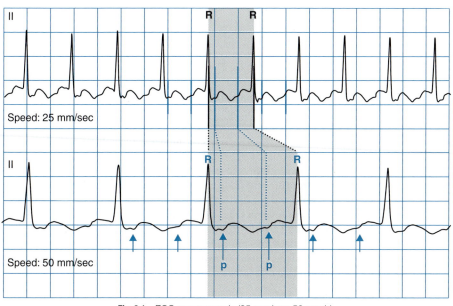

**Fig. 3.1**   ECG paper speeds (25 mm/s vs 50 mm/s).

| | |
|---|---|
| **How to Avoid the Mistake** | ■ Understand the role of ECG paper speeds in defining waveforms. The standard ECG paper moves at 25 mm/s. Speeding up the paper to 50 mm/s spaces out the ECG, allowing better visualization of P waves that may be buried within other waves.<br>■ Before focusing on data interpretation, always think about whether the data can be optimized to allow for more accurate and efficiency interpretation. The interpretation can only be as good as the data! |
| **Antidote** | ■ Not applicable |
| **Common Scenarios** | ■ Not applicable |
| **Note(s)** | ■ Not applicable |

## MISTAKE: OVERLOOKING LIMB LEAD REVERSAL

| | |
|---|---|
| **Case Example** | A 45-year-old female presents with chest pain and receives an ECG that demonstrates sinus tachycardia with some premature atrial complexes. Her episodes resolve within minutes of the ECG. Thirty minutes later, the patient experiences further episodes and another ECG is obtained. This time, you notice that her axis has become rightward and her high lateral leads (I, aVL) demonstrate new T-wave inversions. |
| **Reasoning Error(s)** | ■ Not checking the quality of data prior to interpretation<br>■ Lack of knowledge regarding the ECG presentation of limb lead reversals<br>■ Reliance on memorization of the various ways in which lead misplacement appears on ECG |
| **How to Avoid the Mistake** | ■ For any piece of data, do a quick quality check. Even the most correct clinical decisions may result in unwanted outcomes if the data are incorrect.<br>■ Learn to formally recognize limb lead reversal on ECG:<br>   ■ Suspect left-to-right limb lead reversal if aVR is positive (both QRS and T wave); another trick is to check for complete inversion of lead I (P, QRS, T waves).<br>   ■ A left arm–left leg reversal can be spotted by checking for the presence of complete inversion of lead III (P, QRS, T).<br>   ■ Reversal of the right arm and left leg leads is suspected with when aVR is completely upright.<br>   ■ An isolated near-isoelectric limb lead suggests reversal of an arm lead with the right leg lead.<br>■ Learn a quick trick to suspecting limb lead reversals on ECG. Though not formally validated, in my experience, checking for concordance of QRS and voltage (e.g., the QRS direction and magnitude should be very similar in I and aVL) in a lead distribution identifies all lead placement errors (highly sensitive but less specific—e.g., S1Q3T3 would break this principle). This is an easy way to screen for a potential lead placement error without memorizing the various ways in which lead misplacement manifests on ECG. |
| **Antidote** | ■ Recheck an ECG (preferably yourself) |

| | |
|---|---|
| **Common Scenarios** | ■ Reversal of left and right arm leads<br>■ Reversal of left arm and left leg leads<br>■ Reversal of right arm and left leg leads<br>■ Reversal of either arm lead with the right leg lead |
| **Note(s)** | ■ Limb lead reversal is a very common mistake, occurring in up to 1 in 25 ECGs!<br>■ An important but rare condition that leads to limb lead reversal is dextrocardia. R waves are seen progressively losing amplitude from V1 to V6 because the heart is farther away from the standard precordial lead positions. |

## ECG Components: Rate

### MISTAKE: CALCULATING RATE USING THE BOX METHOD FOR AN IRREGULAR RHYTHM

| | |
|---|---|
| **Case Example** | A 45-year-old female presents to the emergency department with palpitations. An ECG is obtained that demonstrates an irregularly irregular rhythm. You quickly eye two R waves and count the number of small boxes in between: 300—150—not quite 100. You decide that the rate is approximately 100 bpm. Upon looking at the machine read, you notice the rate is deemed 133 bpm. |
| **Reasoning Error(s)** | ■ Lack of identifying the rhythm prior to calculation of the rate<br>■ Not realizing the limitations to the method |
| **How to Avoid the Mistake** | ■ Consider determining rhythm prior to rate. The phrase "rate, rhythm, axis" has become engrained in medical training but may not be the ideal order of ECG interpretation.<br>■ Understand that the "box" (large or small) method relies on the premise that the patient's heart rhythm is regular as you are basing the heart rate calculation off two heartbeats. Get into the habit of understanding the strengths and limitations of each clinical tool. |
| **Antidote** | ■ Calculate the heart rate by using an alternate method, such as by counting the number of QRS complexes and multiplying by 6 (on a standard ECG, which prints at 25 mm/s over 10 seconds of recording). |
| **Common Scenarios** | ■ Not applicable |
| **Note(s)** | ■ Not applicable |

## ECG Components: Rhythm

### MISTAKE: DEFINING SINUS RHYTHM AS "P BEFORE EVERY QRS"

| | |
|---|---|
| **Case Example** | A 25-year-old female presents for a physical and has the following ECG (Fig. 3.2). You note that this is normal sinus given there is a P before each QRS. Your attending frowns and calls it an ectopic atrial rhythm. |
| **Reasoning Error(s)** | ■ Using the term "normal sinus" rhythm without understanding what it means<br>■ Lack of knowledge of criteria to define sinus rhythm<br>■ Not understanding the reason behind the criteria for sinus rhythm |

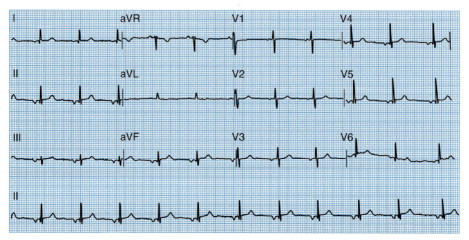

**Fig. 3.2**   Normal sinus rhythm?

**How to Avoid the Mistake**

- Understand that a sinus rhythm refers to one that is generated by the sinoatrial node rather than another area (referred to as an ectopic foci). Other rhythms such as atrial tachycardia also have a "P before every QRS," which really just suggests atrioventricular (AV) synchrony. Thus, what you are conveying by calling a rhythm sinus is the location from which the impulse originates.
- Reason through the axis of the P waves that would suggest a sinus rhythm. Most commonly, check for an upright P wave in I and II followed by a biphasic P wave in V1. This is because the overall direction of the P wave is from the right side of the heart (where the sinoatrial [SA\ node lays) toward the left, creating a positive P in wave I. Lead II is inferior and also positive because the atrial impulse travels downward from the SA node (at the top of the right atrium) toward the AV node. V1 is along the right sternal border and reflects the atrial impulse briefly directed rightward upon creation before heading away toward the left heart.

**Antidote**

- Not applicable

**Common Scenarios**

- Ectopic Atrial Rhythm
- Atrial Tachycardia

**Note(s)**

- The biphasic wave in V1 sometimes appears purely negative due to lead placement (more extreme deviation toward the right precordium). However, this does not preclude conclusion of a sinus rhythm in most cases.

## MISTAKE: CONFUSING SECOND- AND THIRD-DEGREE ATRIOVENTRICULAR BLOCK

**Case Example**     The following (Fig. 3.3) ECG is read as complete heart block.

**Reasoning Error(s)**

- Knowing second- and third-degree heart block as individual entities but lack of experience comparing the key differentiating features

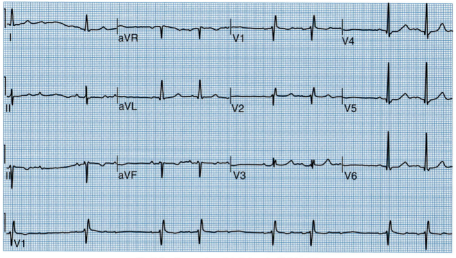

**Fig. 3.3**  Second- or third-degree AV block?

| **How to Avoid the Mistake** | ■ A key feature of complete heart block is a regular but unassociated RR and PP interval (with the exception of ventriculophasic arrhythmia, that is, sinus arrhythmia seen in complete heart block which causes shortening and lengthening of the PP interval). |
| | ■ Second-degree AV block will always feature an irregular RR interval, though Mobitz type 2 can also have a steady PP interval during most beats (but not all because a beat will be dropped at some point). |
| | ■ Grouped beating supports second-degree AV block. |
| **Antidote** | ■ Not applicable |
| **Common Scenarios** | ■ Mobitz type 1 |
| | ■ Mobitz type 2 |
| **Note(s)** | ■ Mobitz type 1 usually occurs at the AV node, whereas type 2 occurs below the AV node. Because AV nodal cells provide stable output, Mobitz type 1 generally does not require a pacemaker. On the other hand, the His-Purkinje system often fails suddenly and thus a pacemaker is recommended for Mobitz type 2. |
| | ■ A rarer mimic of complete heart block is pseudopacemaker syndrome (very prolonged PR interval, defined as >300 ms). Because the PR is so long, the P waves may appear to be dissociated from the QRS complexes. |

## MISTAKE: MISDIAGNOSIS OF PULSELESS ELECTRICAL ACTIVITY AS OTHER RHYTHMS

**Case Example**

A 70-year-old male with ischemic cardiomyopathy (ejection fraction [EF] 30%) suddenly becomes hypotensive and you are called to the bedside. The vitals monitor demonstrates a narrow-complex bradycardia and blood pressure (BP) of 71/40 (from prior 120s–130s systolic BP). You suspect a STEMI versus heart block given the new bradycardia and request a STAT ECG. The ECG demonstrates sinus bradycardia without concern for STEMI. The nurse points out that the patient has no pulse, and you label the patient as in sinus bradycardia. The nurse frantically calls for help, telling you that this is a pulseless electrical activity (PEA) arrest rather than sinus bradycardia given the lack of a pulse.

**Reasoning Error(s)**
- Lack of familiarity with PEA
- Inconsistent identification of patient's pulse
- Considering pulseless ventricular tachycardia as PEA

**How to Avoid the Mistake**
- Understand PEA: the absence of cardiac contractions despite coordinated electrical activity. Any rhythm (whether bradycardic, tachycardic, narrow, or otherwise) that occurs in the absence of a palpable pulse falls under PEA. The exceptions are ventricular fibrillation and pulseless ventricular tachycardia.
- Understand that pulseless ventricular tachycardia results from heart rates that are so rapid that the heart cannot refill, leading to severely diminished cardiac output and an absent pulse. However, the heart is contracting, and this differentiates it from PEA, in which there are no cardiac contractions.
- Learn to rely on the lack of a palpable pulse by honing your ability to palpate pulses. Good locations to palpate pulses include the carotid and femoral arteries.

**Antidote**
- Not applicable

**Common Scenarios**
- Sinus bradycardia
- Supraventricular tachycardia
- Pulseless ventricular tachycardia

**Note(s)**
- About one-third of in-hospital cardiac arrests are due to PEA.

# ECG Components: QRS

## MISTAKE: FORGETTING TO CORRECT THE QTC FOR A PROLONGED QRS

**Case Example**

A 74-year-old female with heart failure with reduced ejection fraction (HFrEF) (EF 25%) with an upcoming cardiac resynchronization therapy defibrillator (CRT-D) upgrade for left bundle-branch block (LBBB) presents with nausea and abdominal pain. Prior to administering ondansetron, you check an ECG, which demonstrates a QTc of 520 ms. You instead provide the patient with lorazepam for his nausea.

**Reasoning Error(s)**
- Lack of understanding regarding what the QTc represents and why it is important
- Taking a machine-generated data point at face value without verification
- Lack of knowledge regarding how to correct the QTc based on the QRS

| How to Avoid the Mistake | ■ Understand that the QTc represents the length of ventricular repolarization and is important as a marker of risk for torsades (acquired long QT syndrome). In other words, the risk of torsades can be viewed as somewhat proportional to the amount of time spent repolarizing the ventricles because a major mechanism for torsades is a ventricular depolarization that occurs during repolarization (R-on-T phenomenon). Thus, other factors such as bradycardia further augment the risk of torsades regardless of QTc. |
|---|---|
| | ■ Always check the accuracy of the machine-determined QTc by checking manually. Machine-derived QTcs usually do not automatically correct for a wide QRS. |
| | ■ Learn common ways of correcting the QTc for a prolonged QRS. Among the more conservative methods is to subtract the QRS width over 120 ms from the QTc. The most liberal method is to divide the QRS width in half and subtract that from the QTc. |
| Antidote | ■ Not applicable |
| Common Scenarios | ■ Not applicable |
| Note(s) Further Reading | ■ Beyond the QTc, take other clinical factors into consideration when determining the risk of torsades in a patient with prolonged QTc. These include bradycardia, electrolyte abnormalities (particularly hypokalemia), and poor myocardial function (e.g., HFrEF). |
| | ■ An excellent primer on key facts about the QTc that every clinician should know is Al-Khatib SM, et al. What clinicians should know about the QT interval. *JAMA*. 2003;289(16):2120-2127. |

## MISTAKE: OVERLOOKING A FRAGMENTED QRS

| Case Example | A 67-year-old male presents with worsening exercise tolerate over the past 3 months. An ECG demonstrates normal sinus rhythm without pathologic Q waves or impressive ST changes. You staff the case with your attending and note a reassuring ECG, upon which the attending frowns and points out fragmentation of the QRS complexes in the inferior coronary territory. |
|---|---|
| Reasoning Error(s) | ■ Lack of awareness of what is a fragmented QRS |
| | ■ Not using a systematic approach to deciphering ECGs |
| How to Avoid the Mistake | ■ Learn about the fragmented QRS. It may be thought about as similar to a Q wave, representing myocardial ischemia or fibrosis/scarring. |
| | ■ Always approach ECGs systematically to avoid missing subtle findings. |
| Antidote | ■ Not applicable |
| Common Scenarios | ■ Not applicable |

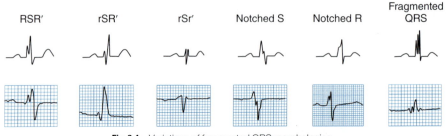

**Fig. 3.4**   Variations of fragmented QRS morphologies.

| Note(s) Further Reading | ■ Fragmented QRS complexes may present in a plethora of ways. The key concept is that one or more parts of the QRS are broken up rather than smooth (Fig. 3.4). |
|---|---|

**Note(s)**
**Further Reading**

- Fragmented QRS complexes may present in a plethora of ways. The key concept is that one or more parts of the QRS are broken up rather than smooth (Fig. 3.4).
- You may be surprised that Q waves are not permanent ECG fixtures after a transmural infarct. On the other hand, fragmented QRS complexes remain longer and have been shown to have higher sensitivity for a prior myocardial infarction (MI).
- An excellent review article on the fragmented QRS, which is a relatively new concept, is Take Y, et al. Fragmented QRS: what is the meaning? *Indian Pacing Electrophysiol J.* 2012;12(5):213-225.

# ECG Components: ST Segment

## MISTAKE: INTERPRETING ALL ST ELEVATIONS AS STEMI

**Case Example**

The following (Fig. 3.5) ECG is read as a STEMI:

**Reasoning Error(s)**

- Well-intentioned but incorrect association of all ST elevations with STEMI
- Skipping a differential diagnosis for all ECG findings
- High-pressure and time-limited situation that pushes STEMI to the top of the differential

**How to Avoid the Mistake**

- Remember to think through a differential for all ECG findings.
- Understand that ST elevations representative of myocardial ischemia generally present in coronary distributions. In other words, diffuse ST elevations spanning multiple coronary distributions are less consistent with transmural ischemia because the probability of a concurrent total occlusion in more than one territory is low.
- Look for reciprocal ST depressions. The primary reciprocal changes occur in the inferior and lateral leads. Anterior STEMIs do not typically have reciprocal changes on a standard 12-lead ECG. Posterior STEMIs demonstrate ST depressions in V1-2 (these are the reciprocal changes).

**Antidote**

- Not applicable

**Common Scenarios**

- Early repolarization
- Pericarditis
- Brugada syndrome
- Abnormal depolarization (LBBB, ventricular pacing)

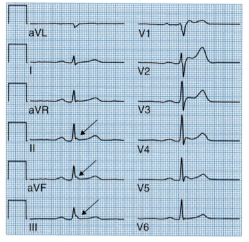

**Fig. 3.5** Early repolarization.

| Note(s) | ■ When in doubt, always call the STEMI. It is far better that an experienced cardiologist rejects the diagnosis of STEMI than to miss a STEMI for academic purposes.<br>■ Trending the ECG is an easy way to improve the certainty of your diagnoses. Ischemic changes usually evolve over time. |

## MISTAKE: IDENTIFYING ST CHANGES RELATIVE TO THE PR INTERVAL

| Case Example | A patient presents with chest pain relieved by sitting forward. An ECG demonstrates diffuse ST elevations. You compare the level of the ST elevations to the PR segment and are alarmed to measure large ST elevations. However, your attending notes that the PR segment is often depressed in pericarditis, the likely diagnosis for the patient. |
| --- | --- |
| Reasoning Error(s) | ■ Lack of understanding regarding the isoelectric portion of the cardiac cycle<br>■ Lack of understanding the pathologies that cause PR- or TP-segment deviation |
| How to Avoid the Mistake | ■ Understand that the ideal baseline for comparing ST changes is a portion of the ECG that is isoelectric (has no electrical activity) and does not change based on any pathology (to avoid confounding).<br>■ Understand that the TP segment defined as from the end of the T wave to the onset of the P wave is a period of electrical neutrality. Notably, there are no cardiac conditions that elevate or depress the TP segment.<br>■ Understand that the PR segment represents the time from the sinus node firing until depolarization of the septum (that is, the time it takes for an impulse to travel from the sinus node to the AV node, the delay experienced in the AV node, and the time that it takes for the impulse to exit the AV node and depolarize the septum) but, importantly, also represents atrial integrity. It may be elevated or depressed in atrial ischemia and depressed in pericarditis. |

| | |
|---|---|
| **Antidote** | ■ Not applicable |
| **Common Scenarios** | ■ Not applicable |
| **Note(s)** | ■ The PR segment has been called the PQ interval by some who believe that the "PR" segment is a misnomer (it ends at the start of the Q wave rather than the R). |

## MISTAKE: USING THE SAME STEMI CRITERIA FOR ALL LEADS AND PATIENTS

| | |
|---|---|
| **Case Example** | A 35-year-old male presents with new-onset chest pain, and an ECG is obtained that demonstrates a 1.8-mm ST elevation in leads V2-3. The STEMI pager is activated and the cardiology attending notes that the patient is unlikely to be experiencing a STEMI, leaving you confused. |
| **Reasoning Error(s)** | ■ Forgetting that the presence of any ST elevation alone does not indicate STEMI <br> ■ Overreliance on memory for STEMI criteria in a high-risk situation |
| **How to Avoid the Mistake** | ■ Understand that ST elevations may be present as a normal variant, depending on the lead or the patient. For STEMI, an elevation of at least 1 mm (in both men and women) is required in at least two contiguous leads, with the exception of leads V2 and V3. Due to the higher voltages seen in V2-3, it is normal to have a nominal ST elevation in these leads, and a STEMI is defined as an elevation of at least 2 mm in men or 1.5 mm in women. Last, in men younger than 40 years, an elevation of 2.5 mm is required in V2-3. <br> ■ Remember that ST elevations are smaller on posterior ECGs due to greater distance from the myocardium. A posterior STEMI is defined as an elevation of only 0.5 mm in two or more leads within V7-9. <br> ■ Refer to the American Heart Association (AHA)/American College of Cardiology (ACC) STEMI guidelines as necessary when in doubt. |
| **Antidote** | ■ Not applicable |
| **Common Scenarios** | ■ STEMI criteria for V2-3 <br> ■ Criteria for women versus men <br> ■ Criteria for young men <br> ■ Posterior STEMI <br> ■ Right ventricular STEMI |
| **Note(s)** | ■ Classic STEMI equivalents include the development of a new Q wave or LBBB (though new evidence suggests that not all LBBB indicates new infarct). New QRS fragmentation may also signal new or recent MI. |

## MISTAKE: OVERLOOKING A POSTERIOR STEMI

| | |
|---|---|
| **Case Example** | The following ECG (Fig. 3.6) is interpreted as an NSTEMI. |
| **Reasoning Error(s)** | ■ Lack of knowledge regarding the existence of posterior infarcts <br> ■ Lack of familiarity and experience with recognizing posterior STEMIs <br> ■ Not obtaining a posterior ECG due to not knowing how or its cumbersome nature |

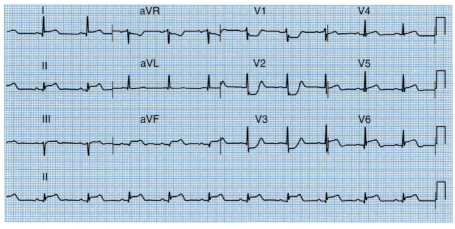

**Fig. 3.6**  Posterior STEMI.

| How to Avoid the Mistake | ▪ Understand that posterior infarcts are often overlooked given the lack of a direct ECG lead visualizing the posterior myocardium. That is, leads V7-9 placed on the patient's back are traditionally used to check for posterior STEMIs but are uncommonly used (thus, many clinicians are unsure how to position them) and may be cumbersome to obtain. |
| --- | --- |
| | ▪ Understand when to suspect a posterior STEMI. The presence of ST depressions or tall R waves in leads V1-4 may actually be reciprocal changes (ST elevation or Q waves) to a posterior STEMI. Another helpful clue is an upright T wave in the presence of ST depressions in leads V1-4. Always check a posterior ECG in these cases. |
| | ▪ Recognize that posterior infarcts compose a significant proportion of STEMIs (up to 20%). |
| Antidote | ▪ Not applicable |
| Common Scenarios | ▪ Not applicable |
| Note(s) | ▪ Leads V7-9 are placed under the left scapula in a horizontal line. |

## MISTAKE: OVERLOOKING A RIGHT VENTRICULAR STEMI

| Case Example | The following ECG (Fig. 3.7) is read as an isolated inferior STEMI. |
| --- | --- |
| Reasoning Error(s) | ▪ Lack of knowledge regarding the existence of isolated right-sided infarcts |
| | ▪ Thinking that a right ventricular (RV) STEMI is the same as an inferior STEMI |
| | ▪ Lack of familiarity and experience with recognizing right-sided STEMIs |
| | ▪ Thinking that an ST elevation in V1 must be isolated for RV STEMI (e.g., no ST elevation in V2) |

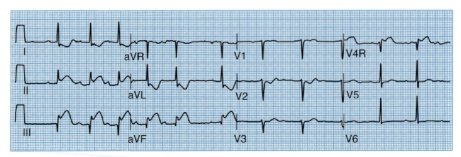

**Fig. 3.7**   Right ventricular STEMI.

**How to Avoid the Mistake**

- Understand the difference between an inferior and RV infarct. An inferior and RV infarct often share the same artery but differ in how proximal the occlusion. An occlusion of the right coronary artery (RCA) proximal to the branching off of the conus and/or acute marginal arteries will lead to both an RV and inferior infarct whereas a more distal occlusion may cause an isolated inferior infarct. Rarely, an RV infarct may occur due to occlusion of the left circumflex artery or left anterior descending coronary artery (LAD) (very rare). Notably, RV infarct occurs in up to 10–50% of inferior infarcts, depending on the study.
- Recognize clues that suggest a right-sided infarct. First, understand that an inferior STEMI accompanies almost all RV infarcts. As such, make it a habit to check for RV infarcts in all inferior STEMIs. Other clues include ST elevation in V1 (the only routine ECG lead that provides a direct view of the RV) and the combination of an ST elevation (or isoelectric ST) in V1 accompanied by ST depression in V2.
- Learn to diagnose a RV STEMI by checking right-sided ECG leads (V3-6R). Lead V4R, when placed correctly along the right midclavicular line, possesses the best sensitivity and specificity for RV STEMI.

**Antidote**

- Not applicable

**Common Scenarios**

- Not applicable

**Note(s) Further Reading**

- Remember that RV infarcts may lead to significant preload dependence and respond well to fluid boluses in the case of hemodynamic compromise. Avoid medications that drop preload such as nitrates (the sublingual nitroglycerin is actually quite a high dose compared to nitroglycerin drip dosing!).
- An old yet excellent review article on RV infarcts is Kinch J, et al. Right ventricular infarction. *N Engl J Med*. 1994;330(17):1211-1217.

## MISTAKE: LOCALIZING ST DEPRESSIONS

**Case Example**

A 70-year-old male with hypertension and hyperlipidemia presents with crushing substernal chest pain. ECG demonstrates ST depressions in V2-4. You call this a likely anterior NSTEMI and send off for troponins. The troponins return significantly elevated. Your colleague suggests checking a posterior ECG, which demonstrates large ST elevations consistent with a posterior STEMI.

| | |
|---|---|
| **Reasoning Error(s)** | ■ Well-intentioned and logical but incorrect interpretation of ST depressions using the same method as for ST elevation |
| | ■ Equating ST depressions as pathognomic of subendocardial ischemia |
| **How to Avoid the Mistake** | ■ Understand that ST segments cannot localize ischemia. In fact, the subendocardial ischemia that we often consider ST depressions to represent actually manifest most commonly in V4-6 and II regardless of where the ischemia is occurring. |
| | ■ Remember that all ECG findings, including ST depression, carry a differential diagnosis. In the case of ST depressions, always consider them as potential reciprocal changes. |
| | ■ Check for ST elevations in the leads opposite (reciprocal) to the coronary distribution with ST depression. In particular, keep a higher suspicion of transmural (STEMI) infarct in ST depressions that are not in leads V4-6 and/or II. |
| **Antidote** | ■ Not applicable |
| **Common Scenarios** | ■ Inferior (II, III, aVF) ST depressions |
| | ■ Anterior (V3-4) ST depressions |
| **Note(s)** | ■ Other ECG changes such as ST elevations, T-wave inversions, and Q waves do localize to the ischemic territory. |
| | ■ The following are the reciprocal leads for common coronary distributions: |
| |   ■ Anterior (V3-4): none (in theory, the posterior leads) |
| |   ■ Inferior (II, III, aVF): I, aVL |
| |   ■ Lateral (V5-6): II, III, aVF |
| |   ■ Posterior: V1-4 |

## MISTAKE: INTERPRETING ST CHANGES IN ABNORMAL DEPOLARIZATION

| | |
|---|---|
| **Case Example** | An ECG is obtained that demonstrates an LBBB and a 2- to 3-mm ST elevations in V2-3. You activate the STEMI pager, and the fellow notes that the ECG is not convincing for a STEMI given a Sgarbossa score of 1 and the lack of active chest pain. |
| **Reasoning Error(s)** | ■ Thinking that all ST changes are interpretable at face value |
| | ■ Lack of understanding the normal and abnormal ECG changes associated with depolarization |
| | ■ Trying to memorize criteria (e.g., Sgarbossa) without understanding the underlying concepts |
| **How to Avoid the Mistake** | ■ Understand that abnormal depolarization is followed by abnormal repolarization. Thus, a left bundle branch block should be followed by an ST segment deviation (such as ST elevation in the anteroseptal leads). In fact, if it is not, that is inappropriately normal and deserves reconciliation. |
| | ■ Learn the principle behind recognizing STEMI in LBBB. Various criteria such as the Sgarbossa criteria exist; however, it is difficult to remember without frequent use. Remember you do not need to memorize these and can always look them up. However, understand that the key principle behind these criteria is looking for inappropriate concordance of the ST segment (i.e., abnormal depolarization followed by normal repolarization). |

| Antidote | ▪ Not applicable |
| --- | --- |
| Common Scenarios | ▪ LBBBs<br>▪ Ventricular pacing<br>▪ Premature ventricular beats |
| Note(s) | ▪ The Sgarbossa criteria are sometimes applied to ventricularly paced rhythms, though this is not well validated. |

## MISTAKE: MISINTERPRETATION OF LATERAL ST OR T-WAVE CHANGES IN THE SETTING OF LEFT VENTRICULAR HYPERTROPHY

| Case Example | The following ECG (Fig. 3.8) is interpreted as an NSTEMI. Comparison to baseline a year ago demonstrates no change. |
| --- | --- |
| Reasoning Error(s) | ▪ Thinking of all ST or T-wave changes as related to ischemia<br>▪ Lack of familiarity and/or experience with repolarization abnormalities in the setting of LVH<br>▪ Not recognizing LVH on ECG |
| How to Avoid the Mistake | ▪ Always consider a differential diagnosis for all ST or T-wave changes.<br>▪ Understand that abnormal myocyte hypertrophy leads to repolarization abnormalities in the form of ST changes and/or T-wave inversions.<br>▪ Be familiar with the key ways to identify LVH on ECG. Consider corroboration with a bedside TTE when in doubt.<br>  ▪ Cornell criteria: R in aVL + S in III >20 (women) or >28 (men)<br>  ▪ Modified Cornell: aVL ≥12 mm<br>  ▪ Sokolow-Lyon: S in V1 + R in V5 or V6 >35 |
| Antidote | ▪ Not applicable |
| Common Scenarios | ▪ LVH |

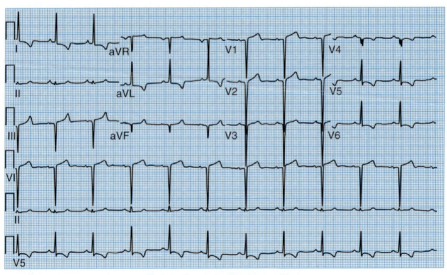

**Fig. 3.8** Repolarization abnormalities.

Note(s)

- The most common cause of lateral ST depressions and T-wave inversions is repolarization abnormality in the setting of LVH.
- LVH may lead to other ECG abnormalities such as a widened QRS and ST elevation (rare).

## MISTAKE: OVERLOOKING A WELLEN PATTERN

Case Example

A patient presents for follow-up after an episode of chest pain (now resolved). The following ECG (Fig. 3.9) is obtained. Troponins are negative twice. The patient is sent home with reassurance that his ECG does not demonstrate recent or active ischemia.

Reasoning Error(s)

- Not exploring an unfamiliar abnormal ECG pattern or dismissal without actually knowing whether the finding is dismissible
- Lack of familiarity or experience with Wellen pattern on ECG
- Forgetting that Wellen syndrome is defined as ECG findings in the absence of symptoms (i.e., mistakenly ruling out the significance of the ECG finding due to lack of chest pain or pressure)
- Thinking that Wellen syndrome on ECG is too rare for it to be real

How to Avoid the Mistake

- Understand Wellen pattern on ECG as a marker of critical LAD stenosis. The pattern consists of either biphasic or deeply inverted T waves in V2 and V3 in the absence of chest pain or pressure. Other precordial leads may be involved though less common.
- Always ask for help from colleagues and consult trusted clinical resources when you see something out of the ordinary (such as large biphasic or inverted T waves in V2-3). You will learn a lot and potentially save a life!

Antidote

- Not applicable

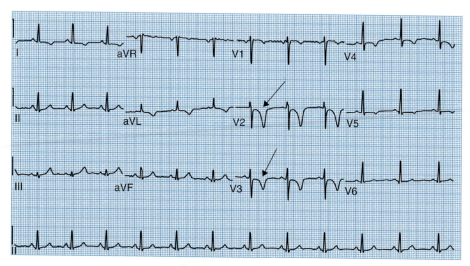
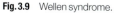

**Fig. 3.9** Wellen syndrome.

| Common Scenarios | ■ Not applicable |
| --- | --- |
| Note(s) | ■ As noted, Wellen pattern is specifically in the absence of chest pain or pressure. |

## MISTAKE: OVERLOOKING A BRUGADA SIGN

| Case Example | The following ECG (Fig. 3.10) is interpreted as normal sinus rhythm. |
| --- | --- |
| Reasoning Error(s) | ■ Not exploring an unfamiliar abnormal ECG pattern or dismissal without actually knowing whether the finding is dismissible<br>■ Lack of familiarity or experience with Brugada sign on ECG |
| How to Avoid the Mistake | ■ Refresh your memory on what Brugada sign appears like on ECG. Type 1 is a coved ST elevation ≥2 mm in V1-3 associated with a T-wave inversion. Previously, types 2 and 3 consisted of a saddleback-shaped ST elevation, though they are now no longer considered Brugada types.<br>■ Always ask for help from colleagues and consult trusted clinical resources when you see something out of the ordinary (such as a coved or saddle-back shaped ST elevation). You will learn a lot and potentially save a life! |
| Antidote | ■ Not applicable |
| Common Scenarios | ■ Coved ST elevation in V1-3 with a T-wave inversion<br>■ Saddleback-shaped ST elevation |
| Note(s) | ■ Brugada syndrome requires both the above ECG criteria and at least one clinical criterion. The clinical criteria are what you would imagine would increase the risk of sudden cardiac death, such as a family history of sudden cardiac death, a prior history of ventricular tachycardia/fibrillation, and prior syncope of unclear etiology. |

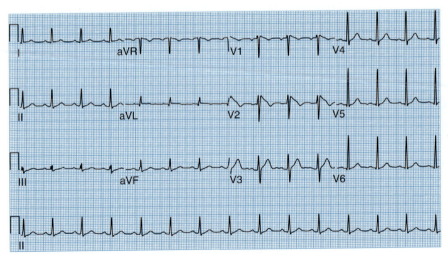

**Fig. 3.10** Brugada pattern ECG.

## MISTAKE: RULING OUT PERICARDITIS IN THE ABSENCE OF DIFFUSE ST ELEVATIONS

| | |
|---|---|
| **Case Example** | A 42-year-old female presents with chest pain radiating to the back that is relieved with sitting up and forward. An ECG is obtained that demonstrates new ST elevations with PR depressions in the inferolateral leads. Though somewhat consistent with typical ECG findings for pericarditis, due to the absence of ST elevations in the anteroseptal leads, you rule out the possibility of pericarditis. The next day, the patient's ECG now also includes ST elevations and PR depressions in the anterior leads. |
| **Reasoning Error(s)** | ■ Reliance on textbook presentations of pericarditis (global inflammation)<br>■ Lack of knowledge of the official criteria for diagnosing pericarditis |
| **How to Avoid the Mistake** | ■ Understand that pericarditis may present focally in which case ST elevations and PR depressions may be in a limited set of leads. Elevation in more than one coronary distribution increases the probability of pericarditis as opposed to ischemia.<br>■ Use clinical context (such as how pain changes with sitting up or laying down) to help inform your probability of a diagnosis of pericarditis.<br>■ Learn the formal criteria for diagnosing pericarditis. Meeting two of following four criteria is required: (1) chest pain (nonischemic and often radiating to the back), (2) friction rub, (3) ST elevation or PR depression, and (4) pericardial effusion. |
| **Antidote** | ■ Not applicable |
| **Common Scenarios** | ■ Not applicable |
| **Note(s)** | ■ You often do not hear a rub on auscultation in pericarditis. In fact, in the presence of a global pericardial effusion (which is not uncommon), you cannot hear a rub because the pericardial layers are not rubbing against one another. |

# ECG Components: T Wave

## MISTAKE: INTERPRETING T-WAVE INVERSIONS AS ACUTE ISCHEMIA IN THE ABSENCE OF ST DEPRESSIONS

| | |
|---|---|
| **Case Example** | A 70-year-old male with no known prior cardiac history presents with worsening shortness of breath over the past 2 weeks. An ECG is obtained that demonstrates T-wave inversions without ST changes in the inferior coronary distribution. You become worried that the T-wave changes reflect ischemia. Troponins are sent, which return negative. |
| **Reasoning Error(s)** | ■ Widespread misbelief that T-wave inversions represent ischemia<br>■ Lack of attention to the absence or presence of ST depressions (i.e., "never thought about that") |
| **How to Avoid the Mistake** | ■ Understand that T-wave inversions are associated with completed ischemia rather than ongoing ischemia. In active ischemia, the accompanying ST-segment deviation represents the ongoing nature of ischemia.<br>■ For patients who present with symptoms compatible with active myocardial ischemia, search for additional clues on ECG beyond T-wave inversions. |

| | |
|---|---|
| **Antidote** | ■ Not applicable |
| **Common Scenarios** | ■ Not applicable |
| **Note(s)** | ■ T-wave inversions that occur after ischemia and then disappear indicates potential recovery of the affected area. |

## MISTAKE: MISDIAGNOSING HYPERACUTE T WAVES

| | |
|---|---|
| **Case Example** | A large T wave is seen on ECG in the context of chest pain, and the ECG is labeled as reflective of a hyperacute T wave. An ECG is repeated 2 hours later, and the same T wave is still present; comparison with prior baseline demonstrates a similar T wave, indicating that the T wave is not hyperacute. |
| **Reasoning Error(s)** | ■ Vague idea of what is a hyperacute T wave<br>■ Overreporting: applying the label "hyperacute T wave" due to a clinical context that fits (i.e., one concerning for ischemia) rather than based on confident interpretation of the ECG<br>■ Lack of effort to verify whether a T wave is truly hyperacute |
| **How to Avoid the Mistake** | ■ Understand how to diagnose a hyperacute T wave: broad and symmetric, amplitude is significant compared with the QRS complex (i.e., >50%) and rarely an isolated finding (i.e., without accompanying ST elevation).<br>■ Trend the ECG serially. Hyperacute T waves are transient and should evolve into ST elevation(s).<br>■ Remember that labels in the medical record are difficult to remove (and thus potentially misleading) even if incorrect. Only interpret ECG findings as you are able, and label uncertainty with appropriate wording. |
| **Antidote** | ■ Not applicable |
| **Common Scenarios** | ■ Not applicable |
| **Note(s)** | ■ A hyperacute T wave is very transient—it often lasts no longer than a few minutes before being replaced by ST elevations. As such, it is rather rare that an ECG would catch the few minutes right after a coronary artery becomes occluded. |

## MISTAKE: LACK OF ATTENTION TO T-WAVE MORPHOLOGY

| | |
|---|---|
| **Case Example** | Refer to some common T-wave morphologies in Fig. 3.11. |
| **Reasoning Error(s)** | ■ Oversimplification of T-wave interpretation, most commonly as normal if upright and pathologic if inverted<br>■ Lack of understanding the possible variations in T-wave morphologies and their significance |

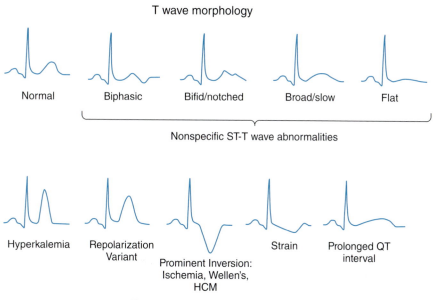

**Fig. 3.11**    Common T-wave morphologies.

| How to Avoid the Mistake | ■ Understand that the T wave can vary in appearance in accordance with the pathophysiology at hand: |
|---|---|

- Understand that the T wave can vary in appearance in accordance with the pathophysiology at hand:
  - Symmetry: normal T waves are asymmetric; pathologic (e.g., ischemia, Wellen's, hypertrophic cardiomyopathy) T waves are usually symmetric
  - Size: hyperkalemia leads to narrow-based but tall peaked T waves; hyperacute T waves are broad and not peaked; hypertrophic cardiomyopathy and elevated intracranial pressures lead to large T waves (inverted)
  - Polarity: most normal T waves are upright; it is normal to have a negative T wave in leads aVR, V1, and sometimes III
- Constantly push yourself to appreciate more and more about routine findings. For example, as your comfort develops with reading ECGs, focus on more subtleties such as the T-wave morphology. Soon, you will be visualizing and interpreting these additional details with minimal additional time.

**Antidote**
- Not applicable

**Common Scenarios**
- Enlargement
- Symmetry
- Inversion

**Note(s)**
- Biphasic T waves confuse many people, but they are actually easy to interpret! Simply look at the terminal portion of the T wave to determine whether a biphasic T wave is positive or negative.

## MISTAKE: OVERLOOKING T-WAVE PSEUDONORMALIZATION

**Case Example**  A 70-year-old male presents with chest pain, and an ECG is obtained, which demonstrates no abnormal-appearing ST segments or T waves. On a prior ECG, there are T-wave inversions in V5-6 but no other notable findings. Given the normal, you opt to let the patient go. An hour later, the patient represents with worsening chest pain and you obtain another ECG to find large ST elevations in leads V5-6.

**Reasoning Error(s)**
- Not comparing an ECG to baseline just because the current ECG appears normal
- Lack of awareness of the pseudonormalization phenomenon for T waves
- Well-intentioned and logical but incorrect thinking that upright T waves are always normal

**How to Avoid the Mistake**
- Remember that pathology on ECG is represented by a deviation from baseline (whether a normal or abnormal baseline)!
- Always compare ECGs with baseline when able, regardless of how normal or abnormal the current ECG is. This is especially true for normal-appearing ECGs in patients with known heart disease and/or a clinical presentation concerning for ischemia.
- Understand that pseudonormalized T waves (previously inverted T waves that become upright) are highly suggestive of myocardial ischemia. This is irrespective of why the T wave was originally inverted on the baseline ECG (e.g., LVH). Immediate workup for ischemia is critical in these cases.

**Antidote**
- Not applicable

**Common Scenarios**
- Not applicable

**Note(s)**
- Although pseudonormalization of T waves is a rare phenomenon (estimated 1% of ECGs in patients with MI), think about how many ECGs you have seen!

# Left Ventricular Hypertrophy

## MISTAKE: RULING OUT LEFT VENTRICULAR HYPERTROPHY IN PATIENTS WITH NORMAL ECG VOLTAGES

**Case Example**  A 55-year-old male with no past medical history presents with syncope, and an ECG is performed. The ECG is notable for bifasicular block (right bundle-branch block [RBBB] + left anterior fascicular block [LAFB]). A TTE demonstrates significant LVH (interventricular septum [IVS] = 1.5 cm, left ventricular posterior wall [LVPW] = 1.3 cm). You attribute the hypertrophy to uncontrolled hypertension despite the patient protesting they have not had hypertension their entire life. A year later, the patient presents with heart failure and a biopsy reveals AL amyloidosis.

**Reasoning Error(s)**
- Lack of understanding the sensitivity and specificity of LVH by ECG criteria; that is, associating ECG criteria for LVH as always concordant with LVH
- Forgetting to consider factors that alter ECG voltages

| | |
|---|---|
| **How to Avoid the Mistake** | ■ Understand that ECG criteria for LVH are limited in sensitivity and specificity. In general, sensitivity is quite low (ranging from 20% to 60% across studies) and specificity is decent (anywhere from 75% to 95% depending on the study). |
| | ■ Think about patient factors that may decrease ECG voltages: obesity, severe lung disease, and infiltrative disease. Even without these factors, the voltages on ECG are not always predictive of LVH! |
| | ■ Assess LVH by the gold standard of visualization (e.g., by echo) when in doubt |
| **Antidote** | ■ Not applicable |
| **Common Scenarios** | ■ Obesity |
| | ■ Severe lung disease |
| | ■ Infiltrative disease |
| **Note(s)** | ■ LVH may be masked or uninterpretable by ECG in patients with prior heart disease (e.g., LBBB, Q waves). |

## MISTAKE: OVERLOOKING ECGS WITH VOLTAGES OUT OF PROPORTION TO HYPERTROPHY

| | |
|---|---|
| **Case Example** | A 70-year-old female with hypertension presents with new shortness of breath. An ECG is notable only for a first-degree AV block. A TTE demonstrates severe LVH (IVS = 1.7 cm, LVPW = 1.3 cm). The medical student on the team is surprised that the ECG did not meet criteria for LVH and asks about infiltrative disorders. A pyrophosphate scan is performed that is positive for transthyretin cardiac amyloidosis. |
| **Reasoning Error(s)** | ■ Widespread yet incorrect teaching that infiltrative cardiomyopathies should be suspected in the presence of low-voltage ECGs |
| | ■ Thinking that infiltrative diseases must have low voltages in all leads |
| | ■ Not checking for concordance between signs of hypertrophy on ECG and cardiac imaging |
| **How to Avoid the Mistake** | ■ Understand that the key clue to infiltrative disease is an ECG voltage that is low out of proportion to the visualized LVH. Because the hypertrophy is not due to myocyte hypertrophy (infiltrates such as amyloid fibrils are electrically inert), the voltages do not increase with hypertrophy. On the other hand, LVH caused by hypertension will usually have large voltages on ECG due to myocyte hypertrophy. |
| | ■ Understand that infiltrative diseases may start focally and demonstrate low voltages only in a few leads. A high degree of suspicion and clinical context is required. |
| **Antidote** | ■ Not applicable |
| **Common Scenarios** | ■ Not applicable |

| | |
|---|---|
| **Note(s)**<br>**Further Reading** | ■ Common infiltrative diseases include AL amyloid, TTR amyloid, hemochromatosis, and sarcoid. Rarer entities include hereditary anomalies such as Fabry disease. |
| | ■ A study from Columbia University demonstrated a fascinating and high incidence of TTR amyloid in patients with severe aortic stenosis: Castano A, et al. Unveiling transthyretin cardiac amyloidosis and its predictors among elderly patients with severe aortic stenosis undergoing transcatheter aortic valve replacement. *Eur Heart J.* 2017;38(38):2879-2887. |

## Supraventricular Tachycardia

### MISTAKE: MISTAKING ATRIAL FIBRILLATION FOR SINUS TACHYCARDIA DURING EXTREME TACHYCARDIA

| | |
|---|---|
| **Case Example** | A patient's heart rate suddenly jumps to the 150s. An ECG is obtained, which demonstrates a rate of 151 bpm with RR intervals that, at quick glance, appear similar. You immediately think of atrial flutter versus atrial tachycardia given the regularity. Your co-fellow points out that the RR intervals are actually irregular but that they appear regular from afar given the fast rate. |
| **Reasoning Error(s)** | ■ Viewing a very fast rhythm from afar (e.g., telemetry or in-room vitals monitor) |
| | ■ Relying on eyes rather than calipers to distinguish regular versus irregular in very fast rhythms |
| **How to Avoid the Mistake** | ■ When in doubt (such as with very fast ventricular rates), use a caliper or increase the ECG paper speed to help determine if the rhythm is truly regular. Adenosine may also help to slow down the rate and reveal clues to the type of arrhythmia. |
| **Antidote** | ■ Not applicable |
| **Common Scenarios** | ■ Not applicable |
| **Note(s)** | ■ There are a limited number of irregular rhythms: atrial fibrillation, atrial flutter with variable block, and multifocal atrial tachycardia. Among these, only atrial fibrillation can occur at potentially very high (>150 bpm) ventricular rates. Thus, an irregular narrow-complex tachycardia at rates >150 bpm is almost always diagnostic of atrial fibrillation. |

### MISTAKE: MISTAKING SUPRAVENTRICULAR TACHYCARDIA AS SINUS TACHYCARDIA DESPITE LACK OF HEART RATE VARIABILITY

| | |
|---|---|
| **Case Example** | A 65-year-old male with HFrEF (EF 30%) is admitted for acute decompensated heart failure (ADHF). The patient improves rapidly with diuresis and is near ready for discharge. On the day of discharge, you are covering for the primary team and notice on telemetry that the patient's heart rate has been constantly around 110 bpm. Despite having been noted as sinus tachycardia, you consider it odd given the lack of heart rate variability, particularly overnight. An adenosine challenge reveals 3:1 flutter, and the patient receives a successful cardioversion prior to discharge. |

| | |
|---|---|
| **Reasoning Error(s)** | ■ Considering all tachycardias with a sinus-appearing P wave to be sinus tachycardia |
| | ■ Lack of attention to heart rate variability |
| **How to Avoid the Mistake** | ■ In patients with significant cardiac history, examine tachycardias closely and refrain from being easily convinced that a tachycardia is sinus. Rule out common possibilities such as atrial flutter. |
| | ■ Understand that heart rate trends and variability (especially a decrease in rate overnight) are powerful predictors of whether a tachycardia is an arrhythmia. Check telemetry when available for heart rate variability and the rate at which heart rate changes (i.e., a gradual increase favors sinus tachycardia versus an abrupt increase). |
| **Antidote** | ■ Not applicable |
| **Common Scenarios** | ■ Not applicable |
| **Note(s)** | ■ Atrial flutter is one of the trickiest arrhythmias to diagnose given its ability to hide flutter waves and mimic sinus tachycardia. A key feature of atrial flutter is its macroentrant circuit, which causes a very stable heart rate. Suspect flutter when the heart rate does not change (or hardly changes). |

## MISTAKE: MISTAKING 2:1 ATRIAL FLUTTER FOR SINUS TACHYCARDIA

| | |
|---|---|
| **Case Example** | A 70-year-old female in septic shock has sustained, very consistently, a heart rate of 120 bpm. Suspecting an arrhythmia, you obtain a 12-lead ECG to better characterize the P waves but are disappointed to see what appears to be a sinus tachycardia. You note that the patient has a reason to be tachycardic and dismiss the idea of an arrhythmia. |
| **Reasoning Error(s)** | ■ Inability to visualize flutter waves, leading to a conclusion that the rhythm is not flutter |
| | ■ Lack of knowledge regarding techniques to better expose atrial flutter on ECG |
| | ■ Not using the clinical picture and other clues such as telemetry |
| **How to Avoid the Mistake** | ■ Slow the rhythm down: vagal maneuvers, adenosine, increasing ECG paper speed |
| | ■ Learn the Lewis lead, a reconfiguration of the limb leads that results in a better view of the atrium than the standard lead placement. Move the Left Arm lead over the lower right sternal border followed by the Left Leg lead over the lower right costal margin. The right arm electrode should be placed upon the manubrium. Observe Lead I for the best view of atrial activity. |
| | ■ Use additional clues such as variability in heart rate (flutter usually has very little heart rate variation) and slope of change in heart rate on telemetry with the onset of tachycardia. |
| **Antidote** | ■ Not applicable |
| **Common Scenarios** | ■ Not applicable |

**Note(s)**
- Consider increasing the ECG paper speed from 25 to 50 mm/s in conjunction with the Lewis lead to even better visualize P waves.
- Another helpful trick is knowing the Bix rule, which states that visualization of a P wave halfway between two RR complexes increases the chances of a P wave buried within the QRS complexes.

## MISTAKE: MISTAKING COARSE ATRIAL FIBRILLATION FOR ATRIAL FLUTTER

**Case Example**   The following ECG (Fig. 3.12) is read as atrial flutter.

**Reasoning Error(s)**
- Associating flutter-like waves on ECG as pathognomonic with atrial flutter
- Checking only one or a few leads rather than the key leads that diagnose atrial flutter
- Not marching out the P (flutter) waves
- Lack of understanding the mechanistic basis for fibrillatory

**How to Avoid the Mistake**
- Understand that atrial fibrillation presents in two ways on ECG: small, "fine" fibrillatory waves and large, "coarse" fibrillatory waves. They are differentiated by the amplitude of the fibrillatory waves (≥ 1 mm for coarse atrial fibrillation).
- Understand why atrial fibrillation may appear coarse. As the left atrium enlarges significantly, the amplitude of the fibrillatory waves may increase. Coarse atrial fibrillation generally indicates left atrial enlargement and a more persistent form of atrial fibrillation.
- Check all ECG leads for consistent flutter waves, in particular the inferior leads (II, III, aVF) and V1, which are the classic leads for visualizing atrial flutter. Coarse atrial fibrillation often is seen in one or two leads (often V1 or V2) rather than in multiple leads.
- March out the flutter waves –they should be regularly spaced and no faster than 300 bpm in flutter.

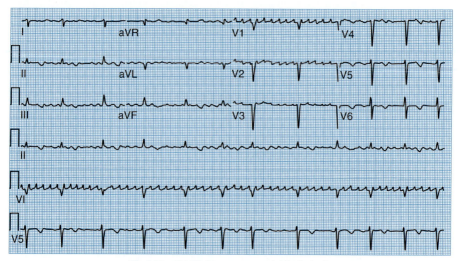

**Fig. 3.12**   Atrial flutter or coarse atrial fibrillation?

| Antidote | ■ Not applicable |
|---|---|
| Common Scenarios | ■ Not applicable |
| Note(s) | ■ In one study of 800 patients, coarse atrial fibrillation was more common in patients with mitral stenosis and associated with a significantly higher risk of stroke compared with fine atrial fibrillation. |

## MISTAKE: MISTAKING MULTIFOCAL ATRIAL TACHYCARDIA FOR ATRIAL FIBRILLATION

| Case Example | The following ECG (Fig. 3.13) is read as atrial fibrillation. |
|---|---|
| Reasoning Error(s) | ■ Thinking that the various P-wave morphologies observed are random fibrillatory waves<br>■ Associating all irregular rhythms with atrial fibrillation |
| How to Avoid the Mistake | ■ Understand that multiple P-wave morphologies may be present on a single ECG. This results from multiple competing atrial foci, similar to atrial fibrillation but in much smaller numbers (e.g., three foci).<br>■ Learn the differential diagnosis for irregular ECG rhythms. Always consider differentials for ECG findings rather than associating any one finding with pathognomonic equivalents. |
| Antidote | ■ Not applicable |
| Common Scenarios | ■ Not applicable |
| Note(s) | ■ Multifocal atrial tachycardia (MAT) is most often associated with marked pulmonary disease, such as severe chronic obstructive pulmonary disease or asthma. It is more commonly found in men and patients >70 years old. Though a high mortality rate is associated with MAT, this is likely secondary to the significant comorbidities that patients with MAT possess. |

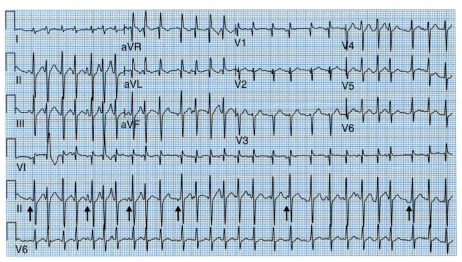

**Fig. 3.13** Atrial fibrillation or multifocal atrial tachycardia?

## MISTAKE: INTERPRETING REGULARIZATION OF CHRONIC ATRIAL FIBRILLATION AS SINUS RHYTHM

**Case Example**    A 45-year-old female with chronic atrial fibrillation is admitted for a severe allergic reaction to poison ivy. One afternoon, she is noted to have a regular narrow-complex rhythm on the in-room monitor, and you celebrate thinking that the patient's atrial fibrillation resolved. However, upon closer inspection, the patient's rhythm is missing sinus P waves, indicating complete heart block with a junctional escape rhythm.

**Reasoning Error(s)**
- Associating sinus rhythm with a regular rhythm and logically assuming that atrial fibrillation that becomes regular signals a return to sinus
- Lack of thorough inspection of the patient's rhythm

**How to Avoid the Mistake**
- Understand that chronic atrial fibrillation by definition will not revert back to sinus rhythm. Thus, a change from atrial fibrillation to a regular rhythm signals complete heart block where impulses are no longer conducted to the ventricles and an escape rhythm (usually junctional) takes over, mimicking sinus rhythm.
- Always inspect all ECGs, telemetry, in-room monitors, and other sources of information toward the patient's rhythm diligently. You will be surprised by what you catch!

**Antidote**
- Not applicable

**Common Scenarios**
- Not applicable

**Note(s)**
- Paroxysmal atrial fibrillation is defined as one that terminates spontaneously within 7 days, though it may terminate much sooner. Persistent atrial fibrillation lasts >7 days but <1 year. Chronic atrial fibrillation lasts >1 year and is usually permanent.

# Wide-Complex Tachycardia

## MISTAKE: MISDIAGNOSING PREEXCITED ATRIAL FIBRILLATION FOR MONOMORPHIC VENTRICULAR TACHYCARDIA

**Case Example**    The following ECG (Fig. 3.14) is read as ventricular tachycardia.

**Reasoning Error(s)**
- Lack of awareness that preexcited atrial fibrillation is a tricky mimic of monomorphic ventricular tachycardia that must be ruled out
- Not knowing the key differentiating feature between preexcited atrial fibrillation and monomorphic ventricular tachycardia

**How to Avoid the Mistake**
- Understand that preexcited atrial fibrillation may share many ECG features with ventricular tachycardia. For example, both rhythms may demonstrate particularly wide monomorphic QRS (>150 ms) and positive precordial concordance (in the case of an accessory pathway located near the left posterolateral region).
- Remember that monomorphic ventricular tachycardia is a regular rhythm. An easy way to distinguish preexcited atrial fibrillation is by checking to see whether the rhythm is irregular.

**Antidote**
- Not applicable

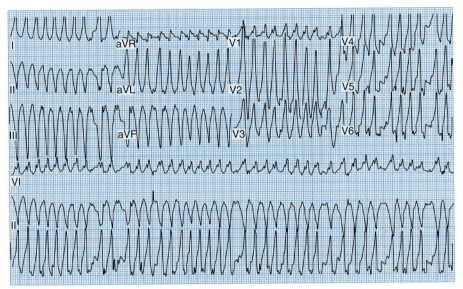

**Fig. 3.14**  Preexcited atrial fibrillation or ventricular tachycardia?

| | |
|---|---|
| **Common Scenarios** | ■ Not applicable |
| **Note(s)** | ■ Given the unique fast, broad, and irregular character of preexcited atrial fibrillation, it has occasionally been referred to as FBI tachycardia. |
| | ■ The other differential for preexcited atrial fibrillation includes atrial fibrillation with aberrancy, which typically demonstrates a baseline bundle-branch block. |
| | ■ Very rarely, in the presence of multiple accessory pathways, preexcited atrial fibrillation may mimic polymorphic ventricular tachycardia given its irregularity and multiple different QRS morphologies. |

## MISTAKE: MISTAKING SINUS TACHYCARDIA IN SEVERE HYPERKALEMIA FOR VENTRICULAR TACHYCARDIA

| | |
|---|---|
| **Case Example** | A 70-year-old female with ESRD who presented to the hospital after missing two dialysis sessions reports frequent palpitations. While awaiting urgent dialysis, you obtain an ECG that demonstrates a wide-complex tachycardia. You become worried about ventricular tachycardia and immediately call your attending, who refers you to her presentation ECG, which was a wide-complex rhythm, albeit not tachycardic. After dialysis, an ECG is reobtained, which demonstrates a narrow QRS. |
| **Reasoning Error(s)** | ■ Lack of understanding the impact of hyperkalemia on ECG findings |
| | ■ Not checking potassium levels during suspected ventricular tachycardia |
| | ■ Lack of a differential diagnosis for a wide-complex tachycardia |

| | |
|---|---|
| **How to Avoid the Mistake** | ■ Understand the impact of hyperkalemia on ECG components. As hyperkalemia progresses, it starts with peaked T waves then progresses to flattening of the P wave and/or PR prolongation before widening of the QRS. At lethal levels of potassium (often >7 mEq/L), sine wave pattern may occur. |
| | ■ Understand that almost all ventricular tachycardias will be at rates of 120 bpm or higher, especially in the lack of ventricular antiarrhythmics such as amiodarone or mexiletine. Slower rates (as is often the case with sinus tachycardia in the setting of a wide QRS due to hyperkalemia) should be a red flag against the rhythm being ventricular tachycardia. |
| | ■ Check potassium levels in the setting of a wide-complex tachycardia. Not only does it help rule out a sinus tachycardia in the setting of hyperkalemia, but it also exposes a correctable risk factor in the setting of true ventricular tachycardia. |
| **Antidote** | ■ Not applicable |
| **Common Scenarios** | ■ Hyperkalemia (leading to widened QRS) |
| | ■ Post-MI reperfusion arrhythmias |
| | ■ Tricyclic antidepressant overdose |
| **Note(s)** | ■ The widened QRS in the setting of hyperkalemia does not appear morphologically similar to bundle-branch blocks. Instead, it appears as a nonspecific intraventricular conduction delay (IVCD). |
| | ■ Very rarely, in the presence of multiple accessory pathways, preexcited atrial fibrillation may mimic polymorphic ventricular tachycardia given its irregularity and multiple different QRS morphologies. |

## MISTAKE: MISTAKING A VENTRICULARLY PACED RHYTHM FOR VENTRICULAR TACHYCARDIA

| | |
|---|---|
| **Case Example** | A 75-year-old male with HFrEF (EF 15%) and sick sinus syndrome presents with shortness of breath. An ECG is obtained that demonstrates a slow wide-complex tachycardia around 60 bpm. You diagnose the patient with slow ventricular tachycardia and administer an amiodarone bolus and drip. The patient's rhythm does not budge, and you add high doses of lidocaine and procainamide to no avail. |
| **Reasoning Error(s)** | ■ Assuming that all pacemaker impulses are always visible on ECG |
| | ■ Lack of knowing the type of pacemaker the patient has and/or inability to determine whether a patient has a unipolar or bipolar lead |
| | ■ Failure to reassess key assumptions when treatment is not working |

| | |
|---|---|
| **How to Avoid the Mistake** | ■ Understand that not all pacing discharges are visible on ECG. In particular, unipolar pacing usually has easily visible large pacing spikes, whereas bipolar pacing may leave extremely small spikes that may or may not be visible (or thought to be artifact). Furthermore, epicardial leads produce smaller pacing spikes than endocardial leads. |
| | ■ Understand how to check for paced rhythms in the absence of obvious pacing spikes on ECG. First, focus on the rate—it is very rare for a ventricular tachycardia to be as slow as the backup rate of a paced rhythm. Second, assess the morphology of the supposed ventricular complex. An RV-paced rhythm takes the shape of an LBBB and an LV-paced rhythm appears as an RBBB. Thus, if a patient has only RV leads, then an RBBB-morphology wide-complex cannot be from the pacemaker. Last, look for ectopic ventricular beats, which would signal that the rhythm is not coming from the ventricles (a true ventricular tachycardia is not interrupted by another ectopic ventricular foci). |
| | ■ Learn how to determine whether a pacemaker is using unipolar or bipolar leads. Refer to the amplitude of pacing spikes on prior ECGs or read the original PPM implantation note. Most PPM leads can be programmed to be either unipolar or bipolar. |
| | ■ Remember to occasionally take a step back and restart from the beginning, assessing for potential misunderstandings that may heavily influence clinical decisions. |
| **Antidote** | ■ Not applicable |
| **Common Scenarios** | ■ Not applicable |
| **Note(s)** | ■ A unipolar lead is one that has only a positive or negative pole in contact with the myocardium. A bipolar lead has both positive and negative poles in contact with the myocardium. |
| | ■ RV-paced rhythms may appear similar in morphology to a rhythm with an LBBB. The key difference is in the lateral leads (V5-6)—a paced rhythm will usually not have a positive QRS (broad R wave). |

# Cardiac Imaging

Bliss J. Chang

Mistake: Using Pressure Half-Time Without Considering Left Ventricular Compliance or Afterload

**Echocardiography: Pericardial Disease**

Mistake: Mistaking Pleural Effusions or Ascites for Pericardial Effusions

Mistake: Thinking That Pericardial Effusions Are Only Fluid

**Echocardiography: Mass Mimics**

Mistake: Left Atrial Mass Mimics

Mistake: Left Ventricular Mass Mimics

Mistake: Right Atrial Mass Mimics

Mistake: Right Ventricular Mass Mimics

Mistake: False Ascending Aortic Dissection

**Cardiac Computed Tomography: Quality**

Mistake: Inadequate Patient Preparation for Coronary Computed Tomography Angiography

Mistake: Breathing During a Cardiac Computed Tomography Scan

Mistake: Poor-Quality Electrocardiogram for the Gated Cardiac Study

Mistake: Drawing Formal Conclusions From a Raw Coronary CT Scan

# Echocardiography: Quality

## MISTAKE: OVERCONFIDENT REPORTING IN THE FACE OF UNCERTAINTY

**Case Example**   You read a transthoracic echocardiogram (TTE) (echo) for a "cardiac complaint" and notice very limited imaging windows. Despite this, you see an echogenic area moving vigorously up and down in the lower left corner of the apical four-chamber view; you assume it is the tricuspid annulus and call the right ventricular (RV) size and function as normal. The ordering clinician reads your report and deems a massive pulmonary embolism less likely in a patient with hypoxia, tachycardia, and borderline soft blood pressures. The patient's oxygen saturation does not improve, and a computed tomography (CT) chest angiogram (CTA) is finally obtained, which demonstrates a saddle pulmonary embolism with an RV:left ventricular (LV) ratio of 1.7:1. Just as the CTA read comes back, the patient has a cardiac arrest.

**Reasoning Error(s)**
- Pressure to report something for every parameter on an echo report
- Lack of knowledge regarding the patient's clinical presentation
- Aversion to seeking help or second opinions
- Overconfidence
- Lack of adequate clinical context provided by ordering clinicians

**How to Avoid the Mistake**
- Always interpret only as much as you can with a good degree of confidence. Well-intentioned yet incorrect reporting can turn into a vicious cycle of propagation and clinical mismanagement.
- Report uncertainty when present (i.e., using words such as "probably" and "unclear"); can suggest repeat imaging, imaging with contrast, and even transesophageal echocardiography (TEE)
- Compare to prior images when able
- Seek a second opinion or help when needed
- Use clinical history and context to help define possibilities (i.e., suggesting that a mass is likely a vegetation in the context of bacteremia)
- Encourage clinicians to order imaging studies with the correct indications rather than vague diagnoses suggested by the electronic medical record system such as "cardiac complaint." More helpful indications include information such as "rule out pericardial effusion." This helps the interpreting physician to contextualize the study.

| | |
|---|---|
| **Antidote** | ■ Not applicable |
| **Common Scenarios** | ■ Lack of adequate imaging windows<br>■ Lack of necessary imaging data<br>■ Lack of experience with a particular image finding<br>■ Unusual image findings |
| **Note(s)** | ■ Medical errors are the third leading cause of mortality in the United States. Notably, this is a huge underestimate of the number of clinical errors that are caught before they affect clinical outcomes or do not tangibly affect outcomes. One key source of error is unreliable or incorrect clinical information.<br>■ You are not bound to the information fields suggested by echo reading software. When exceptions occur, you should include information that will help nonspecialty teams care for the patient receiving a cardiac imaging study. For example, patients with severe mitral regurgitation may have what appears to be a "normal" LV ejection fraction (LVEF), though understanding that the LVEF should be "hyperdynamic" in the setting of severe mitral regurgitation should be conveyed in the report as the patient may already meet criteria for mitral valve repair/replacement. |

## MISTAKE: IMAGING WITHOUT CONSIDERING THE EFFECT OF RESPIRATION

| | |
|---|---|
| **Case Example** | You are obtaining a routine echocardiogram on a patient admitted for shortness of breath. You successfully obtain the parasternal views and move on to the apical views but have significant difficulty finding a good window. You impatiently move around the probe trying to find a good window but are unable to do so; your colleague is walking by and asks the patient to hold her breath in end-expiration and is able to obtain diagnostic apical views. |
| **Reasoning Error(s)** | ■ Lack of knowledge regarding the impact of lung volumes on image quality<br>■ Lack of use of respiratory holds to optimize image quality<br>■ Forgetting to pay attention during the respiratory phase when optimizing imaging windows<br>■ Patient lacks ability to volitionally control respiration (e.g., on respiratory support) |
| **How to Avoid the Mistake** | ■ Understand the impact of lung volumes on image quality. Generally, larger lung volumes hinder image quality, and most views (particularly parasternal and apical) improve if done during expiration, particularly end-expiration. However, image quality can actually improve with inspiration when visualizing the subxiphoid view or the inferior wall in the two-chamber view.<br>■ Use respiratory holds to optimize image quality. Ask the patient (if they are able) to perform expiratory or inspiratory holds while you record a certain window. Importantly, hold your breath along with them so you do not forget how they are feeling!<br>■ When searching for nice image windows, factor in the respiratory phase. For example, if the patient is inspiring, consider waiting until they expire to see if the window improves. |
| **Antidote** | ■ Not applicable |

| **Common Scenarios** | ▪ Not applicable |
|---|---|
| **Note(s)** | ▪ Inspiration increases the anteroposterior diameter of the chest, causing the heart to move farther away from the sternum in addition to adding more air that ultrasound has great difficulty penetrating, thereby decreasing image quality. Conversely, expiration brings the heart closer to the thoracic wall, reduces air that needs to be penetrated, and improves image quality.<br>▪ For the subxiphoid view, consider asking the patient to take only a half-breath. You obtain the benefit of some inspiration that pushes down the diaphragm to allow a better window into the heart, and the patient's abdomen does not become as tense as when a full deep breath is taken.<br>▪ When the endocardial borders are not easily visualized, intravenous contrast such as Definity (perflutren lipid microsphere; non–blood-based ultrasound contrast agent that is not renally cleared) may help. Per the American Society of Echocardiography (ASE) guidelines, contrast may be used when unable to clearly visualize two or more endocardial border cardiac segments. |
| **Further Reading** | ▪ An excellent review of respiratory mechanics and maneuvers in echocardiography is given in Ginghina C, et al. Respiratory maneuvers in echocardiography: a review of clinical applications. *Cardiovasc Ultrasound.* 2009;42(7). |

## MISTAKE: SHADOWING ARTIFACT

| **Case Example** | A patient who had a transaortic valve replacement (TAVR) procedure 1 week ago presents with jaundice. Lab results are worrisome for hemolysis. A TTE demonstrates no evidence of paravalvular leak around the aortic bioprostheses. An extensive workup for other causes of hemolysis is undertaken without success. |
|---|---|
| **Reasoning Error(s)** | ▪ Lack of awareness of shadowing artifact in ultrasound<br>▪ Lack of experience with the clinical relevance of shadowing artifact |
| **How to Avoid the Mistake** | ▪ Understand shadowing artifact: reflection and blocking of ultrasound sound waves by a dense material, resulting in diminished echogenicity behind the culprit density<br>▪ Understand that shadowing prevents the clear visualization of any type of ultrasound signal beyond the culprit density. For example, paravalvular leak (not necessarily just visualization of an anatomic structure) may be difficult to visualize in the presence of significant shadowing.<br>▪ Try alternate windows to avoid shadowing artifact |
| **Antidote** | ▪ Not applicable |
| **Common Scenarios** | ▪ Heavily calcified aortic or mitral valve<br>▪ Prosthetic material (e.g., mechanical valves)<br>▪ Intracardiac calcifications (e.g., large calcified thrombus)<br>▪ Bone |
| **Note(s)** | ▪ Shadowing is the reason why we find imaging windows between the ribs!<br>▪ Pearl: Use off-axis imaging to find paravalvular regurgitant leaks.<br>▪ Recommend alternative imaging in the report such as TEE if clinically indicated |

## MISTAKE: USING A LARGE AREA OF INTEREST FOR COLOR DOPPLER

**Case Example**      You are performing an echocardiogram of a patient who presented for acute-onset shortness of breath and was found to have moderate pulmonary edema on chest imaging. While obtaining color Doppler scans of the parasternal long-axis view, you increase the size of the color box to include both the mitral and aortic valves.

**Reasoning Error(s)**
- Desire to be "maximally efficient" resulting in attempt to image two areas (e.g., two valves) with one color box
- Lack of knowledge regarding the correlation of the size of the region of interest to the frame rate and resolution

**How to Avoid the Mistake**
- Understand that the larger the region of interest, the lower are the resolution and frame rate. Apply only the minimal box size required to visualize the blood flow over a particular structure.
- Maximize depth setting prior to "zooming in."
- Image patiently when able and you will be rewarded with superior image quality.

**Antidote**
- Decrease the box width to the minimal area required.

**Common Scenarios**
- Not applicable

**Note(s)**
- Learning occurs with experience. Try adjusting the size of the color Doppler box in both directions and observe what happens with the quality of the imaging including the Nyquist range!

## MISTAKE: ALIASING DUE TO IMPROPER NYQUIST LIMITS DURING JET QUANTIFICATION IN COLOR DOPPLER

**Case Example**      You are evaluating a middle-aged female for mitral regurgitation after hearing a holosystolic murmur at the apex with radiation to the axilla. As you perform color Doppler over the mitral valve, you are confused by the velocity peaks appearing "cut off" and "wrapping around" in the opposite direction. You determine the mitral regurgitation to be mild, but your attending notes that this is actually an underestimation due to an improper Nyquist limit selection.

**Reasoning Error(s)**
- Lack of awareness or knowledge about the phenomenon of aliasing
- Inability to recognize aliasing
- Forgetting or inadequate adjustment of Nyquist limit prior to imaging
- Not checking and/or adjusting Nyquist baselines between studies

**How to Avoid the Mistake**
- Understand aliasing. In simple terms, aliasing occurs when the velocity of blood flow exceeds a certain threshold termed the Nyquist limit, resulting in display of the blood flow "wrapping around" and going opposite in addition to the true direction.
- Set your imaging up for success (just as you would prior to a procedure) by checking and adjusting key parameters such as the Nyquist limit as needed.
- Note that when the scale of the color Doppler requires adjustment, the wrong button may be adjusted causing the baseline to shift leading to an incorrect color Doppler setting. Another common mistake is using a baseline shift to assess the proximal isovelocity surface area (PISA) and then accidentally leaving the baseline at the new settings, thus causing an incorrect remainder of the study. Always remember to return the baseline back to normal if it is adjusted!

| | |
|---|---|
| **Antidote** | ■ Adjust the Nyquist limit for goal range between 50 and 70 cm/s. |
| **Common Scenarios** | ■ Not applicable |
| **Note(s)** | ■ You cannot add the velocities together when aliasing is present as a portion of the signal is lost because it is unable to be measured.<br>■ Aliasing is a phenomenon that occurs because Nyquist the echo machine is trying to image something that is occurring much faster than at the rate that the images are acquired (i.e., undersampling). It is found with both color Doppler and pulsed-wave Doppler because they both acquire data in pulses (frequent sampling). It does not occur in continuous-wave Doppler because the data acquisition is constant. |

## MISTAKE: CONFUSING PULSED-WAVE DOPPLER WITH CONTINUOUS-WAVE DOPPLER

| | |
|---|---|
| **Case Example** | You are evaluating an older male for aortic stenosis after hearing a harsh, late-peaking systolic murmur at the base radiating to the carotids. As you perform pulsed-wave Doppler imaging over the aortic valve, you are confused by the velocity peaks appearing "cut off" and "wrapping around" in the opposite direction. You decide to add the velocities together to determine the aortic jet velocity. Your attending is alarmed at your lack of knowledge between pulsed-wave and continuous-wave Doppler and refer you to this book. |
| **Reasoning Error(s)** | ■ Lack of understanding the difference between pulsed-wave and continuous-wave Doppler<br>■ Not understanding the proper mode to obtain a maximal velocity for aortic valve assessment |
| **How to Avoid the Mistake** | ■ Pulsed-wave Doppler examines the velocity found in a small gated region of your choosing, whereas continuous-wave Doppler determines the maximum velocity along the entire cursor line. This means that while pulsed-wave Doppler has signal aliasing, continuous-wave Doppler is not affected by aliasing. On the other hand, pulsed-wave Doppler is able to provide information at a specific area (known as depth acuity), whereas continuous-wave Doppler measures the highest velocity anywhere along the cursor line (depth ambiguous).<br>■ Remember that continuous-wave Doppler must be used for assessment of a maximal aortic valve jet velocity because it does not lead to aliasing and it is not possible to determine the exact location to place the small gating to obtain the maximal jet velocity. |
| **Antidote** | ■ Not applicable |
| **Common Scenarios** | ■ Not applicable |
| **Note(s)** | ■ The maximum velocity measurable with pulsed-wave Doppler lessens as the depth increases. This is because the maximum velocity measurable is no more than half of the pulse repetition frequency (PRF), which decreases as the depth increases (an inverse relationship). |

## MISTAKE: FORESHORTENING

**Case Example**

You are imaging the apical four-chamber view for a patient who recently had a distal left anterior descending coronary artery (LAD) ST-segment elevation myocardial infarction (STEMI) complicated by a stroke 1 week later. You notice that the apex is contracting well and send those images to your attending, who swings by and checks for herself. You now incredulously visualize an apical area of akinesis with a mobile, apical thrombus.

**Reasoning Error(s)**

- Lack of knowledge of the foreshortening phenomenon
- Inability to recognize foreshortening
- Improper probe positioning (typically too high and/or medial)
- Difficult patient positioning due to anatomy or clinical condition

**How to Avoid the Mistake**

- Understand foreshortening. Foreshortening means that the LV appears more spherical than bullet-shaped and the ventricle has been erroneously "short-ened." This can lead to several problems, such as inability to clearly visualize the apical myocardium (e.g., miss an apical LV thrombus) and overestimation of EF (foreshortening cuts out portions of the LV that do not move and "brings" the endocardium closer together, thus causing the overestimation).
- Always assess the integrity of each image you obtain. Check for and recognize foreshortening of the LV (Fig. 4.1).
- When encountering foreshortening, adjust the probe positioning (typically api-cally and laterally)
- Position the patient as optimally as able (lateral decubitus, expiration)

**Antidote**

- Move the probe apically (down one or two intercostal spaces) and/or laterally

**Common Scenarios**

- Not applicable

**Note(s)**

- Foreshortening occurs due to the ultrasound beam slicing through at the incor-rect level of the heart (Fig. 4.1), hence missing the true apex of the LV.
- Foreshortening may also negate the benefit of echo contrast such as Definity. For example, if the goal of using contrast was to rule out an LV thrombus, foreshortening will prevent adequate visualization of the apex regardless of whether contrast is used.

**Fig. 4.1**   Foreshortening.

# Echocardiography: Left Ventricular Structure

## MISTAKE: IMPROPER POSITIONING OF M-MODE LINE FOR MEASURING LEFT VENTRICULAR DIAMETER

**Case Example**    You are learning to read standard TTEs and measure the LV end-diastolic diameter (LVEDD) by using M-mode. You measure a dilated 5.9 cm, but your attending physician notes that the correct diameter is only 5.4 cm.

**Reasoning Error(s)**
- Lack of knowledge regarding proper boundaries for measuring LV diameter
- Mistaking the chordae for the posterolateral wall when measuring the diameter
- Imaging without consideration of the probe position (which influences the imaging plane)—that is, measurements at an oblique angle to the papillary muscle and mitral valve
- Measuring during the wrong part of the cardiac cycle
- Measuring with M-mode despite inadequate image quality or M-mode cursor orientation

**How to Avoid the Mistake**
- Understand the proper positioning of the M-mode cursor: in parasternal long-axis view, perpendicular to the LV long axis. The line should be measured at the level of the mitral valve leaflet tips (per the 2015 ASE's recommendations for cardiac chamber quantification in adults by Lang et al).
- Position the probe ideally between the third and fourth intercostal spaces to obtain the highest chance of positioning the M-mode cursor perpendicular to the LV.
- Only perform M-mode measurements if able to obtain a good position with the M-mode cursor. You will not be able to obtain a high-fidelity measurement in many patients.
- Understand the anatomic structures that define the endocardial boundaries for LV diameter measurement. The superior boundary is straightforward: the interventricular septum. The inferior boundary may be trickier if chordae are seen; ensure that the posterior wall thickens and comes inward (unlike the chordae).
- Recognize the part of the cardiac cycle that corresponds to the end-diastolic and end-systolic diameters. The end-diastolic diameter is when the ventricle is at its largest and occurs at the beginning of the QRS complex. The end-systolic diameter is usually the smallest diameter (exception may be if dyskinetic wall present) measured at the end of the T wave.

**Antidote**
- Not applicable

**Common Scenarios**
- Cutting through the improper anatomic structures
- Nonorthogonal M-mode cursor in relation to LV structures
- Confusing the chordae for the posterolateral LV wall
- Measuring during the wrong part of the cardiac cycle

**Note(s)**
- The advantage of an M-mode measurement over two-dimensional (2D) measurement is the increased resolution of time, whereas the advantage of 2D measurement is more freedom to measure in various orientations (the M-mode cursor is a fixed straight line that does not always coincide with the desired plane of the heart). For example, nonorthogonal cuts may lead to either overestimation or underestimation of the diameter.
- Another easy way to tell whether the M-mode cursor is well positioned over the LV in parasternal long-axis view is to see if the interventricular septum and aorta are nearly parallel.

## MISTAKE: IMPROPER TWO-DIMENSIONAL MEASUREMENT OF THE LEFT VENTRICULAR DIAMETER

**Case Example**

You are learning to read standard TTEs and measure the LVEDD parasternal long view. You obtain 5.9 cm, but your attending notes that the diameter is only 5.4 cm.

**Reasoning Error(s)**

- Poor image quality (e.g., cannot visualize the endocardial borders)
- Improper measurement technique (e.g., measuring from the myocardium rather than the endocardium)
- Measuring during the wrong part of the cardiac cycle
- Measuring after a premature contraction, whether premature ventricular contraction (PVC) or premature atrial contraction (PAC)

**How to Avoid the Mistake**

- Optimize image resolution prior to measurement. Consider the use of LV contrast (Definity) to enhance endocardial border delineation. Definity is recommended when unable to adequately visualize at least two contiguous endocardial segments.
- Ensure measurement begins and ends at the endocardial surface
- Recognize the part of the cardiac cycle that corresponds to the end-diastolic and end-systolic diameters. The end-diastolic diameter occurs at the beginning of the QRS complex and is typically when the ventricle is at its largest, though this may not hold true in cardiomyopathy and/or the presence of dyskinetic segments. The end-systolic diameter (when the LV is smallest) is measured just prior to the opening of the mitral valve. The T wave representing repolarization does not always precisely correspond to the end of systole.

**Antidote**

- Not applicable

**Common Scenarios**

- Measuring from the pericardium or myocardium
- Inclusion of papillary muscles or chordae
- Views that underestimate LV dimensions
  - Two-chamber view
  - Three-chamber view
- Very small ventricles
- Foreshortening
- Inadequate image quality

**Note(s)**

- LV dimensions can be variable on apical views. The parasternal long-axis view is considered the standard 2D view for measuring the LVEDD.
- The length (not diameter) of the ventricle can be measured from the apical four-chamber view.

## MISTAKE: IMPROPER MEASUREMENT OF THE INTERVENTRICULAR SEPTUM

**Case Example**

A 22-year-old female soccer player undergoes health screening prior to signing with the professional team of her dreams. Her physical exam is unremarkable, but her TTE at outside hospital reveals concentric LVH with an interventricular septum of 1.3 cm. Based on this finding, the patient is diagnosed with hypertrophic cardiomyopathy and told that she cannot play competitive soccer. The patient is devastated and comes to see you for a second opinion. You look at the images from her recent TTE and notice that most image frames show a septal thickness of 1.1 cm. It appears that certain frames may have provided an appearance of a thicker LV wall due to oblique slicing from an off-axis image and premature beats. Given the patient's supernormal exercise tolerance, you discuss with your attending and clear the patient for competitive soccer. She is elated and goes on to have a stellar career over nearly two decades without any cardiovascular issues.

| | |
|---|---|
| **Reasoning Error(s)** | ▪ Inadequate image quality (e.g., off-axis imaging for the parasternal view, heart movement during respiration, premature beats) |
| | ▪ Excessive focus on a single part of the septum |
| **How to Avoid the Mistake** | ▪ Ensure that the image quality is appropriate for interpretation. Be sure to recognize off-axis imaging for the parasternal views, which are used for measuring the septal thickness. Helpful clues for an off-axis parasternal long view include closed mitral/aortic valves and visualization of the LV apex. Image quality may also vary frame by frame if the probe shifts position during recording, in the presence of a premature beat, or with heart movement during respiration. |
| | ▪ Understand that septal thickness should be measured at end-diastole in a parasternal view (usually long axis). It should not include any structures that may be seen adjacent in the RV. |
| | ▪ Sometimes it may be helpful to visualize the hypertrophy in corresponding views such as parasternal short-axis or apical imaging. |
| | ▪ Describe any significant variations in septal thickness (such as by denoting the specific location of septal hypertrophy like basal). This provides the clinician with more context. For example, a report with an interventricular septum (IVS) of 1.5 cm is usually interpreted as LV hypertrophy (LVH), whereas if the patient has only a 1.5-cm basal septum but has a thickness of 1.0 cm elsewhere, the patient may not have what we classically think of as LVH and/or hypertrophic cardiomyopathy (HCM) but rather has a sigmoid septum (frequently in older patients). |
| **Antidote** | ▪ De-training (though often devastating career-wise for competitive athletes) |
| | ▪ Consider strain imaging with cardiovascular magnetic resonance imaging (CMR) |
| **Common Scenarios** | ▪ Off-axis imaging for the parasternal view |
| | ▪ Movement of the heart in respiration |
| | ▪ Premature beat (compensatory squeeze after the extrasystolic beat leading to increased septal thickening) |
| **Note(s)** | ▪ Patients often vary in their heart axis and the textbook description of probe manipulation may not work well. When off-axis, first focus on identifying the center of the image (i.e., the aortic and mitral valves); this is often done via moving intercostal spaces, angling, and tilting of the probe. Once the mitral and aortic valves are centered, rotate the probe clockwise or counterclockwise without changing the angle to open up the valves into an on-axis image. |
| | ▪ Competitive athletes with physiologic thickening of the heart will have supernormal exercise capacity. This is a quick and easy first screen for whether the patient's hypertrophied heart may likely be physiologic versus genetic. |
| | ▪ A sigmoid septum refers to relatively isolated hypertrophy at the basal portion of the IVS. While the clinical significance of it is unclear, there is some thought that it may reflect an early precursor to concentric LVH (i.e., the basal septum is the most prone and thus earliest place to hypertrophy). |

## MISTAKE: ONLY CHARACTERIZING SEPTAL HYPERTROPHY

**Case Example**   A 20-year-old male basketball player presents for a physical evaluation prior to signing with your city's professional team. Exam demonstrates normal S1 and S2 with no extra heart sounds. ECG demonstrates large T-wave inversions in the precordial leads. A TTE to follow-up the ECG changes demonstrates a 1.1-cm IVS with normal mitral valve function, and you clear the patient for basketball. The patient is elated and signs a large player's contract. A month later, the patient can hardly make it through half of the game due to shortness of breath. You review the TTE again and notice a severely hypertrophied LV apex, likely signaling apical HCM. Though the patient is started on metoprolol and subsequently disopyramide, the patient is unable to meet the expectations of the basketball team and loses his contract.

**Reasoning Error(s)**
- Reflex to only measure or consider the IVS as the sole and definitive measurement for LVH
- Lack of awareness of other presentations of LVH
- Oversight in LVH by using only the parasternal long-axis view

**How to Avoid the Mistake**
- Understand that any segment of the LV may be hypertrophied, either in an asymmetric and isolated fashion or in a symmetric and concentric manner. Though the septum is usually the first (and sometimes, incorrectly, the only) segment checked for hypertrophy, it is critical to consider the possibility of hypertrophy in other LV segments. Hypertrophy usually suggests a pathologic state.
- Search all LV segments for evidence of LVH. This cannot be done solely using the parasternal long-axis view because the apex should be out of the window when the view is properly acquired.
- If not well visualized by echo, consider cardiac magnetic resonance imaging (MRI [CMR]) for alternative imaging assessment.

**Antidote**
- Not applicable

**Common Scenarios**
- Septal hypertrophy
- Apical hypertrophy

**Note(s)**
- Apical hypertrophy is often associated with a particular form of HCM that is seen most commonly in Japanese patients (up to 15% of Japanese patients with HCM).
- If visualization of the apex is difficult, consider using contrast to better outline the endocardial border.
- Note that not all types of HCM are obstructive!

# Echocardiography: Ejection Fraction

## MISTAKE: VISUALLY ESTIMATING EJECTION FRACTION DURING BRADYCARDIA OR TACHYCARDIA

**Case Example**   You are reading a routine TTE and calculate the LVEF to be 45%. Compared with prior reports, there appears to be a new reduction in the EF. The primary team initiates a new workup for a new cardiomyopathy.

**Reasoning Error(s)**
- Not considering heart rate during calculation of EF
- Forgetting to provide a caveat in LVEF interpretation in the setting of bradycardia or tachycardia
- Lack of understanding the impact of heart rate on EF

| **How to Avoid the Mistake** | ■ Always measure and note the heart rate during the study; this is a requirement by the ASE. You may also consider noting a particularly fast heart rate (e.g., >120 bpm) in the LV function section of the report. |
| --- | --- |
| | ■ Understand the impact of heart rate on EF. As heart rate increases, the stroke volume may decrease unless there is a concurrent increase in inotropic response. The greatest change in stroke volume would occur due to a decrease in the diastolic filling time and, hence, preload. As such, the EF (difference between the end-diastolic volume and end-systolic volume) may appear to decrease when measured by visual estimate, leading to underestimation of the LVEF. The calculated LVEF (e.g., via the Simpson biplane method) would not change. Similarly, during bradycardia (especially heart rate <40 bpm), diastolic filling time increases significantly and stroke volume increases, which can also lead to an inaccurate visual estimation of LVEF. Thus, it is recommended that LVEF be reported after formal computation using a method such as the Simpson biplane method. |
| | ■ Separately be aware that a true reduction in EF can occur in the setting of prolonged tachyarrhythmias (i.e., heart rate >120–130 bpm for >24 hours); this case would be referred to as a tachycardia-induced cardiomyopathy. |
| **Antidote** | ■ Revisit study at a different time |
| | ■ Though ideally the heart rate is controlled through addressing the etiology of bradycardia or tachycardia, if needed can consider atrioventricular (AV) nodal blockade or vagal maneuvers for persistent tachycardia |
| | ■ Formally calculate LVEF (e.g., via Simpson biplane method) |
| **Common Scenarios** | ■ Tachycardia |
| | ■ Bradycardia |
| **Note(s)** | ■ Clinical Pearl: Always compare the current images to prior images yourself rather than simply reading the report as you may interpret the prior study differently from the prior read and there may not actually be a significant change in LVEF. |
| | ■ Often in tachycardia, the heart is moving more out of a perfect image plane which may cause measurement errors. This is also seen with increased respiratory movement, which further decreases image quality as the heart may move farther from the probe and become "shielded" by air. |
| | ■ Tachycardia may affect the visual assessment of EF more significantly in the setting of less passive diastolic filling (i.e., time in diastole). |

## MISTAKE: CALCULATING EJECTION FRACTION DURING IRREGULAR RHYTHMS

| **Case Example** | A 78-year-old female with nonischemic cardiomyopathy (NICM) and long-standing atrial fibrillation presents for a routine TTE. You trace the endocardial borders perfectly on the apical two- and four-chamber views and calculate the EF to be 27%. Comparing this to the prior TTE, you notice a significant decrease (from 38%). You note this decrease, and the primary team initiates a workup for worsening EF. |
| --- | --- |
| **Reasoning Error(s)** | ■ Lack of understanding of how the Simpson method calculates EF |
| | ■ Not considering the pathophysiologic impact of irregular beats |

| | |
|---|---|
| **How to Avoid the Mistake** | ■ Understand the principle behind the Simpson method: calculating the difference in volume between diastole and systole based on volumes derived by division into numerous discs. |
| | ■ Understand that an irregular rhythm leads to beat-to-beat variation in the EF due to the differing preload and systolic time. In these cases, the EF should be averaged over multiple beats. |
| **Antidote** | ■ Average measurements over multiple beats |
| **Common Scenarios** | ■ Irregular rhythm |
| |    ■ Premature beats (PACs and, more significantly, PVCs) |
| |    ■ Atrial fibrillation |
| |    ■ Multifocal atrial tachycardia |
| |    ■ Any arrhythmia with variable block |
| | ■ Regional wall motion abnormalities (WMAs) |
| | ■ Poor image quality |
| **Note(s)** | ■ Regional WMAs may alter the EF calculated using the Simpson method given the Simpson method uses only the four-chamber view (or the biplane Simpson method, which uses the two-chamber view as well) which may not demonstrate regional WMAs found on other views. |
| | ■ The Simpson biplane plane method is superior to the single-plane method, which should usually be avoided. |

## MISTAKE: END-POINT SEPTAL SEPARATION IN VALVULAR DISEASE AND LEFT VENTRICULAR HYPERTROPY

| | |
|---|---|
| **Case Example** | A patient with longstanding uncontrolled hypertension presents to the emergency department with new shortness of breath and tachycardia. On bedside ultrasound, you note that the E-point septal separation (EPSS) is 6 mm and conclude that the EF is normal. Assuming that the tachycardia is from hypovolemia, you administer fluids and the patient develops worsening heart failure symptoms. |
| **Reasoning Error(s)** | ■ Not thinking through the physiology that influences end-point septal separation on a case-by-case basis |
| | ■ Lack of attention to structural heart disease, in particular mitral/aortic valve pathology and hypertrophy |
| **How to Avoid the Mistake** | ■ Understand that EPSS is dependent on two factors beyond LV function: the mobility of the anterior mitral leaflet and the thickness of the IVS (particularly the basal septum) |
| | ■ Rule out limitations to use of EPSS such as significant mitral/aortic valve disease, the two most common being mitral stenosis and LVH. |
| **Antidote** | ■ Characterize LVEF using a more suitable method. |

| | |
|---|---|
| **Common Scenarios** | ■ Overestimation of EPSS (lower LVEF)<br>   ▪ Restricted leaflet motion<br>■ Mitral stenosis<br>■ Prosthetic valves<br>■ Aortic regurgitation<br>   ▪ Increased distance between anterior mitral leaflet and septum<br>■ Extreme LV dilation<br>■ Underestimation of EPSS (higher LVEF)<br>   ▪ Decreased distance between anterior mitral leaflet and septum<br>■ LVH<br>■ Asymmetric IVS hypertrophy (e.g., hypertrophic obstructive cardiomyopathy [HOCM], sigmoid septum) |
| **Note(s)** | ■ EPSS is a quick and easy method to objectively discriminate normal from significantly reduced EF. A normal EPSS is <7 mm, whereas >12 mm indicates severely reduced EF. The EF is likely decreased for EPSS between 7 and 12 mm.<br>■ EPSS is overestimated in the presence of any process that contributes to decreasing the mobility of the anterior mitral valve leaflet. Conversely, EPSS is underestimated in the presence of any process that increases the mobility of the anterior mitral valve leaflet. |

## MISTAKE: FRACTIONAL AREA/SHORTENING IN REGIONAL WALL MOTION ABNORMALITIES

| | |
|---|---|
| **Case Example** | A 65-year-old female with a recent inferior STEMI presents for a routine echocardiogram. To teach the new first-year cardiology fellow, you demonstrate estimation of the LVEF using fractional shortening (50%). You then calculate the LVEF to be 30% by using the Simpson biplane method. The fellow asks why there is such a large discrepancy in the LVEF estimates. |
| **Reasoning Error(s)** | ■ Not considering the presence of abnormal wall motion as a limiting factor to fractional shortening measurement of LVEF<br>■ Poor image quality that hides abnormal wall motion |
| **How to Avoid the Mistake** | ■ Always consider the limitations of each clinical tool. Fractional shortening is one of the first methods devised for estimating LV function and is generally no longer used to determine reportable LV function because it visualizes only the septum and posterolateral LV walls through the point the M-mode cursor passes, assuming that the rest of the LV is similar in function.<br>■ Ensure adequate image quality for tracing the endocardial border |
| **Antidote** | ■ Characterize LVEF using a more suitable method |
| **Common Scenarios** | ■ Regional WMAs<br>■ Abnormal septal activation (e.g., left bundle-branch block [LBBB])<br>■ Poor image quality |
| **Note(s)** | ■ Regional WMAs may both underestimate or overestimate the LVEF. Underestimation occurs when the WMAs are present in the segments through which the M-mode cursor passes. Overestimation occurs when the WMAs are outside of the M-mode cursor. |

## MISTAKE: COMMON TRACING ERRORS FOR THE SIMPSON METHOD

| | |
|---|---|
| **Case Example** | A patient with a prior large anterior myocardial infarction undergoes a follow-up TTE a month after revascularization. The echo demonstrates a large anterior aneurysm that is akinetic, though without thrombus in addition to several other severely hypokinetic segments. You calculate the EF to be 29% using the biplane Simpson method. Given the LVEF will affect the recommendation for possible automated implantable cardioverter-defibrillator (AICD), your colleague orders a CMR, which shows an EF of 37%. The patient is grateful she did not unnecessarily receive an AICD. |
| **Reasoning Error(s)** | ■ Lack of knowledge or experience with common tracing errors<br>■ Using poor image quality |
| **How to Avoid the Mistake** | ■ Understand the proper method of tracing the LV for the Simpson method. The endocardial borders should be traced carefully after verification on multiple frames. Care should be taken to exclude the papillary muscles and any significant geometrical disturbances such as LV aneurysm in the tracing.<br>■ Check to avoid foreshortening the ventricle during scanning.<br>■ Ensure the best image quality possible. Consider patient positioning, respiratory maneuvers, and contrast (e.g., Definity).<br>■ Do not use the method if image quality is inadequate. A visual estimate may be better. |
| **Antidote** | ■ Not applicable |
| **Common Scenarios** | ■ Inaccurate endocardial borders<br>■ Foreshortening<br>■ Inclusion of papillary muscles<br>■ Inclusion of trabeculations<br>■ Inclusion of pathologic variations in LV geometry (e.g., LV aneurysm)<br>■ Poor image quality |
| **Note(s)** | ■ The modified or biplane Simpson method is the most widely used method of assessing EF by echocardiography due to better characterization of the LV geometry (using oval-shaped discs).<br>■ Because the Simpson method uses the four- and two-chamber views, the LVEF will not account for regional wall motion abnormalities in LV segments not visualized by those views (e.g., the posterolateral LV wall). |

## MISTAKE: "EYEBALLING" EJECTION FRACTION WITHOUT A SYSTEMATIC APPROACH

| | |
|---|---|
| **Case Example** | A 75-year-old female presents with new shortness of breath and you perform a bedside echocardiogram. You begin with the parasternal long-axis view and decide that the patient's LVEF is likely normal based on a quick glance at the screen. |
| **Reasoning Error(s)** | ■ Thinking of "eyeballing" as a "1-second shortcut"<br>■ Overeagerness to determine the LVEF quickly, leading to rushing and errors<br>■ Not considering as many LV segments as possible<br>■ Looking at only one view (e.g., longitudinal) of the heart's contraction |

| | |
|---|---|
| **How to Avoid the Mistake** | ■ Consider "eyeballing" as one technique of many, with its own pros and cons<br>■ Take your time and use a systematic approach each time<br>■ Understand that a complete echocardiographic study provides multiple views of the ventricle, some views visualizing the same LV wall segment although from a different perspective/plane. This approach is needed to more confidently support or exclude regional WMAs.<br>■ Understand that the heart contracts in multiple dimensions (longitudinal, circumferential, and radial) and that accurate estimation of EF is dependent on considering all dimensions. |
| **Antidote** | ■ Use a formal calculation to verify the visually estimated EF. |
| **Common Scenarios** | ■ Not applicable |
| **Note(s)** | ■ Generally, experienced echocardiographers are able to achieve good agreement between a visually estimated EF and one that is computed, such as through the biplane Simpson method, although the more technically limited the image quality can reduce both visual and semiquantitative assessment accuracy.<br>■ Be aware that a very dilated ventricle's true function can be underestimated by visual estimation of the EF; conversely, a very small ventricle's function can be overestimated more by visual assessment than by a more semiquantitative method (i.e., biplane Simpson) |

## MISTAKE: CROSS-INTERPRETATION OF EJECTION FRACTION AMONG DIFFERENT IMAGING MODALITIES

| | |
|---|---|
| **Case Example** | A patient presents to your office and wants to discuss his TTE results. He says that his CMR only a month ago showed an EF of 65% and is now worried that his TTE estimates LVEF at 55%. |
| **Reasoning Error(s)** | ■ Less familiarity with the relative differences in EF by imaging modality, and even by method within one imaging modality |
| **How to Avoid the Mistake** | ■ Understand that it is important to note the imaging modality used to estimate an EF as they vary somewhat between imaging modalities. For example, an EF will typically be greater on CMR compared with echocardiography due to better visualization of the apex on MRI (even without foreshortening). The normal LVEF by CMR is >54% for men and >56% for women (Gelfand et al, *JCMR* 2006). Contrast this with the normal LVEF by echocardiography in men of >52% and in women of >54% (per the ASE).<br>■ Understand that EFs vary even within one modality based on the calculation method used (e.g., biplane versus volumetric echocardiographic estimates).<br>■ Trend changes in EF using a consistent modality and calculation method |
| **Antidote** | ■ Not applicable |
| **Common Scenarios** | ■ Not applicable |

**Note(s)**
- The LVEF is underestimated by approximately 7%–9% on average by echo compared with CMR, even when stratified by various LVEF ranges (Simpson et al, Heart 2018).
- CMR is usually considered the most accurate test for EF.
- The left ventriculogram (based on catheter-based injection of contrast into the LV cavity) is crude estimate of LVEF, and a confirmatory echocardiogram should always be obtained for suspected abnormalities.
- Importantly, situations such as whether a patient has an inotrope like dobutamine or milrinone infusing at the time of the echo can yield very significant differences in LVEF in the same patient. Always ensure context for the test is provided!

**Further Reading**
- Comparison of EF among several imaging modalities and among different echocardiographic methods: Pellikka PA, et al. Variability in ejection fraction measured by echocardiogram, gated single-photon emission computed tomography, and cardiac magnetic resonance in patients with coronary artery disease and left ventricular dysfunction. *JAMA Network Open.* 2018;1(4):e181456.

# Echocardiography: Diastology

## MISTAKE: OMITTING DIASTOLOGY ASSESSMENT IN THE ROUTINE ECHOCARDIOGRAM

**Case Example**
A 78-year-old female presents for worsening dyspnea. A TTE is obtained that demonstrates normal EF. There is no comment on diastology. The patient undergoes an extensive workup that rules out infectious and pulmonary causes. Suddenly, the patient becomes even more hypoxic, requiring intubation. Chest imaging demonstrates severe pulmonary edema. A TTE is repeated that demonstrates grade III diastolic dysfunction, supporting flash pulmonary edema.

**Reasoning Error(s)**
- Thinking that diastolic dysfunction is rare or less useful information
- Lack of comfort with methods to assess diastology
- Lack of desire to analyze data on diastolic dysfunction (from the reader's perspective)

**How to Avoid the Mistake**
- Understand the prevalence of diastolic dysfunction. For example, over the past few decades, as revascularization methods and medical therapy of heart failure with reduced ejection fraction (HFrEF) have improved while the population continues to age, heart failure with preserved ejection fraction (diastolic heart failure) (HFpEF) accounts for a slight majority of cases of heart failure in patients >60 years old in the United States.
- Familiarize yourself with the most common methods of screening for diastolic dysfunction. These include the E/A (mitral inflow) and E/e' (tissue Doppler) ratios, as well as searching for evidence of structural heart disease (i.e., left atrial enlargement and tricuspid regurgitation).

**Antidote**
- Not applicable

**Common Scenarios**
- Not applicable

**Note(s)**
- The mitral inflow velocities provide a visualization of the two key parts of diastole: early passive diastolic filling and late diastole (the atrial kick), referred to E and A, respectively. With normal ventricular relaxation, there is relatively much more early passive diastolic filling; as filling pressures rise, passive filling decreases and thus the contribution of the atrial kick to preload increases. The atrial kick may account for up to 20% of the preload, reaching 35%–40% of total atrial filling by the eighth decade of life (due to age-related diastolic dysfunction).
- Tissue-wave Doppler imaging analyzes the movement of myocardial tissue. For assessment of LV diastolic dysfunction, this is performed at the mitral annulus (both averaging the E/e' from the lateral and septal mitral annuli and interpreting the separate e').
- HFpEF is increasingly viewed as a heterogeneous entity with numerous etiologies. This may explain the wider variability in speed of onset and response to treatments.
- The presence of LVH does not automatically confer a diagnosis of HFpEF. Diastolic dysfunction must be assessed to diagnose HFpEF.
- The last decade has been an exciting period for HFpEF as we now have formally approved treatments, namely sodium-glucose cotransporter 2 (SGLT2) inhibitors (regardless of diabetes status) and spironolactone (largely based on a reanalysis of the 2014 Treatment of Preserved Cardiac Function Heart Failure with an Aldosterone Antagonist (TOPCAT) trial, which excluded treatment arms discovered to be missing the expected urinary metabolites of spironolactone, calling into question adequate medication administration). The Prospective Comparison of ARNI with ARB Global Outcomes in HF with Preserved Ejection Fraction (PARAGON-HF) study also demonstrated the potential benefit of Entresto (sacubitril/valsartan) in HFpEF with LVEF <57%, leading to Entresto being the first FDA-approved treatment in the US for HFpEF.
- Some patients may have exercise-induced diastolic dysfunction and should undergo exercise stress echocardiography to best make the diagnosis.

**Further Reading**
- The ASE's most recent suggested approach to assessment of diastolic function: Nagueh SF, et al. Recommendations for the evaluation of left ventricular diastolic function by echocardiography: an update from the American Society of Echocardiography and the European Association of Cardiovascular Imaging. *J Am Soc Echocardiogr*. 2016;29:277-314.

## MISTAKE: MISTAKING SUPERNORMAL FILLING FOR DIASTOLIC DYSFUNCTION

**Case Example**
A 27-year-old male soccer player presents to your outpatient clinic for a routine physical including an echocardiogram. While reading the echo, you notice a markedly high E/A ratio (2.3) and become concerned about diastolic dysfunction. You refer the patient to a heart failure specialist, who concludes the patient is healthy and normal.

**Reasoning Error(s)**
- Lack of differential diagnosis on high E/A ratios
- Lack of knowledge of supernormal filling
- Interpreting all high E/A ratios (≥2) as restrictive filling/diastolic dysfunction
- Not considering patient characteristics and clinical context

| | |
|---|---|
| **How to Avoid the Mistake** | ■ Always contextualize diastology. Consider the patient's age, clinical presentation, and presence of structural heart disease (e.g., LVH, left atrial enlargement, reduced EF). Restrictive filling (grade III) is almost always accompanied by structural changes. |
| | ■ Learn the concept of supernormal filling: a physiologic adaptation of the heart to strenuous aerobic exercise that induces a suction effect in the LV during diastole, increasing passive diastolic filling (and the E, hence the E/A ratio). Consider supernormal filling as a differential for high E/A ratios. |
| | ■ Understand how to differentiate supernormal filling from restrictive filling using echocardiographic parameters (in addition to clinical context). Start with the ASE guidelines, which state that positivity for three of the four following criteria indicate diastolic dysfunction: (1) average E/e' >14, (2) septal e' velocity <7 cm/s or lateral e' velocity <10 cm/s, (3) tricuspid regurgitation jet velocity >2.8 m/s, and (4) left atrial volume index >34 mL/m$^2$. If indeterminate, can consider additional parameters such as isovolumetric relaxation time (IVRT), DT (deceleration time of E) and pulmonary vein flow to support or refute an increased E/A (e.g., IVRT is less in supernormal filling compared with restrictive filling). |
| **Antidote** | ■ Not applicable |
| **Common Scenarios** | ■ Not applicable |
| **Note(s)** | ■ IVRT is the amount of time it takes for the LV to begin filling after the onset of diastole (time from aortic closure to mitral valve opening). With beginning stages of diastolic dysfunction, the IVRT increases (the ventricle takes longer to relax and accommodate filling) to >110 ms. The extreme values are the most useful (<60 ms or >110 ms). A value of <60 ms can happen with young healthy patients or those with elevated left atrial pressures (with other anatomical and Doppler findings helping differentiate). For >110 ms, mitral valve opening is delayed and is seen in early stages of diastolic dysfunction with normal mean left atrial pressures. |

## MISTAKE: OVERLOOKING PSEUDONORMAL FILLING IN THE PRESENCE OF A NORMAL E/A RATIO

| | |
|---|---|
| **Case Example** | An 80-year-old female presents for worsening dyspnea. A TTE is obtained, which demonstrates normal EF. You glance at the E/A ratio (1.3) and deem it to be normal. The patient undergoes an extensive workup. Suddenly, the patient becomes even more hypoxic requiring intubation. Chest imaging demonstrates severe pulmonary edema. Looking back at the diastology, the patient turns out to have grade II pseudonormal diastolic dysfunction. |
| **Reasoning Error(s)** | ■ Lack of knowledge/consideration of pseudonormal (grade II) diastolic dysfunction |
| | ■ Cursory glance over normal-appearing data without considering an inappropriately normal appearance (misinterpreting pseudonormal E/A ratio as normal E/A ratio) |
| | ■ Lack of knowledge on how to differentiate between normal relaxation and pseudonormal filling |

**How to Avoid the Mistake**

- Always consider context when assessing diastology. Consider the patient's age, presence of LVH, left atrial and ventricular chamber sizes. These are likely to be present to a mild to moderate degree in grade II diastolic dysfunction.
- Check tissue-wave Doppler of the mitral annulus. True diastolic dysfunction will have a lower velocity given increased LV stiffness.
- Use ASE criteria to determine the grade of diastolic function including left atrial volume, tricuspid regurgitant jet velocity, and tissue Doppler along with mitral valve inflow (Fig. 4.2).
- Consider a Valsalva maneuver to unmask true diastolic dysfunction. Because Valsalva decreases preload, the left atrial pressure temporarily decreases, in turn leading to decreased early diastolic filling (a decrease in the E and, hence, E/A ratio).
- Check for the presence of an L wave on the mitral inflow signal. Though rare, the presence of an L wave represents diastolic dysfunction.

**Antidote**

- Not applicable

**Common Scenarios**

- Not applicable

**Note(s)**

- Memory Aid: Recall the LV moves away from the probe during diastole on apical views. Think about the ventricle expanding to accommodate filling.
- The L wave represents residual blood flow from the pulmonary vein after early diastole. It is more commonly seen with slower heart rates that allow for longer diastasis and better separation of the E and A waves.

## Diastolic Dysfunction Classification

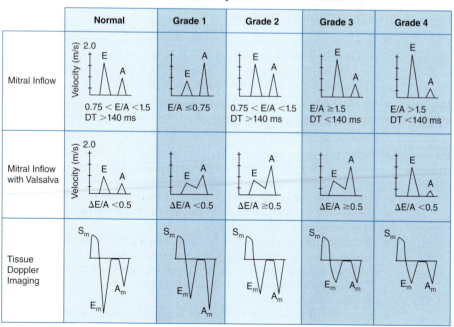

**Fig. 4.2** Grades of diastolic dysfunction.

## MISTAKE: ASSESSMENT OF FUSED E/A WAVES

**Case Example**

You obtain a mitral inflow signal. Despite the fused E and A waves, you attempt to calculate the E/A ratio. Later, you repeat the mitral inflow measurements when the patient is not tachycardic and obtain a very different E/A ratio.

**Reasoning Error(s)**

- Attempting to use data that are suboptimal for diagnosis
- Lack of understanding the physiology that leads to fusion of E and A waves
- Thinking that the fusion of E and A waves cannot be unfused

**How to Avoid the Mistake**

- Always ensure the integrity of the data you are analyzing. If the E and A waves are fused and difficult to discern, do not attempt calculation of the E/A ratio, and diastolic assessment could be indeterminate at that period in time (ASE reference).
- Understand that the fusion of E and A waves typically occurs in the setting of tachycardia due to lack of adequate diastolic filling time.
- Come back at a later time when patient is less tachycardiac if data necessary for diagnosis. Can consider trying to separate out the E and A waves by speeding up the sweep speed on the machine to separate out the mitral valve inflow.

**Antidote**

- Maneuvers or medications that slow heart rate
  - Vagal maneuvers
  - β-Blockers

**Common Scenarios**

- Not applicable

**Note(s)**

- The lack of an A wave in conditions that lack atrial kick (e.g., atrial fibrillation, atrial flutter, AV dyssynchrony, paced rhythms) prevents use of mitral inflow velocities for the assessment of diastolic dysfunction.

## MISTAKE: INTERPRETING MITRAL INFLOW AND TISSUE DOPPLER IN MITRAL OR AORTIC VALVE DISEASE

**Case Example**

A 56-year-old female with severe rheumatic mitral stenosis presents for her annual TTE. On pulsed-wave Doppler, you notice that the E/A ratio is 3, concerning for severe restrictive filling. You refer the patient to a heart failure specialist, who is puzzled at how you arrived to that conclusion.

**Reasoning Error(s)**

- Lack of understanding the physiology that affects common measurements of diastolic function, including mitral inflow velocities and tissue Doppler
- Incomplete understanding of a patient's comorbidities

**How to Avoid the Mistake**

- Understand that any pathology that alters pressure gradients across the mitral valve may affect the validity of the E/A ratio derived from mitral inflow veloci-ties. For example, mitral stenosis may falsely decrease the mitral inflow during early diastole due to increased resistance at the mitral opening. Likewise, aortic insufficiency may decrease the early diastolic gradient across the mitral valve due to an increase in LVEDP.
- Understand the physiology behind E/e' ratios. Simply put, the mitral inflow E veloc-ity represents early diastolic filling, which is sensitive to changes in LV filling pressure (and diastolic dysfunction); the e' velocity on tissue Doppler corrects the mitral inflow E for any effects of impaired LV relaxation. Remember to average the septal e' veloc-ity with that of the lateral wall
- Ensure adequate knowledge of at least the major confounding comorbidities when performing a test. For example, this can be done by looking for particular information first within a study you are currently interpreting, such as calculating diastology toward the end of reading a TTE once you have analyzed valvular and systolic function.

**Antidote** ▪ Not applicable

**Common** ▪ Moderate-severe mitral valve disease
**Scenarios**
    ▪ Mitral stenosis: inflow velocities not accurate for diastology
    ▪ Mitral regurgitation: use additional criteria to assess diastology
  ▪ Severe aortic insufficiency: careful positioning of the sample volume is needed to avoid contamination of the mitral inflow aortic regurgitation jet (also during diastole!)
  ▪ Moderate-severe mitral annular calcification (MAC): may prevent use of mitral annular tissue Doppler assessment
  ▪ Prosthetic mitral valves, valve repairs with annular ring, Alfieri repair
  ▪ Pericardial disease (e.g., large effusion even if not tamponade)
  ▪ Heart transplantation: generally, interferes with accurate diastolic assessment
  ▪ LV assist device (e.g., LVAD or Impella): precludes assessment
  ▪ Post-cardioversion (i.e., from atrial fibrillation or flutter): atria may still be stunned resulting in low A velocity; use other parameters besides the E/A ratio

**Note(s)** ▪ Ensure correct positioning of the pulsed-wave Doppler cursor—exactly at the level of the fully open mitral valve leaflet tips.
  ▪ Do not use continuous-wave Doppler for assessment of diastology.
  ▪ In most hearts, the septal e' velocity is normally lower relative to the lateral e' velocity due to more limited motion of the septal annulus given its position amidst the interatrial/ventricular septum. Averaging the septal and lateral e' velocities is recommended.
  ▪ In constrictive cardiomyopathy, the lateral e' velocity is lower than the septal e' velocity. This is a unique characteristic that can be very helpful in distinguishing constrictive from restrictive cardiomyopathy.
  ▪ E/e' <8 typically reflects normal LV filling pressures (including lack of diastolic dysfunction), whereas values >14 signify likely diastolic dysfunction. Values in between suggest the need for further evaluation.
  ▪ Many patients with systolic dysfunction will have diastolic dysfunction. Thus, use systolic dysfunction as a reminder to check diastology!

**Further** ▪ Great reads to help refresh your knowledge of cardiac pathophysiology: Lilly
**Reading** LS. *Pathophysiology of Heart Disease.* 7th ed. Wolters Kluwer; 2021.

# Echocardiography: Right Heart Disease

### MISTAKE: TRICUSPID ANNULAR PLANAR SYSTOLIC EXCURSION AS DEFINITIVE MEASURE OF RIGHT VENTRICULAR SYSTOLIC FUNCTION

**Case** A patient with a BMI of >40 presents with worsening dyspnea on exertion. You
**Example** perform a TTE and, despite optimizing the windows, image quality is markedly poor. However, you see an echogenic density near the area of the tricuspid annulus that appears to be moving up and down robustly. Based on the tricuspid annular planar systolic excursion (TAPSE), you conclude that the patient has normal RV function. When the patient's oxygen requirements acutely worsen later, he is intubated but arrests during the intubation.

**Reasoning** ▪ Lack of understanding what TAPSE represents or the contractile mechanism of
**Error(s)** the RV
  ▪ Estimating TAPSE visually rather than measuring through M-mode
  ▪ Overreporting or assuming function based on limited information
  ▪ Lack of understanding the limitations to TAPSE

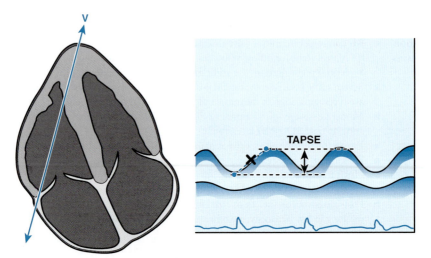

**Fig. 4.3**    TAPSE measurement: vertical distance, not slope.

**How to Avoid the Mistake**
- Understand that TAPSE represents the longitudinal function of the right ventricle, which is one component to RV systolic motion (longitudinal and transverse motion)
- Remember that TAPSE is an M-mode measurement and that it is not meant to be a visual estimation from the apical four-chamber view (though in practice it is a quick gestalt). Also remember that the measurement is done vertically (it is not the slope, which is a mistake frequently made), as shown in Fig. 4.3.
- If the image quality is suboptimal, report what you can and do not use TAPSE; instead, use other parameters that assess RV function.
- Understand the limitations of TAPSE. It depends significantly on the angle at which it is measured and is load dependent, meaning that it is unreliable in conditions such as significant tricuspid regurgitation.

**Antidote**
- Confirm RV systolic function based on alternate methods (e.g., RV systolic tissue Doppler imaging [i.e., S'-wave measurement])

**Common Scenarios**
- Not applicable

**Note(s)**
- Normal TAPSE is >1.7 cm.
- A normal peak RV systolic velocity (S'wave) measured by tissue Doppler is >9.5 cm/s.
- The S'wave is the tissue Doppler–derived tricuspid lateral annular velocity, similar to the e'wave used in assessment of LV filling pressures. It should correlate well (>9.6 cm/s is normal while <9.6 cm/s is consistent with a depressed RV function) with the TAPSE. A limitation of the RV systolic tissue Doppler imaging is that it is measuring only at the base of the RV and extrapolating to apply to the entire RV so visual assessment should correlate. If visual assessment does not correlate, the most accurate interpretation would be of focal RV function (e.g., that of the RV base).
- A common error with measuring RV systolic tissue Doppler imaging is using the first systolic spoke rather than the second. Always use the second systolic spike.

# Echocardiography: Aortic Stenosis

## MISTAKE: ATTRIBUTING ALL HIGH AORTIC JET VELOCITIES TO AORTIC STENOSIS

**Case Example**   You measure the aortic velocity to be 4.4 m/s and annotate aortic stenosis in the report. However, the intrepid intern notes that the patient's aortic leaflets appear to have full unrestricted range of motion. You look back at the 2D images and realize that the patient likely has a subvalvular membrane causing the high velocities.

**Reasoning Error(s)**
- Premature closure (not thinking of a differential for a finding)
- Lack of contextualization based on the 2D images and clinical presentation

**How to Avoid the Mistake**
- Place the velocity measured in context. Is the aortic valve well visualized, and does the aortic valve appear calcified and/or restricted? Is there significant septal hypertrophy? Systolic anterior motion of the mitral valve? How old is the patient?
- Think through a differential for each piece of data. For a high velocity measured near the aortic valve, this includes HOCM and a subvalvular membrane and, less commonly, a supravalvular obstruction. Also, continuous-wave imaging can show mid-cavitary gradient in hyperdynamic LV function and sometimes with apical HCM.
- Pay attention to the shape of the measured jets. Certain pathologies have unique jet shapes; for example, HOCM presents with a late-peaking dagger-shaped jet or mitral regurgitation starting earlier in relation to the QRS compared with aortic valve flow.

**Antidote**
- Not applicable

**Common Scenarios**
- HOCM
- Nonvalvular aortic stenosis (e.g., subvalvular membrane)
- Eccentric mitral regurgitation jet

**Note(s)**
- Fun Fact: HOCM has been described by >75 different names throughout history, including "idiopathic hypertrophic subaortic stenosis" when Drs. Eugene Braunwald and Andrew Morrow first released a modern description of the disease in 1960. The first known description of HCM was called "cardiac sub-aortic stenosis" and dates back to 1869 by Henri Liouville.

**Further Reading**
- Interesting paper on the history of HCM: Braunwald E. Hypertrophic cardiomyopathy: the first century 1869–1969. *Glob Cardiol Sci Pract*. 2012;1(5).

## MISTAKE: SUBOPTIMAL ALIGNMENT OF DOPPLER FOR AORTIC JET VELOCITY MEASUREMENT

**Case Example**   A 79-year-old male presents with dyspnea on exertion and is found with a 4/6 systolic ejection murmur best heard at the right upper sternal border. You perform a TTE and measure the aortic jet velocity to be 3.7 m/s on the short-axis view at the level of the RVOT. However, you are surprised to find that the aortic jet measures 4.6 m/s on the apical five-chamber view and 4.9 m/s on the apical three-chamber view.

**Reasoning Error(s)**
- Measuring the jet velocity in a single view and not from ideal views
- Lack of knowledge regarding the significant variation in aortic jet velocity based on the fidelity of Doppler signal alignment
- Suboptimal imaging windows

| | |
|---|---|
| **How to Avoid the Mistake** | ■ Measure the aortic jet velocity on multiple views to find the highest velocity. |
| | ■ Adjust the angle of the probe even within one window to check for the maximum velocity. |
| | ■ Obtain adequate windows and velocity tracings prior to measuring. |
| | ■ Consider using a Pedoff probe (a probe that provides only velocities but does so exceptionally well given its small size and ability to be put between rib spaces). In addition, measure from alternative views such as right sternal border (RSB), suprasternal notch (SSN), and subcostal. |
| **.Antidote** | ■ Not applicable |
| **Common Scenarios** | ■ Not applicable |
| **Note(s)** | ■ An incorrect aortic jet velocity leads to magnified errors of the aortic valve pressure gradient because the gradient is derived exponentially by the Bernoulli equation (gradient = 4v2, where v is the peak velocity). |
| | ■ When the angle of insonation and the flow of blood deviate by >20 degrees, the measured value becomes progressively underestimated. |

## MISTAKE: CALCULATION OF THE AORTIC VALVE AREA BASED ON INCORRECT LEFT VENTRICULAR OUTFLOW TRACT MEASUREMENTS

| | |
|---|---|
| **Case Example** | You are tasked with confirming the aortic valve area for a patient with presumed severe aortic stenosis. You grab the echo machine and excitedly head over to the patient's room. You proceed to measure the left ventricular outflow tract (LVOT) diameter and LVOT velocity. You then successfully obtain the peak aortic jet velocity with a Pedoff probe. You calculate the aortic valve area (AVA) by plugging the radius of the LVOT into the continuity equation ($A_1V_1 = A_2V_2$). To your surprise, the AVA significantly differs from previously reported value. |
| **Reasoning Error(s)** | ■ Not knowing or considering the position of the Doppler signal relative to the aortic valve when measuring the LVOT velocity |
| | ■ Calculating the AVA using velocities (which are highly dependent on high-quality images and appropriate beam positioning) |
| | ■ Lack of attention to position of the Doppler signal within the LVOT (i.e., how close to the aortic valve) |
| | ■ Forgetting to convert the LVOT diameter to radius when using the continuity equation |
| **How to Avoid the Mistake** | ■ Ensure that the Doppler signal is not placed too close to the aortic valve as flow acceleration takes place in that region. Also, avoid placing the signal too far away and into the LV (ideally at mid-systole and inner edge to inner edge 3–5 mm from the aortic valve plane between septal endocardium and anterior mitral valve leaflet). |
| | ■ Consider using velocity-time integrals (VTIs) rather than velocities for calculating the AVA as the VTI is dimensionless. |
| | ■ When measuring the LVOT diameter, take your time to obtain a high-fidelity measurement. Double check the measurement as this measurement becomes squared ($A = \pi r^2$) in the continuity equation further adding error if your measurement is incorrect. |
| **Antidote** | ■ None |

| Common Scenarios | ■ None |
|---|---|
| Note(s) | ■ The three most common locations for using the Pedoff probe are the apical, suprasternal, and right parasternal windows. |

## MISTAKE: INCONSISTENT OR EXAGGERATED TRACING OF AORTIC JET VELOCITY

| Case Example | You trace the aortic jet velocity, computing a maximum velocity of 5.1 m/s, which is then used to derive a mean aortic gradient of 60 mmHg. As a budding interventionalist, you are ecstatic to see a patient qualify for TAVR, but your attending frowns at your tracing. |
|---|---|
| Reasoning Error(s) | ■ Well-intentioned but incorrect method of achieving maximal velocities from the tracing<br>■ Inconsistent tracing methodology to achieve maximal velocities |
| How to Avoid the Mistake | ■ Trace the aortic jet only using well-defined (the brightest, nonhazy) contours<br>■ Always trace aortic jets in a consistent manner. Even if your measurements are slightly off, they will be fairly reproducible, which is essential to monitoring progression of disease. Otherwise, you would be "gaming" the measurements to be as high as possible. |
| Antidote | ■ Not applicable |
| Common Scenarios | ■ Not applicable |
| Note(s) | ■ Remember, even small variations in the aortic jet velocity measurements can lead to large differences in the mean pressure gradient. |

## MISTAKE: AORTIC VELOCITY AND GRADIENT MEASUREMENT DURING HIGH- OR LOW-FLOW STATES

| Case Example | A 72-year-old female with moderate aortic stenosis and a new AV fistula presents for an echocardiogram to monitor her aortic stenosis. You calculate the peak aortic velocity to be 4.0 m/s, significantly increased from the 2.8 m/s last year. Interestingly, the aortic valve leaflets do not appear to be more restricted than last year. |
|---|---|
| Reasoning Error(s) | ■ Performing measurements in the presence of an obvious confounder<br>■ Not contextualizing the measurements<br>■ Lack of follow-up testing to verify questionable measurements (e.g., dimensionless index) |
| How to Avoid the Mistake | ■ In general, avoid obtaining measurements when clear confounders are present (e.g., a high-output state in the above example). Use alternatives such as the dimensionless index, which is a ratio between the VTIs of the LVOT and aortic valve jet, meaning that the most common source for significant error (i.e., inaccurate measurement of the LVOT cross-sectional area via the continuity equation) is avoided.<br>■ Contextualize the measurements. Is there anything that can be causing the measurements to be artificially high or low? What is the clinical status of the patient during the TTE?<br>■ If in doubt, perform a repeat TTE or further studies (e.g., dobutamine stress echo in setting of low LVEF, TEE, cardiac CTA, and/or cardiac catheterization to better assess the aortic valve). |

| | |
|---|---|
| **Antidote** | ■ Not applicable |
| **Common Scenarios** | ■ High-flow states |
| |    ■ Aortic regurgitation |
| |    ■ Arteriovenous fistula |
| |    ■ Severe anemia |
| |    ■ Severe hyperthyroidism |
| |    ■ Low-flow states |
| |    ■ Depressed LV function |
| |    ■ Low-flow low-gradient aortic stenosis |
| |    ■ Paradoxical low-flow low-gradient aortic stenosis |
| |    ■ Sepsis |
| |    ■ Cardiogenic shock |
| |    ■ Hypovolemic shock |
| **Note(s)** | ■ AVA is fairly flow independent and may be a better surrogate for aortic stenosis severity in the presence of a significant flow-influencing state. |
| | ■ Though not a high- or low-flow state, be aware that the aortic pressure gradient may be overestimated in the presence of a small ascending aorta due to the pressure recovery phenomenon (pressure increases as velocity decreases). This is particularly important when there is moderate aortic stenosis along with a small ascending aorta (<2 cm). Normally when blood enters the ascending aorta, kinetic energy is converted into heat and prevents a "pressure recovery," though this does not occur with a small aorta and kinetic energy is converted into pressure. This increase in ascending aortic pressure, therefore, results in an increase in the peak-peak gradient (compared with catheterization) and therefore an incorrectly, smaller calculated AVA (i.e., turning moderate aortic stenosis into severe aortic stenosis). |
| | ■ Remember the dimensionless index is particularly helpful in low- and high-flow states. It is calculated by dividing the LVOT VTI by the AV VTI. A value <0.25 suggests severe aortic stenosis. |

## MISTAKE: AORTIC VELOCITY AND GRADIENT MEASUREMENT DURING ARRHYTHMIAS

| | |
|---|---|
| **Case Example** | An 80-year-old male with chronic kidney disease and atrial fibrillation presents with dyspnea, angina, and syncope. You order a TTE after hearing a loud systolic crescendo-decrescendo murmur that radiates to the carotids. The TTE reveals severely restricted aortic valve leaflets and you measure the peak aortic velocity in the three-chamber view over a single RR interval. To your surprise, the peak aortic velocity is only 3.7 m/s despite preserved EF and no evidence of diastolic dysfunction. |
| **Reasoning Error(s)** | ■ Forgetting that arrhythmias disrupt the preload and stroke volume, thus influencing the aortic valve measurements |
| | ■ Not averaging measurements in the presence of arrhythmia |

| | |
|---|---|
| **How to Avoid the Mistake** | ■ Understand that all arrhythmias distort the aortic valve measurements via various mechanisms. Irregular arrhythmias may produce wide beat-to-beat variability in measurements due to varying preload and stroke volume. Even regular arrhythmias such as atrioventricular nodal reentrant tachycardia (AVNRT) may lead to decreased preload and hence ejected stroke volume due to decreased diastolic filling time and/or AV dyssynchrony.<br>■ Average measurements over multiple beats (minimum 5 beats) unless using the single-cycle method, which involves matching the RR intervals for the aortic valve VTI and LVOT VTI (Esquitin et al, 2018) |
| **Antidote** | ■ Not applicable |
| **Common Scenarios** | ■ Irregular rhythms (e.g., atrial fibrillation, variable block)<br>■ Regular rhythm arrhythmias (e.g., AVNRT, multifocal atrial tachycardia)<br>■ PACs<br>■ PVCs |
| **Note(s)** | ■ Remember in general to not use the compensatory beat following a premature beat since these beats are delayed generally resulting in a higher single-beat velocity and can alter diagnostic measurements. |
| **Further Reading** | ■ Esquitin KA, et al. Accuracy of the single cycle length method for calculation of aortic effective orifice area in irregular heart rhythms. *J Am Soc Echocardiogr*. 2018;11(18):344-350. |

# Echocardiography: Valvular Regurgitation

## MISTAKE: CHARACTERIZATION OF REGURGITANT LESIONS WITHOUT OPTIMIZING HEMODYNAMICS

| | |
|---|---|
| **Case Example** | A 73-year-old female with mitral regurgitation and HFrEF (EF 30%) is admitted for decompensated heart failure. The TTE demonstrates severe mitral regurgitation and you refer the patient for a MitraClip (transcatheter mitral valve repair). However, because the patient cannot lie flat, her procedure is deferred until after volume optimization. Prior to her MitraClip, another TTE is performed and the mitral regurgitation only appears at most moderate. |
| **Reasoning Error(s)** | ■ Not considering the effect of hemodynamics on valvular regurgitation<br>■ Forgetting to optimize hemodynamics |
| **How to Avoid the Mistake** | ■ Remember that pressure gradients due to LV filling conditions and other hemodynamic parameters such as afterload all influence the degree of regurgitation (significantly!). In other words, regurgitation is dynamic!<br>■ Ideally, optimize the patient as close to euvolemic state prior to analyzing regurgitant valvular lesions and making decisions on therapeutic referrals. |
| **Antidote** | ■ Not applicable |
| **Common Scenarios** | ■ Volume overload<br>■ Hemodynamic support (e.g., pressors)<br>■ β-Blockade in aortic regurgitation and aortic stenosis<br>■ Poorly controlled hypertension |
| **Note(s)** | ■ A limitation to the MitraClip is a potential to cause mitral stenosis if too many clips are placed or the clips are placed with inadequate spacing. |

## MISTAKE: COLOR-FLOW DOPPLER FOR ECCENTRIC OR MULTIPLE JETS

| | |
|---|---|
| **Case Example** | A patient presents with shortness of breath and a 3/6 blowing systolic murmur at the left upper sternal border. You perform a TTE and discover an eccentric mitral regurgitant jet. You decide that your auscultation overestimated the possible mitral regurgitation compared with the TTE and decide that the patient has only mild mitral regurgitation. After going home and having difficulty sleeping because the murmur was out of proportion to the discovered mitral regurgitation, you decide to order a TEE. You are glad you did so when the TEE demonstrates severe mitral regurgitation, visualizing a large eccentric jet wrapping into the back of the atrium. |
| **Reasoning Error(s)** | ■ Inadequate understanding the principle of color-flow Doppler<br>■ Lack of knowledge of the Coanda effect<br>■ Obtaining a single window to characterize the jet(s)<br>■ Not pursuing additional imaging when there is discordance between symptoms and physical exam and the TTE |
| **How to Avoid the Mistake** | ■ Understand that color-flow Doppler (and all other types of Doppler) most accurately measure flow that is parallel to the sound beam. In other words, perpendicular flow (i.e., part of eccentric jets) will not be seen well with color Doppler.<br>■ Learn the Coanda effect, which causes eccentric jets to hug the atrial wall and lose their energy, leading to a smaller jet.<br>■ Use multiple windows to determine the direction and origin of the regurgitant jet(s).<br>■ Look for other associated findings of severe mitral regurgitation, such as pulmonary vein flow reversal, increased peak E wave across the mitral valve with increased gradient without evidence of mitral stenosis, or increased estimated pulmonary artery systolic pressure in the setting of mitral regurgitation. |
| **Antidote** | ■ Confirmatory Imaging (e.g., TEE) |
| **Common Scenarios** | ■ Multiple regurgitant jets (regardless of which valve)<br>■ Eccentric regurgitant jets (regardless of which valve) |
| **Note(s)** | ■ The degree to which a regurgitant jet extends into the preceding heart chamber may be a quick estimate of the severity of regurgitation. However, it is influenced by many factors, such as the angle of the probe and the hemodynamics. Hence, it is important to remember that color Doppler can better at indicating the presence of regurgitation than quantifying it. |

## MISTAKE: LIMITATIONS OF PROXIMAL ISOVELOCITY SURFACE AREA

| | |
|---|---|
| **Case Example** | A patient presents for evaluation of her mitral regurgitation secondary to mitral valve prolapse. You use the PISA to estimate the severity of her regurgitation as severe, but your colleague notes that the PISA is inaccurate in this case. |
| **Reasoning Error(s)** | ■ Not considering the limitations to using a method<br>■ Lack of understanding of the physical principles underlying PISA |
| **How to Avoid the Mistake** | ■ Understand that the PISA is based on the conservation of mass. In other words, the regurgitant flow corresponds to the flow convergence zone (which is ideally a hemispheric shape given PISA = $2\pi r^2$). Learn the scenarios in which PISA should not be used: calcified or prosthetic valves, eccentric jets, multiple jets, nonholosystolic jets, noncircular orifice. |

| | |
|---|---|
| **Antidote** | ■ Not applicable |
| **Common Scenarios** | ■ Nonholosystolic jets<br>■ Noncircular orifice<br>■ Eccentric jets<br>■ Multiple jets<br>■ Calcified valves<br>■ Prosthetic valves |
| **Note(s)** | ■ The PISA is based on a single frame. Thus, the assumption is that the severity of the regurgitation is constant. If the jet is not holosystolic, the PISA may overestimate the regurgitant jet.<br>■ Small errors in the measurement of the PISA radius can lead to large differences in the effective regurgitant orifice area. |
| **Further Reading** | ■ Great article on how to define severe functional mitral regurgitation: Graybum PA, et al. Defining "severe" secondary mitral regurgitation. *JACC.* 2014;64(25):2792-2801. |

## MISTAKE: USING PRESSURE HALF-TIME WITHOUT CONSIDERING LEFT VENTRICULAR COMPLIANCE OR AFTERLOAD

| | |
|---|---|
| **Case Example** | A patient with NICM (EF 20%) and grade IV diastolic dysfunction presents to clinic for worsening shortness of breath. A diastolic rumble is head on exam near the apex; initial TTE demonstrates only mild mitral stenosis based on the pressure half-time. However, given the severe diastolic dysfunction, you perform further assessment of the mitral valve by measuring the mean gradient and three-dimensional (3D) planimetry, both which support a diagnosis of moderate to severe mitral stenosis. |
| **Reasoning Error(s)** | ■ Forgetting factors that affect the pressure half-time<br>■ Lack of understanding about the concept of pressure half-time<br>■ Lack of knowledge about relevant comorbidities |
| **How to Avoid the Mistake** | ■ Understand that pressure half-time refers to the amount of time it takes for a pressure gradient across a valve to decrease to half of its maximum. Thus, the measurement is dependent on a patient's current hemodynamics.<br>■ Recognize conditions that alter the pressure half-time: LV compliance, preload, afterload, and chronic aortic regurgitation (if over time, LV pressures have increased and aortic pressures decreased, the pressure half-time may be compensated).<br>■ Obtain as much information on potentially confounding comorbidities as possible. |
| **Antidote** | ■ Not applicable |
| **Common Scenarios** | ■ LV compliance (diastolic dysfunction)<br>■ Afterload<br>■ Atrial fibrillation (must average multiple pressure half-time values) |
| **Note(s)** | ■ Pressure half-time is most often used to characterize the severity of mitral stenosis and acute (rather than chronic) aortic regurgitation.<br>■ Consider additional echo-derived variables such as possible diastolic flow reversal in the thoracic aorta (moderate) or abdominal aorta (severe), assess the vena contracta, area of the color jet in short-axis view of the aortic valve, jet width in LVOT, quantitative flow measurements with calculation of regurgitant volume/fraction, premature closure of the mitral valve in diastole (severe), and use of 3D echo. |

# Echocardiography: Pericardial Disease

## MISTAKE: MISTAKING PLEURAL EFFUSIONS OR ASCITES FOR PERICARDIAL EFFUSIONS

**Case Example**

You obtain a parasternal long-axis view and notice a 1.5 cm of free-flowing fluid near the inferolateral wall of the heart. You then shift to the subcostal view and notice a significant pocket of fluid next to the RV. You conclude that the patient has a significant pericardial effusion without chamber compromise. Images in Fig. 4.4. Your attending notes that these represent a small left-sided pleural effusion and small ascites, respectively.

**Reasoning Error(s)**

- Bias toward diagnosing a pericardial effusion by virtue of using a cardiac test (echocardiography)
- Lack of knowledge on anatomic distinctions when assessing fluid adjacent to the heart
- Not thinking through a differential diagnosis for imaging findings
- Technical limitations of study potentially caused by lack of experience of sonographer, patient body habitus, postsurgical bandaging, etc.

**How to Avoid the Mistake**

- Recognize that echocardiography windows may also reveal noncardiac structures.
- Maintain a differential diagnosis for findings surrounding the heart: pericardial effusion, pleural effusion, ascites, prominent pericardial fat pad, and mediastinal collections.
- Familiarize yourself with the anatomy in each imaging view, with attention to the anatomic landmarks that distinguish various body compartments. For example, on a parasternal long-axis view, fluid around the heart that resides anterior to the descending thoracic aorta would be a pericardial effusion, whereas fluid posterior to the thoracic aorta correlates with pleural effusions. Ascites on the subcostal view can be recognized by the presence of a floating falciform ligament within the fluid anterior to the RV in addition to seeing perihepatic fluid.
- Report uncertainty in the face of poor image quality

**Antidote**

- None

**Common Scenarios**

- Pleural effusions
- Ascites
- Prominent pericardial fat pad

**Note(s)**

- Clinical Pearl: When imaging larger, predominantly fluid pericardial effusions, place the patient supine with the head of the bed at 45 degrees, which would simulate how a pericardiocentesis would be set up. This allows for the fluid to accumulate anteriorly and apically where an interventionist could insert a needle or drain. Remember that not all pericardial effusions can be easily accessed and that confirming accessibility is important.
- To distinguish a pericardial fat pad from a pericardial effusion, check for movement of the "fluid" with changes in patient position. Pericardial effusions (if only fluid) can be completely anechoic/echolucent, whereas pericardial fat pads appear more heterogeneous and moves along with the typically RV chamber from beat to beat. Look for other collections and consider clinical context if patient is postsurgical or postprocedure; consider whether the collection represents thrombi.
- A prominent pericardial fat pad, usually seen anterior to the RV, has long been considered to be of little clinical significance, but more recent data demonstrate an association with increased risk of atrial fibrillation.
- A close look at pericardial fluid may reveal additional details such as small strands that correspond to septations, cellular debris, pus, or thrombus.

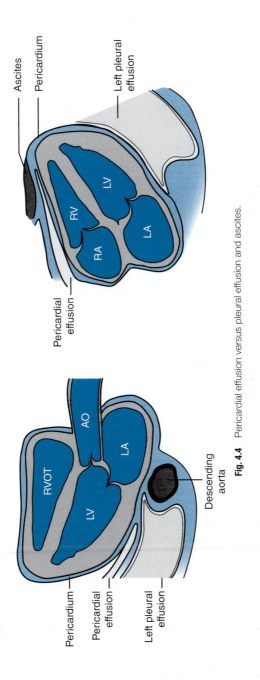

**Fig. 4.4**  Pericardial effusion versus pleural effusion and ascites.

## MISTAKE: THINKING THAT PERICARDIAL EFFUSIONS ARE ONLY FLUID

**Case Example**    A 70-year-old female undergoes a dual-chamber permanent pacemaker placement without obvious complications. The postoperative chest radiograph and ECG appear normal, and she returns to the floor. She suddenly has difficulty breathing with a drop in blood pressure, and a STAT TTE is performed, which you interpret as reassuringly having a small pericardial effusion and some pericardial fat and determine no tamponade physiology is present. Your attending is alarmed, noting there is mixed blood and thrombus, and in the clinical context cardiac tamponade is present; the patient is emergently sent to the operating room.

**Reasoning Error(s)**
- Lack of viewing all data (i.e., pericardial effusions) with a differential diagnosis (e.g., fluid, blood, etc.)
- Lack of clinical context
- Not considering that cardiac tamponade can be present in the setting of a small pericardial effusion if the effusion has accumulated rapidly

**How to Avoid the Mistake**
- Understand that the term "pericardial effusion" simply refers to what is in the pericardial space. It does not necessarily mean it is a homogeneous free-flowing fluid. For example, it may be a mix of fluid and echogenic material or completely echogenic material without free-flowing fluid. Common nonfluid possibilities include blood/thrombus, bacteria (or other infection), and mixed etiologies.
- Always interpret pericardial effusions within the clinical context. For example, a patient who is status post endocardial biopsy would be at risk for tamponade from perforation and bleeding.

**Antidote**
- None

**Common Scenarios**
- Fluid
- Blood
- Infection
- Echogenic material
- Mixed (two or more of the above)

**Note(s)**
- The pericardium usually contains <50 mL of free-flowing fluid that acts as a lubricant to facilitate movement of the heart within the sac.

# Echocardiography: Mass Mimics

## MISTAKE: LEFT ATRIAL MASS MIMICS

**Case Example**    You visualize an echogenicity in the left atrium and start the patient on apixaban for a left atrial appendage thrombus.

**Reasoning Error(s)**
- Lack of a differential for echodense structures in the left atrium and jumping to the idea of a thrombus, vegetation, or malignancy
- Lack of familiarity with the appearance on echocardiography caused by the coumadin ridge, a large hiatal hernia compressing the left atrium, or lipomatous hypertrophy
- Lack of clinical context
- Overconfident reporting (e.g., not considering technical limitations)

**How to Avoid the Mistake**

- Use language that most accurately describes the limitations of your study. For example, rather than stating "No LV apical thrombus" on a noncontrast TTE, it may be better to note "Cannot be excluded" or "Not clearly seen … consider further characterization with contrast."
- Remember that every imaging finding has a differential diagnosis just like any other symptom or sign. Reason through the differential each time rather than prematurely closing.
- Remember that a bandlike structure may be present near the left atrial appendage frequently referred to as the "coumadin ridge" that often gets confused for a mass/left atrial appendage thrombi.
- Learn that a natural variant of the interatrial septum is to contain excess fat termed "lipomatous hypertrophy," which contributes to a dumbbell-like shape at the interatrial septum.
- Understand that a large hiatal hernia compressing on the left atrium may mimic a left atrial mass.
- Always apply clinical context to imaging findings. For example, is the patient at risk of a thrombus, vegetation, or malignancy? Do they have a known large hiatal hernia?
- Determine the need for further confirmation of the potential mass based on clinical context. Perform a TEE, CMR, or CT as needed to confirm your suspicions.

**Antidote**

- Not applicable

**Common Scenarios**

- Coumadin ridge
- Lipomatous hypertrophy
- Hiatal hernia

**Note(s)**

- The most common cardiac mass is thrombus (excluding mass mimics).
- Sometimes in close proximity to the echodensity caused by compression of the left atrium there may appear to be a moving smoky-appearing or swirling structure—this represents gastric contents/bubbles (e.g., depends what they recently had to eat) and supports a hiatal hernia.
- The presence of thrombi should always prompt consideration of cause whether an arrhythmia such as atrial fibrillation causing a left atrial appendage thrombus, an LV apical thrombus caused by an ischemic cardiomyopathy, or an RV apical thrombus caused by eosinophilic heart disease. Other right-sided thrombi may also result from the presence of a central catheter or pacemaker lead.

## MISTAKE: LEFT VENTRICULAR MASS MIMICS

**Case Example**

You visualize an echogenicity in the LV and alert the primary team to the presence of a pathologic LV mass.

**Reasoning Error(s)**

- Lack of a differential for echodensities in the LV and jumping to the idea of a thrombus, vegetation, or malignancy
- Lack of familiarity with a false tendon or significant mitral annular calcification and its appearance on echocardiography
- Lack of clinical context
- Overconfidence reporting findings (e.g., definitely excluding the possibility of a LV mass)

**How to Avoid the Mistake**
- Remember that every imaging finding has a differential diagnosis just like any other symptom or sign. Reason through the differential each time rather than prematurely closing.
- Learn about LV bands, which are fibromuscular bands that may connect between the interventricular septum, free wall, and papillary muscle(s).
- Remember that the mitral annulus may undergo significant calcification as well as develop caseous necrosis, particularly in patients with end-stage renal disease and in older women.
- Always apply clinical context to imaging findings. For example, is the patient at risk of a thrombus, vegetation, or malignancy?
- Determine the need for further confirmation of the potential mass based on clinical context. Perform a TEE, CMR, or CT as needed to confirm your suspicions.

**Antidote**
- Not applicable

**Common Scenarios**
- LV band (false tendon)
- Ruptured false tendon (may closely mimic the chaotic motion of vegetation)
- Papillary muscles
- Chordae
- Significant mitral annular calcification
- Degenerative stands (also called Lambl excrescences) commonly seen on the atrial side of the mitral valve or LV side of the aortic valve cusps

**Note(s)**
- False tendons may closely mimic chordae. However, the trick to differentiating them is to observe whether they attach to the mitral valve itself. False tendons do not touch the valve.
- Lambl excrescences are very thin filamentous strands that most commonly appear on the mitral (atrial side) and aortic valves (ventricular side). They are differentiated from vegetations by their very thin and delicate appearance.

## MISTAKE: RIGHT ATRIAL MASS MIMICS

**Case Example**
You visualize an echogenicity in the right atrium and alert the primary team to the presence of a pathologic right atrial mass.

**Reasoning Error(s)**
- Lack of a differential for echodensities in the right atrium and jumping to the idea of a thrombus, vegetation, or tumor
- Lack of familiarity with the Eustachian valve, Chiari network, or crista terminalis as anatomic structures and their appearance on echocardiography
- Lack of clinical context
- Overconfidence reporting findings (e.g., definitely excluding the possibility of a right atrial mass)

| | |
|---|---|
| **How to Avoid the Mistake** | ■ Remember that every imaging finding has a differential diagnosis just like any other symptom or sign. Reason through the differential each time rather than prematurely closing. |
| | ■ The Eustachian valve is an embryological, functionless remnant of the inferior vena cava (IVC). Similarly, the Chiari network is the embryological remnant of the sinus venosus. The crista terminalis is a well-defined fibromuscular ridge along the lateral right atrium extending from the superior vena cava (SVC) to the IVC. All three may rarely be prominent in adults and mimic a right atrial mass. |
| | ■ Always apply clinical context to imaging findings. For example, is the patient at risk of a thrombus, vegetation, or malignancy? |
| | ■ Determine the need for further confirmation of the potential mass based on clinical context. Consider performing a 3D TTE, TEE, CMR, or CT as needed to confirm your suspicions. |
| **Antidote** | ■ Not applicable |
| **Common Scenarios** | ■ Crista terminalis |
| | ■ Eustachian valve |
| | ■ Chiari network |
| | ■ Prominent AV groove fat |
| | ■ Lipomatous hypertrophy |
| | ■ Central catheter |
| | ■ Pacing wire |
| **Note(s)** | ■ The crista terminalis, Eustachian valve, and Chiari network do not have well-defined, postembryologic functions. |
| **Further Reading** | ■ Excellent article on common mass mimics on TTE: Malik SB, et al. Transthoracic echocardiography: pitfalls and limitations as delineated at cardiac CT and MR imaging. *RadioGraphics*. 2017;37(2):383-406. |

## MISTAKE: RIGHT VENTRICULAR MASS MIMICS

| | |
|---|---|
| **Case Example** | You visualize an echogenicity in the RV and alert the primary team to the presence of a pathologic RV mass. |
| **Reasoning Error(s)** | ■ Lack of a differential for echodensities in the RV and jumping to the idea of a thrombus, vegetation, or tumor |
| | ■ Lack of familiarity with the moderator band and/or atrioventricular groove fat as an anatomical structure and its appearance on echocardiography |
| | ■ Lack of clinical context |
| | ■ Overconfidence reporting findings (e.g., definitely excluding the possibility of an RV mass) |

| | |
|---|---|
| **How to Avoid the Mistake** | ■ Remember that every imaging finding has a differential diagnosis just like any other symptom or sign. Reason through the differential each time rather than prematurely closing. |
| | ■ Learn about the moderator band. It is a structure that carries a large segment of the right bundle branch from the interventricular septum to the right anterior papillary muscle. |
| | ■ Learn about the AV groove fat. It insulates the right and left circumflex coronary arteries that course through the AV groove. |
| | ■ Always apply clinical context to imaging findings. For example, is the patient at risk of a thrombus, vegetation, or malignancy? |
| | ■ Determine the need for further confirmation of the potential mass based on clinical context. Perform a 3D TTE, TEE, CMR, or CT as needed to confirm your suspicions. |
| **Antidote** | ■ Not applicable |
| **Common Scenarios** | ■ Moderator band |
| | ■ Prominent AV groove fat |
| | ■ Central catheter |
| | ■ Pacemaker or defibrillator wire |
| | ■ Prominent RV trabeculations |
| **Note(s)** | ■ The moderator band provides electrical impulses to the more remote portion of the RV, thus allowing for coordinated contraction of the LV and RV. |
| | ■ Less commonly, true masses (rather than mass mimics) to avoid overlooking on TTE include an RV thrombus, metastatic cancer, primary cardiac sarcoma, and eosinophilic heart disease. |

## MISTAKE: FALSE ASCENDING AORTIC DISSECTION

| | |
|---|---|
| **Case Example** | A patient undergoes a routine echo as part of the preop for bariatric surgery. You notice what you believe to be a false lumen concerning for an ascending aortic dissection. Alarmed, you send the patient to the emergency department for further evaluation. The patient undergoes CTA, which rules out dissection. |
| **Reasoning Error(s)** | ■ Lack of knowledge or experience with reverberation artifact that may create artifact that appears to be an ascending aortic dissection |
| | ■ Not taking clinical context into consideration |
| | ■ Reporting with too much confidence |

| | |
|---|---|
| **How to Avoid the Mistake** | ■ Understand that artifacts (things that are not actually there) may be created on images. One type is reverberation artifact, which occurs when the ultrasound beam bounces strongly between two parallel surfaces. This is particularly common in patients with obesity, and an already poor imaging window may further increase the likelihood of seeing artifact.<br><br>■ Change the angle of the echo probe to limit the reverberation effect from occurring. Consider using alternate views. A true reverberation effect should disappear or at least change if the angle of the probe is changed.<br><br>■ Interpret images with clinical context. What is the habitus of the patient? Are they experiencing chest and/or back pain?<br><br>■ Report findings with room for diagnostic uncertainty. While clinical context and experience may lead to the right answer most of the time, leave the possibility of dissection on the table because it is a life-changing mistake if missed. Based on clinical context, the clinical team can decide the level of suspicion and need for further imaging.<br><br>■ If available, always closely compare prior echocardiogram to the current study to see if the finding was previously seen. |
| **Antidote** | ■ Even patients who undergo TEE to better assess the aorta can have misdiagnoses either by confusing artifact or misinterpreting anatomical variants of normal structures. Patients have undergone TEE with "confirmation of aortic dissection" only to be reinterpreted as the "dissection flap" being a longitudinal cut of the azygous or hemiazygos veins that course in close proximity to the descending thoracic aorta and aortic arch before emptying into the SCV. |
| **Common Scenarios** | ■ Not applicable |
| **Note(s)** | ■ Missing a diagnosis is usually worse than a false diagnosis that causes an extra diagnostic study (e.g., CTA). When in doubt, given the magnitude of the diagnosis, further workup should be performed. |

# Cardiac Computed Tomography: Quality

## MISTAKE: INADEQUATE PATIENT PREPARATION FOR CORONARY COMPUTED TOMOGRAPHY ANGIOGRAPHY

| | |
|---|---|
| **Case Example** | A 45-year-old female is admitted for further evaluation of chest pain. A coronary CTA is ordered, and the patient is NPO overnight. At the CT scanner, she appears nervous with dry mucous membranes, heart rate of 89 bpm, and blood pressure of 98/60. The technologist proceeds with the scan, and much of the study is deemed to be nondiagnostic due to motion artifact. |
| **Reasoning Error(s)** | ■ Inexperience or lack of thought regarding optimal patient preparation for coronary CTA, including optimizing hydration and intravenous (IV) access (18-gauge IV line is the standard)<br><br>■ Lack of understanding of the influence of heart rate on the temporal resolution and thereby cardiac CT image quality<br><br>■ Forgetting to administer the appropriate agents (i.e., β-blocker) to control heart rate prior to imaging<br><br>■ Forgetting that nitroglycerin (which is standardly used for most coronary CTA protocols) can lead to a reflex tachycardia especially if the patient is relatively hypotensive and not adequately hydrated at the time of the scan |

**How to Avoid the Mistake**

- Understand that CT image quality frequently decreases with higher heart rates due to motion artifact (related to underlying temporal resolution of the cardiac CT scanner). Hydration and premedication with (either β-blocker or calcium channel blocker) are paramount. In particular, a notably more significant rebound in heart rate may occur in the setting of sublingual nitroglycerin use when dehydrated.
- Remember to administer oral β-blockers or calcium channel blockers ideally 30–60 minutes prior to imaging. Target a heart rate of 55 bpm, though this is not an absolute threshold and results may vary by patient and CT scanner. Once the patient is on the CT table, consider giving IV β-blocker to reach target heart rate prior to administering nitroglycerin.
- Patients frequently are incorrectly kept NPO prior to a cardiac CT. In general, a patient may have a light meal 2 hours prior to the scan and then should be keep hydrated by encouraging drinking of water (up to the time of the scan) or IV hydration (if clinically appropriate) to lower resting heart rate, reduce the likelihood of compensatory heart rate increase, or drop in blood pressure after administration of nitroglycerin. Ease the placement of a larger-bore IV line, and reduce the risk of contrast nephropathy in select patients. Avoid the patient consuming caffeine or stimulants (e.g., Adderall [amphetamine and dextroamphetamine]) and even albuterol inhalers on the morning of the test.
- Remember that patients require at least an 18-gauge IV line as contrast injection typically occurs at 5 mL/s. A lower contrast flow rate may affect the image quality. A 20-gauge IV line is perhaps the most common yet generally an inadequate IV line size in hospitalized patients. Ensure that the IV line is placed in the right arm to ensure avoidance of possible streak artifact when placed in the left arm, which may lead to premature triggering/scanning.

**Antidote**

- Do not scan until appropriate patient prep and institutional CT protocol lowering of the heart rate have been accomplished (may try IV β-blocker or calcium channel blocker).
- You may attempt to improve image quality by prolonging the scanning exposure window, changing the target cardiac phase range for prospective-gated studies, and using all available phases for of reconstruction in addition to newer AI reconstruction algorithms.

**Common Scenarios**

- Not applicable

**Note(s)**

- Remember to check for contraindications to β-blocker (e.g., high-degree AV block or significant asthma) or calcium channel blockers (e.g., systolic dysfunction)!
- Ideally, provide an oral heart rate control (better results) prior to arrival at the scanner. Alternatively, give the patient an oral agent and wait for heart rate to be achieved prior to putting patient in the scanner.
- Check for contraindications to sublingual nitroglycerin use (Viagra [sildenafil], Levitra [vardenafil], Cialis [tadalafil], etc.) to allow for optimal image acquisition. This may require not giving a patient's home medication(s) (when clinically appropriate) or not giving sublingual nitroglycerin at the time of the scan.

## MISTAKE: BREATHING DURING A CARDIAC COMPUTED TOMOGRAPHY SCAN

| | |
|---|---|
| **Case Example** | A 47-year-old female is admitted for evaluation of acute chest pain and shortness of breath. At the CT scanner, she appears visibly tachypnic and saturating 91% on room air. You obtain the images with the patient's best efforts at breath holding but notice that the images are quite blurry. |
| **Reasoning Error(s)** | ■ Lack of understanding the influence of breathing on CT image quality <br> ■ Lack of clear instructions to the patient on performing a breath hold <br> ■ Not targeting the underlying mechanism for the patient's inability to perform an adequate breath hold |
| **How to Avoid the Mistake** | ■ Understand that breathing induces significant motion artifact that degrades image quality <br> ■ Provide clear instructions to patients who are able to perform a breath hold <br> ■ Clarify and fix the etiology preventing a proper breath hold. Decrease the drive to breathe by providing supplemental oxygen if needed. Also, do not forget to identify the etiology of true hypoxia (it may be overlooked in the setting of focusing on the effect of tachypnea on image quality). |
| **Antidote** | ■ Reattempt scan with clear instructions to pause breathing during image acquisition |
| **Common Scenarios** | ■ Not applicable |
| **Note(s)** | ■ Patients should also be positioned in such a way that is comfortable and minimizes the likelihood of movement during the scan. |

## MISTAKE: POOR-QUALITY ELECTROCARDIOGRAM FOR THE GATED CARDIAC STUDY

| | |
|---|---|
| **Case Example** | A 44-year-old female is admitted for evaluation of acute chest pain and shortness of breath. You ensure that the patient is able to hydrate overnight and eat a light breakfast. You also confirm that the patient has an 18-gauge IV line. Metoprolol tartrate 50 mg is administered 1 hour prior to the scan. When the patient is brought down and transferred onto the CT table, your attending beams. A short way through the scan, you notice that the ECG tracing on the CT scanner becomes quite noisy. Your attending stops the scan, and you ask why. |
| **Reasoning Error(s)** | ■ Lack of understanding the influence of a poor-quality ECG on cardiac CT scans <br> ■ Not optimizing patient factors that contribute to a poor-quality ECG tracing |

**How to Avoid the Mistake**

- Understand that the scanner recognizes when to scan or not based on the interpretation of where the patient is in the cardiac cycle. This interpretation is based on the ECG; thus, a low-quality tracing may lead to scanning in the incorrect part of the cardiac cycle or not scanning at all. Ideally, the scan should occur during mid-diastole (when ideal heart rate has been achieved) to limit coronary artery motion.
- Prepare for a high-quality ECG tracing by ensuring that the patient understands not to move (this will also affect the entire study severely!) as well as the ECG leads have been well secured in the appropriate locations. In cases of involuntary tremors such as in Parkinson disease or essential tremors of the head/chest, ensure that appropriate medications (e.g., carbidopa-levodopa) are administered beforehand.

**Antidote**

- Reattempt scan with high-quality ECG

**Common Scenarios**

- Patient movement
- Poor ECG lead setup
- Parkinson disease

**Note(s)**

- Gating and appropriate timing of the scanning can significantly alter image quality and interpretation. For example, a CTA PE protocol study may provide some preliminary insight into coronary calcifications but would be inappropriate for drawing formal conclusions given the gating is incorrect.

## MISTAKE: DRAWING FORMAL CONCLUSIONS FROM A RAW CORONARY CT SCAN

**Case Example**

A 50-year-old female presents with atypical chest pain and elevated troponins. A coronary CT scan is finished after perfect patient preparation. You read the coronary scan immediately after the scan using the axial slices. Your curious resident inquires eagerly about the results. You note that the patient appears to have non-obstructive coronary arteries. The patient is discharged, but when you later perform a complete and thorough read using orthogonal imaging assessment and curved reformatted images, you realize the patient has a significant stenosis. Unfortunately, the patient has already been discharged and a few days later presents with typical chest pain with a STEMI and is urgently taken for a coronary angiogram, which reveals a sub-totally occluded LAD.

**Reasoning Error(s)**

- Pressure (often time pressure) to provide clinical information
- Not realizing that the images must be reconstructed
- Not following the full and standard approach to image analysis before providing a result to the ordering team

**How to Avoid the Mistake**

- Remember to take your time and provide accurate information rather than sacrifice accuracy for speed. If a preliminary read is required urgently, provide a clear disclaimer that the information provided is preliminary and subject to significant change based on proper processing software (note the limitations of the preliminary read).
- Reconstruct images and read them on a standard cardiac/coronary CTA reading software.

**Antidote**
■ Review images after reconstruction to ensure preliminary impression is correct.

**Common Scenarios**
■ Not applicable

**Note(s)**
■ A thoughtful coronary CTA protocol and image reconstruction has a large role in determining image quality at a particular radiation dose. Good image processing can significantly reduce the radiation dose needed for a particular quality of image.
■ In cases where the typical coronary anatomy is not well visualized, think about what vessel is supplying a specific territory. For example, a patient may be missing the mid to distal LAD because there is a proximal stenosis.

# Devices

Bliss J. Chang

## Right Heart Catheterization

### MISTAKE: IMPROPER POSITIONING AND ZEROING OF THE PRESSURE TRANSDUCER

**Case Example**
A patient with severe World Heart Organization Group I pulmonary hypertension diagnosed last year at an outside hospital presents to you for a transplant workup. During the right heart catheterization (RHC), you are pleased to find that the pulmonary artery (PA) systolic pressure is now significantly improved. However, your elation soon abates as you notice the pressure transducer is perched atop an elevated stand.

**Reasoning Error(s)**
- Focusing on the main task at hand (often the more interesting aspect), without adequate attention to foundational principles (often less interesting)
- Lack of knowledge regarding how proper positioning and setup of the pressure transducer affect zero leveling
- Not realizing that positioning and, hence, zero levels may easily vary between catheterization laboratories and centers without a system of standardization

**How to Avoid the Mistake**
- Understand that the pressure transducer position directly correlates with accurate pressure measurements on RHC. The measured pressure would be overestimated if the pressure transducer is lower than the level of the mid-right atrium and underestimated if the transducer is below the mid-right atrium. Hence, the best level with which to align the transducer is the mid-thoracic level (midway between the table and top of patient's sternum).
- Ensure there are no filling defects (e.g., bubbles) or kinks in the tubing of the pressure transducer system and PA catheter. This avoids issues with underdampening/overdampening of the pressure tracing. If defects are present, re-flush the catheter.
- Maintain equal focus and meticulousness to all parts of a procedure, from start to finish. Do not be tempted to relax and lose focus on "easier" segments.

| | |
|---|---|
| **Antidote** | ■ Repeat measurements after adjusting the position of the pressure transducer. |
| **Common Scenarios** | ■ Not applicable |
| **Note(s)** | ■ Approximately 2-mmHg change occurs for each 1 inch of deviation in the level of the pressure transducer relative to the mid-right atrium. |

## MISTAKE: REPEATED WEDGING AND/OR OVERWEDGING IN THE PULMONARY ARTERIES

| | |
|---|---|
| **Case Example** | An RHC is performed in a patient with known severe PA hypertension (PAH). The operator recognizes the tricky nature of obtaining accurate measurements in severe long-standing PAH given the propensity of PAs to abruptly narrow, causing difficulty with achieving a good seal with the balloon. He attempts multiple wedges, deflating and reinflating, and, after getting frustrated at inconsistent pressure readings, inflates the balloon to its maximal capacity. Soon, the patient becomes hemodynamically unstable with massive hemoptysis. |
| **Reasoning Error(s)** | ■ Tunnel vision on a goal (i.e., obtaining a good pulmonary capillary wedge pressure [PCWP]) without thinking of complications<br>■ Lack of experience of knowledge regarding consequences of repeated wedging |
| **How to Avoid the Mistake** | ■ Understand that the PAs are limited in their elasticity and ability to tolerate acute changes in pressure. Both repeated wedging (deflating and inflating the balloon) or overwedging (inflating the balloon excessively) can result in large unnecessary increases in pressure on the PAs, rarely resulting in rupture.<br>■ Remember to generally inflate the balloon when in the right atrium, prior to crossing the native tricuspid valve. The safest way of reinflating a balloon is to first withdraw the catheter out of the position from which you were formerly trying to obtain a PCWP. |
| **Antidote** | ■ Emergent intubation<br>■ Consider temporizing the bleed through tamponade with balloon inflation and/or vascular plugs (e.g., Amplatzer)<br>■ Immediate cardiothoracic surgery consultation<br>■ Consider interventional radiology embolization |
| **Common Scenarios** | ■ Not applicable |
| **Note(s)** | ■ PA rupture is associated with a very high mortality rate (some estimates are up to 50%). Symptoms include acute chest pain, cough, shortness of breath, and hemoptysis. |

## MISTAKE: UNDERWEDGING/OVERWEDGING AND INACCURATE PRESSURE READINGS

| | |
|---|---|
| **Case Example** | An RHC is performed by a first-year cardiology (heart failure) attending in a patient with known severe PAH. Despite multiple careful attempts at wedging in end-expiration, the operator is unable to achieve precise pressure measurements. She is confused because her technique was praised for its consistency during fellowship. |

| | |
|---|---|
| **Reasoning Error(s)** | ■ Lack of knowledge of anatomic differences in PA structure in severe PAH |
| | ■ Repeated attempts at consistency rather than attempting to figure out the source of error |
| **How to Avoid the Mistake** | ■ Understand that patients with severe PAH may have PAs that narrow or taper rapidly, causing an inconsistent and/or ineffective seal with the balloon. If an unusually high diastolic pressure is visualized on initial wedging, consider the possibility of a partial wedge (seal that is not tight). Try deflating the balloon slightly and let the swan wedge inward more. Similarly, if the PCWP appears unusually high, the balloon may be overwedged, and one may try deflating it somewhat. |
| | ■ Use the $SpO_2$ to help distinguish a partial from ideal wedge. The $SpO_2$ at the tip of the PA catheter should be high if a tight seal is achieved and lower with partial wedging. |
| **Antidote** | ■ When in doubt, remeasure |
| **Common Scenarios** | ■ Not applicable |
| **Note(s)** | ■ Normal venous $SpO_2$ ranges around 65–70%. This is maintained until blood is oxygenated, resulting in $SpO_2$ of approximately 95% in the left heart, as well as a partial but noticeable increase in the $SpO_2$ measured when a nice wedge is obtained. |

## MISTAKE: OBTAINING A WEDGE PRESSURE DURING INSPIRATION ON AN INTUBATED PATIENT

| | |
|---|---|
| **Case Example** | You are called to the bedside to measure the PCWP on an intubated patient in cardiogenic shock. As a first-year fellow, you astutely remember that PCWP should be obtained at end-expiration to minimize the influence of intrathoracic pressure swings. Given that the intrathoracic pressure swings are reversed in positive pressure ventilation, you confidently obtain the PCWP at maximal inspiration. Your attending solemnly pats you on the back. |
| **Reasoning Error(s)** | ■ Lack of understanding regarding the impact of the respiratory cycle on intrathoracic pressures and, hence, PCWP |
| | ■ Confusing the goal point for measuring PCWP as the most negative intrathoracic pressure rather than neutral (ambient) pressure |
| **How to Avoid the Mistake** | ■ The simple rule is that regardless of the type of respiratory support, PCWP should always be measured at end-expiration. |
| | ■ Understand the impact of the normal respiratory cycle on PCWP. During inspiration, the intrathoracic pressure decreases; conversely, it increases during expiration. The ideal measurement of PCWP would be when the intrathoracic pressure is closest to zero—that is, there is equalization of pressure inside the lungs with the outside world (no air movement). This is in end-expiration. |
| | ■ In positive pressure ventilation, the lowest intrathoracic pressure continues to occur during end-expiration. The difference is that the end-expiratory pressure is non-zero because there is a constant pressure maintained to keep the alveoli open. |

| | |
|---|---|
| **Antidote** | ■ Not applicable |
| **Common Scenarios** | ■ Positive pressure ventilation |
| |     ■ High-flow nasal canula |
| |     ■ Continuous positive airway pressure (CPAP) |
| |     ■ Bilevel positive airway pressure (BiPAP) |
| |     ■ Mechanical ventilation |
| **Note(s)** | ■ One proposed method of eliminating the effect of positive pressure ventilation on PCWP has been use of an expiratory hold maneuver. |
| | ■ Remember that positive end-expiratory pressure (PEEP) increases right ventricular afterload, which may transiently dilate the right ventricle into the left ventricle (ventricular interdependence), leading to a higher than true PCWP. |
| **Further Reading** | ■ "Expiratory hold" approach to measuring PCWP in intubated patients: Yang W, et al. "Expiratory holding" approach in measuring end-expiratory pulmonary artery wedge pressure for mechanically ventilated patients. *Patient Prefer Adherence*. 2013;7:1041-1045. |

## MISTAKE: RIGHT HEART CATHETERIZATION IN MECHANICAL RIGHT-SIDED VALVES

| | |
|---|---|
| **Case Example** | An RHC is performed as part of a transplant workup for a patient with arrhythmogenic right ventricular dysplasia complicated by severe tricuspid regurgitation and a mechanical tricuspid valve placed 2 years ago. The PA catheter is advanced from the right atrium to the right ventricle against the severe tricuspid regurgitation and over the mechanical valve without much trouble. With a sigh of relief, the operator obtains some wedge pressures. When retrieving the catheter, the operator suddenly feels resistance and is unable to withdraw the catheter. |
| **Reasoning Error(s)** | ■ Lack of experience and/or recognition that passing a PA catheter over a mechanical valve has a unique set of considerations |
| | ■ Lack of planning with regard to necessary but tricky and/or low-volume procedures |
| | ■ When possible, not involving other more experienced operators to help oversee and guide |
| **How to Avoid the Mistake** | ■ Understand the possible complications of passing a PA catheter and/or inflated balloon past a mechanical valve. The catheter may become entrapped, and attempted removal may lead to unnecessary stress on the valve leaflets, leading to damage and changes in blood flow, which may then lead to increased risk of valve thrombosis and bacterial seeding. |
| | ■ When attempting rare, low-volume, unfamiliar, and/or tricky procedures, plan out each step in advance and rehearse as much as possible. Contingency planning is extra important in these cases, since many reflexes may be absent or diminished due to lack of experience. For the passage of a PA catheter over a mechanical tricuspid valve, the ideal preparation would include an ex vivo simulation using the exact catheter and valve involved. |
| | ■ If possible, particularly at large medical institutions, try to ask colleagues for help when attempting low-volume and/or unfamiliar procedures. |

| | |
|---|---|
| **Antidote** | ■ Not applicable |
| **Common Scenarios** | ■ Mechanical tricuspid valve |
| | ■ Mechanical pulmonic valve |
| | ■ Right-sided endocarditis |
| | ■ Right heart thrombus |
| **Note(s)** | ■ In the presence of a mechanical valve that is much less deformable, there is usually more catheter-related regurgitation. This may decrease the utility of certain techniques, such as thermodilutional measure of cardiac output. |

## MISTAKE: SINGLE MEASUREMENTS OF PULMONARY PRESSURES AND CARDIAC OUTPUT

| | |
|---|---|
| **Case Example** | You are called to the bedside to measure the cardiac output on an intubated patient in cardiogenic shock. As a first-year fellow, you astutely remember that PCWP should be obtained at end-expiration to minimize the influence of intrathoracic pressure swings, regardless of respiratory mechanics (e.g., intubation). You confidently report the first measured value as the Fick cardiac output. Your attending solemnly pats you on the back. |
| **Reasoning Error(s)** | ■ Lack of experience or knowledge regarding the variation in readings produced by catheters used for pressure and pulmonary pressure measurements |
| | ■ Overly trusting machines and protocols without verifying and/or trying to optimize their reliability and utility (e.g., "This PA catheter was designed for measuring pressures, of course it would provide a reliable measurement"). |
| **How to Avoid the Mistake** | ■ Understand that PA catheter design has improved over the past decade but that there still may be significant variation from sampling to sampling, in part due to the nature of measurement techniques. In particular, thermodilution catheters are less precise (wider range of numbers, though accurate) compared with other catheter types. |
| | ■ To improve accuracy of the reported cardiac output or pulmonary pressures, consider averaging several measurements. A common recommendation is taking three high-fidelity measurements, particularly when in doubt (e.g., measurement value seems unusual for the particular patient). That is, the measurements being averaged should ideally be within 10% of each other; values that are clearly off may require consideration of exclusion. |
| **Antidote** | ■ Average three measurements |
| **Common Scenarios** | ■ Not applicable |
| **Note(s)** | ■ Precision refers to how tight a series of measurements are (regardless of how close to the true value), whereas accuracy refers to how close the measurement is to the true value. |

## MISTAKE: CARDIAC OUTPUT VIA THERMODILUTION IN SEVERE TRICUSPID REGURGITATION

**Case Example**

A 60-year-old with long-standing ischemic cardiomyopathy, severe tricuspid regurgitation, and morbid obesity is admitted with acute decompensated heart failure. On admission, she is on 4 L nasal cannula and without easily visible jugular venous distention; legs are warm and notable for 1+ tense edema to the knees. Despite a valiant effort at diuresis, her volume exam remains difficult and oxygen requirements persist. The patient undergoes RHC, which reveals a wedge pressure of 20 mmHg. The cardiac output is also measured via thermodilution, and you are alarmed to see a cardiac index of 2.0, signifying a low-output state. An urgent transthoracic echocardiogram demonstrates no change from prior.

**Reasoning Error(s)**

- Lack of knowledge regarding the limitations of cardiac output by thermodilution
- Not thinking about the principles behind measuring cardiac output via thermodilution
- Incomplete information about patient comorbidities

**How to Avoid the Mistake**

- Understand that thermodilution relies on cold injectate traveling forward and being detected by the thermistor of the PA catheter. Conditions that disrupt the usual flow of blood forward may decrease the accuracy of measured cardiac output. For example, severe tricuspid regurgitation causes the cold injectable to flow backward, delaying the detection by the thermistor and, hence, underestimating the cardiac output. Similarly, a left-to-right shunt would increase the flow of blood, leading to an overestimate of the cardiac output.
- Collect enough information to reassure yourself that the diagnostic test you perform (e.g., measurement of cardiac output by thermo-dilution) is accurate. For example, an echocardiogram would be prudent prior to RHC. Validate the test with alternate methods.

**Antidote**

- Validate with alternate method of measuring cardiac output (e.g., Fick)

**Common Scenarios**

- Severe tricuspid regurgitation (underestimates carbon dioxide [CO])
- Left-to-right shunt (overestimates CO)
- Low cardiac output (especially <2.5 L/min; overestimates CO)

**Note(s)**

- The Fick method of calculating cardiac output also has its own limitations. In particular, watch out for severe anemia and conditions that increase pulmonary oxygen consumption (e.g., severe pneumonia), which would overestimate cardiac output.

# Coronary Artery Disease

Yonatan Mehlman

# General Principles

## MISTAKE: LACK OF ASCVD RISK ASSESSMENT

**Case Example**        A 50-year-old male presents for a yearly visit with you as his primary care physician complaining of back pain and erectile dysfunction. You address his primary concern each year, yet each year he returns with a similar but new (and important to him!) complaint. You rarely have a chance to have a deliberate discussion regarding his atherosclerotic cardiovascular disease (ASCVD) risk.

**Reasoning Error(s)**
- Culture and/or prioritization of treatment over prevention
- Bias of tackling concrete medical issues rather than estimating and treating risk
- Lack of time to focus on ASCVD risk characterization (particularly in primary care: screening, immunizations, social determinants of health, mental health, and so forth)

**How to Avoid the Mistake**
- Develop a habit of organizing patient visits into prevention and treatment—for example, considering using standard built-in electronic medical record (EMR) functions to track and address gaps in prevention.
- Value the prevention of disease equally as treatment of disease.
- Use a multidisciplinary team–based approach to educate and engage patients regarding their ASCVD risk.
- Assess and reassess all adult patients' ASCVD risks, including those younger than 40 years, routinely and deliberately, and engage in active primary prevention, including addressing risk factors such as lifestyle and lipids discussed in this chapter.

**Antidote**            - Not applicable

**Notes**
- ASCVD refers to disease resulting from atherosclerotic plaques in blood vessels that supply the heart (coronary artery disease [CAD]), brain (cerebrovascular disease), and limbs (peripheral arterial disease).
- Proper ASCVD assessment includes not only using the ASCVD risk calculator but also considering socioeconomic factors, family history of premature ASCVD, and the presence of any risk-enhancing factors. Furthermore, adjunct lipid measurements or coronary artery calcium (CAC) score may be valuable.
- Consider using a 30-year ASCVD risk calculator for patients at lower overall risk (age <40 or ASCVD risk <7.5%), especially as having a number to quantify lifetime or 10-year risk can be a powerful motivating factor for patients when coupled with dedicated counseling of the devastating nature of ASCVD events.
- The most used ASCVD risk calculator is based on the Pooled Cohort Equation (PCE, 2013). Know that this may underestimate or overestimate risk for those other than non-Hispanic Whites and non-Hispanic Blacks living in the United States. Many alternate calculators are available.

# MISTAKE: FORGETTING TO RECOMMEND LIFESTYLE MODIFICATIONS

**Case Example**

A 50-year-old male presents to your office to establish care with you as his primary care physician. In the middle of your discussion, he tells you that he smokes three packs of cigarettes per day. He has obesity and hypertension, in addition to a family history of hyperlipidemia, and wants to know whether you would recommend any medications for his health. You order a lipid panel and tell him you will call him back with the results. Based on the lipid panel, you calculate his 10-year ASCVD risk to be 21% and prescribe atorvastatin 80 mg nightly.

**Reasoning Error(s)**

- Thinking of ASCVD as an illness treatable only with medications
- Forgetting to consider complimentary, less invasive, modifiable risk factors for intervention (e.g., diet, weight loss, smoking cessation)
- Assuming that counseling is ineffective and a "low yield" use of office time
- Incorrect belief that lifestyle modifications are effective only if at a high level (e.g., running several miles, achieving a BMI <25)
- Lack of knowledge regarding the full modifiable risk factor profile of a patient
- Lack of knowledge that smoking cessation counseling is a valuable service that is actually reimbursable
- Lack of access or knowledge of smoking cessation resources for the patient

**How to Avoid the Mistake**

- Take a thorough history on each patient, ensuring you elucidate modifiable risk factors such as smoking, alcohol use, physical inactivity, and poor diet.
- Recommend practical and achievable lifestyle interventions, even if modest. Inquire, counsel, and use motivational interviewing on small steps each visit.
- Approach lifestyle modifications as an interdisciplinary team; consider referrals to nutritionists, bariatric surgeons, and therapists. Prepare yourself to provide optimal patient care by informing yourself of common resources such as those concerning smoking cessation.

**Antidote**

- Not applicable

**Common Scenarios**

- Smoking
- Obesity
- Unhealthy diet
- Sedentary lifestyle
- Excess stress

**Notes**

- While the diets with the most evidence for reducing ASCVD are the DASH (Dietary Approaches to Stop Hypertension), vegetarian, and Mediterranean diets, encouraging small changes in a patient's diet (e.g., cutting out butter with dinner rolls) can be a great start.
- Consider medical interventions to aid with certain modifiable risk factors. For example, consider bariatric surgery for weight loss and pharmacotherapy for smoking cessation (e.g., nicotine patches or varenicline).

**Further Reading**
- Ever wondered what the evidence was for reducing coronary events with walking? An example is Manson JE, et al. A prospective study of walking as compared with vigorous exercise in the prevention of coronary heart disease in women. *N Engl J Med.* 1999;341:650-658.

## MISTAKE: ROUTINE USE OF DAILY ASPIRIN FOR PRIMARY PREVENTION OF ASCVD

**Case Example**

A 50-year-old male with hypertension, hyperlipidemia, and a history of gastrointestinal bleed presents to your office saying that he just had a grandchild; congratulations! His father had a heart attack at the age of 65, so your patient wants to do everything he can to be heart healthy. His 10-year ASCVD risk is 7.5%. He asks you: What about taking a daily aspirin? You prescribe aspirin given his risk and age. Two years later, the patient is admitted with melena and hypotension.

**Reasoning Error(s)**
- Using outdated guidelines or evidence
- Forgetting to individualize the risk-benefit of aspirin for patients
- Lack of frequent reevaluation of a patient's continued need for primary prevention with aspirin as their profile (age, comorbidities) evolves

**How to Avoid the Mistake**
- Learn the new evidence for and against primary prevention with aspirin. Three big trials (ASPREE [A Study of Cardiovascular Events in Diabetes], ASCEND [Aspirin in Reducing Events in the Elderly], and ARRIVE [Aspirin to Reduce Risk of Initial Vascular Events]) published in 2018 called into question the net benefit of aspirin monotherapy for primary prevention. Specifically, the investigations focused on three key populations: (1) those with type 2 diabetes, (2) patients at intermediate risk for cardiovascular events, and (3) patients ≥70 years old. Despite a modest reduction in serious vascular events in some patients, there was no net benefit given an increase in major bleeding. Taken together, these studies call into question the benefit of aspirin for primary prevention in patients who are not at significantly increased risk of ASCVD.
- Explore individual comorbidities that may increase the risk of aspirin use (e.g., bleeding history and use of other medications) or increase the benefit of aspirin (high ASCVD risk such as those with significant family history or severe hyperlipidemia).
- No matter how routine a medication, always consider the risks and benefits in a patient-centered discussion. For example, myocardium is often unsalvageable, whereas a gastrointestinal bleed may resolve (other bleeds such as intracranial hemorrhage may be devastating); patients may weight these consequences differently.
- For patients on aspirin (or any other medication), reevaluate the indication frequently, especially if their medical problems change or evolve. Deescalation of medications is very important and helps combat polypharmacy, which not only provides potentially unnecessary side effects but also decreases medication adherence.

**Antidote**
- Not applicable

**Notes**

- The most recent American College of Cardiology (ACC)/American Heart Association (AHA) guidelines as of this publication now recommend against routine use of aspirin in primary prevention. Suggested patient populations for use include those at high risk of ASCVD (suggested ASCVD >10%) and between the ages of 40 and 70.
- Other common comorbidities that should give you pause regarding daily aspirin include presence of other agents that include bleeding risk (anticoagulants), low ASCVD risk, chronic liver disease, and a high 5- to 10-year mortality risk
- For patients with aspirin allergies, the first-line alternative is clopidogrel 75 mg daily. The bleeding risk of clopidogrel is greater than that of aspirin, whereas the primary prevention utility is thought to be similar.
- Likewise, it is reasonable to consider substituting clopidogrel for aspirin in patients who have experienced a cardiovascular event on aspirin.

**Further Reading**

- Excellent summary of the ARRIVE, ASCEND, and ASPREE trials and a discussion of their implications on the role of aspirin in primary prevention: Marquis-Gravel G, et al. Revisiting the role of aspirin for primary prevention of cardiovascular disease. *Circulation*. 2019;140:1115-1124.

# Lipid Management

## MISTAKE: MANDATING FASTING LIPID PANELS

**Case Example**

A 65-year-old patient presents to your clinic for follow-up after a recent hospitalization for a complicated UTI. You notice a lipid panel was among the labs run in their hospitalization that showed high-density lipoprotein (HDL) of 40 mg/dL, low-density lipoprotein (LDL) of 170 mg/dL, and triglycerides (TG) of 140 mg/dL. Noting that the lab was drawn at 3 p.m. on the day before discharge, you presume it was not a fasting panel, so you send another lipid panel before determining whether to start a statin.

**Reasoning Error(s)**

- Lack of knowledge or forgetting that a fasting lipid panel does not usually improve the ability to calculate ASCVD risk
- Lack of knowledge regarding key patient comorbidities that may warrant the utility of a fasting lipid profile
- Not considering the logistical burden to the health care system and patients by mandating a fasting lipid profile

**How to Avoid the Mistake**

- Understand that the evidence comparing the prognostic value of fasting and nonfasting LDL demonstrates no significant difference in most cases.
- Remember common scenarios where a fasting lipid profile is beneficial: TG ≥400 mg/dL, chronic inflammatory conditions (particularly HIV infection), familial history of lipid disorders (including apolipoprotein [apo]E).
- Recognize the logistical barriers and burdens associated with each clinical action.

| | |
|---|---|
| **Common Scenarios** | ■ Unclear timing of lab draws<br>   ▪ During hospitalization<br>   ▪ By another provider |
| **Notes** | ■ Most laboratory-derived LDL levels are an indirect calculation based on the Friedewald equation rather than a direct measurement. This limits the ability to accurately estimate LDL in the setting of significant hypertriglyceridemia (≥400 mg/dL): |

$$LDL = Total\ Cholesterol - HDL - \left( \frac{Triglycerides}{5} \right)$$

■ TG are significantly affected by recent food intake, particularly carbohydrates. Thus, if an initial nonfasting lipid panel is unable to calculate an LDL due to significantly elevated TG, a fasting lipid panel should be performed. Alternatively, a direct LDL measurement may be considered.

■ Patients with HIV infection often demonstrate significant hyper-triglyceridemia with a low HDL and may be good candidates for fasting lipid panels.

## MISTAKE: FORGETTING TO CONSIDER RISK-ENHANCING FEATURES IN ASCVD RISK ASSESSMENT

| | |
|---|---|
| **Case Example** | A 48-year-old male with long-standing HIV infection and rheumatoid arthritis presents to your office wanting to know if there are any medications he should be taking for his heart, especially since his father had a heart attack at age 50. You calculate his ASCVD risk to be 7% and defer treatment with statins. Three years later, the patient has a posterior myocardial infarction (MI). |
| **Reasoning Error(s)** | ■ Limited knowledge of what contributes to ASCVD risk<br>■ Limited knowledge of potential gaps in the ASCVD risk calculators<br>■ Lack of knowledge regarding patient comorbidities |
| **How to Avoid the Mistake** | ■ Recognize common ASCVD risk enhancers. These include chronic inflammatory conditions (e.g., rheumatoid arthritis or HIV), family history of premature ASCVD, significant chronic kidney disease, and ethnicity (e.g., South Asian).<br>■ Understand when risk-enhancing factors influence clinical decision-making. Patients with borderline ASCVD risk (defined as 5–7.4%) may benefit from statins in the presence of risk-enhancing features; those with intermediate risk (7.5–20%) are more likely to benefit and should receive at least moderate-intensity statins.<br>■ Conduct a patient-centered discussion regarding statin initiation in patients with significant risk-enhancing features. Patients hesitant to initiate statins based on their ASCVD risk alone may benefit from understanding the broader context of the decision to initiate statins. |
| **Antidote** | ■ Not applicable |
| **Common Scenarios** | ■ Borderline ASCVD risk (5–7.4%)<br>■ Intermediate ASCVD risk (7.5–20%) |

**Notes**

- The intensity of statin therapy corresponds to the predicted LDL-lowering effects:
  - Low intensity: <30%
  - Moderate intensity: 30–49%
  - High intensity: ≥50%
- High-intensity statins from most to least potent: Rosuvastatin 40 mg (~60% LDL reduction) > atorvastatin 80 mg (~55%) > rosuvastatin 20 mg = atorvastatin 40 mg
- Due to significantly increased rates of rhabdomyolysis, high-intensity simvastatin is no longer recommended.
- Some experts believe that rosuvastatin 40 mg should not be recommended over atorvastatin 80 mg, given the limited additional increase in lipid-lowering effect.

## MISTAKE: OVERLOOKING ADJUNCT LIPID PARTICLES SUCH AS APOLIPOPROTEIN B AND LIPOPROTEIN(A)

**Case Example**

A 28-year-old female patient with hypertension presents to your office for her annual visit. She has a family history of early ASCVD (father and older brother died from MI at ages 35 and 33, respectively), but her 10-year ASCVD risk is 0.5%. A fasting lipid profile demonstrates LDL 120, HDL 40, and TG 125. Given her low ASCVD, you withhold any lipid management and reassure her that her risk of 10-year ASCVD is very low. When the patient does not show up for her next annual visit, you are devastated to see that she died from a large anterior MI.

**Reasoning Error(s)**

- Lack of awareness of adjunct lipid markers
- Lack of understanding when to use adjunct lipid markers when assessing ASCVD risk and statin initiation

**How to Avoid the Mistake**

- Consider apoB and lipoprotein(a) [Lp(a)] protein measurements in patients who may be borderline for initiation of statin, have a family history of premature ASCVD, or have a personal history of ASCVD not explained by major risk factors.

**Antidote**

- Not applicable

**Common Scenarios**

- Borderline ASCVD risk (5–7.4%)
- Intermediate ASCVD risk (7.5–20%)

**Notes**

- According to the 2018 AHA guidelines, TG >200 is a relative indication for measurement of apoB, wherein apoB ≥130 mg/dL constitutes a risk-enhancing factor.
- Further in the 2018 guidelines, elevated Lp(a) can constitute a risk-enhancing factor when >50 mg/dL or >125 nmol/L. Family history of premature ASCVD is a relative testing indication.
- In women, Lp(a) was only associated with CVD if the women had a total cholesterol >220 mg/dL.

**Further Reading**

- An excellent review of Lp(a) and its role in ASCVD is available in Kaiser Y, et al. Association of lipoprotein(a) with atherosclerotic plaque progression. *JACC.* 2022; 9(3):223-233.

## MISTAKE: UNDERUSE OF CORONARY ARTERY CALCIUM SCORING

**Case Example**

A 47-year-old male patient with hypertension presents to your office to establish care. His father had a heart attack at age 43, and mother has hyperlipidemia. Between his lipid panel and other risk factors, you note that he should begin a statin. The patient is reluctant to start a statin, and you have difficulty convincing the patient.

**Reasoning Error(s)**

- Forgetting CAC is an available test given its relative lack of use at many institutions as compared with other CAD assessment modalities
- Fear of a false-negative test
- Overlooking the value of visualization to patients during counseling

**How to Avoid the Mistake**

- Understand when to use CAC scoring. CAC is most useful in those who have a borderline risk for CAD or who are borderline for initiation of a statin. It is not recommended in those who are high (≥20% 10-year ASCVD risk) or low (<5% 10-year ASCVD risk) risk, as it may yield a false-negative or false-positive result, respectively.
- Understand that a zero CAC score means a very low 10-year ASCVD risk. Scores of 1–99 favor statin initiation, and statins should certainly be started for scores of ≥100.
- Show patients their calcium plaques! Many patients who are reluctant will be convinced to undertake pharmacologic and lifestyle changes once they visualize plaque in their coronaries.

**Antidote**

- Not applicable

**Notes**

- For patients reluctant to initiate a statin, CAC scoring may help by providing the patient a visualization of the abstract ASCVD risk we discuss so frequently.
- CAC scoring of zero can still be associated with significant 10-year ASCVD risk in select populations, including patients who smoke, have diabetes, have a strong family history of ASCVD, or have chronic inflammatory conditions such as HIV infection.
- CAC scoring has no use in patients already treated with statins (i.e., those with established ASCVD).
- CAC should be reassessed every 5–10 years if the patient's pretest probability of ASCVD continues to be borderline.

**Further Reading**

- 2018 ACC/AHA Cholesterol Guidelines
- 2018 United States Preventive Services Task Force Recommendations on Cardiovascular Risk Assessment
- HNR Study on the Value of Monitoring CAC Progression: Lehmann N, et al. Value of progression of coronary artery calcification for risk prediction of coronary and cardiovascular events. *Circulation.* 2018;137(7):665-679.

## MISTAKE: INADEQUATE ASSESSMENT AND TREATMENT OF HYPERTRIGLYCERIDEMIA

**Case Example**  A patient on high-dose statin with LDL of 80 and HLD of 50 has a fasting TG of 175. He says that he noticed the red exclamation point next to his TG value and wants to know what this means for him. You reassure him that TG do not affect ASCVD risk; after all, it is not an explicit value in the Pooled Cohort Equations (PCE), and he thanks you before leaving. Later that night, you listen to a podcast by a lipid expert about the concept of residual ASCVD risk with hypertriglyceridemia.

**Reasoning Error(s)**
- Anchoring on HLD and LDL within the lipid panel and underappreciating TG as a contributor to ASCVD risk
- Older school of thought that TG play little to no role in ASCVD

**How to Avoid the Mistake**
- Understand that hypertriglyceridemia (defined as ≥150 mg/dL) contributes to ASCVD risk as evidenced by several contemporary studies.
- Consider fasting lipid panels for patients with hypertriglyceridemia to better quantify TG and ASCVD risk.
- The most recent 2018 ACC/AHA guidelines suggest consideration of statins (in addition to lifestyle modifications) as a cornerstone for ASCVD risk reduction in TG ≥150 mg/dL. Statins should be maximized prior to alternate TG-lowering therapies.
- Avoid fibrate therapy unless severe hypertriglyceridemia is uncontrolled with statins, ezetimibe, and lifestyle management due to the lack of benefit beyond reducing TG levels (no firm evidence of improved clinical outcomes). The exception is in the setting of hypertriglyceridemia so severe that it causes pancreatitis (usually >800 mg/dL).

**Antidote**
- Not applicable

**Notes**
- The Reduction of Cardiovascular Events With EPA (REDUCE-IT) Intervention Trial provides recent evidence supporting icosapent ethyl (a highly concentrated omega-3 derivative) for reduction of cardiovascular events in patients with hypertriglyceridemia, although trials at lower doses have generated controversy. While we await further studies, there is little evidence of adverse events from icosapent ethyl other than a small signal that it may marginally increase the incidence of atrial fibrillation.
- The risk of myopathy and rhabdomyolysis increases with combined statin and fibrate therapy. If this combination must be used, avoid fenofibrate, which has the highest risk.
- Address common concomitant medical conditions that may cause hypertriglyceridemia, including thyroid disease, alcoholism, and obesity.
- Notable common and unique manifestations of severe hypertriglyceridemia include xanthomas and recurrent pancreatitis.

## MISTAKE: UNDERUSE OF ADJUNCT LIPID-LOWERING THERAPIES IN ADDITION TO MAXIMALLY TOLERATED STATIN THERAPY

**Case Example**  A 57-year-old male with diabetes and hypertension walks into your office to establish care. His fasting LDL is 210. You start a statin, but even with rosuvastatin 40 mg, his LDL falls to only 110.

| | |
|---|---|
| **Reasoning Error(s)** | ■ Anchoring on statin therapy to the exclusion of other well-evidenced therapies of additional LDL lowering and ASCVD risk reduction |
| | ■ Lack of knowledge regarding appropriate LDL goals for various populations |
| | ■ Lack of knowledge regarding alternate lipid-lowering therapies |
| **How to Avoid the Mistake** | ■ After a patient is on maximally tolerated statin therapy, consider adjunct therapies if not meeting goal LDL or ASCVD risk. |
| | ■ Understand the appropriate LDL goals for various populations: |
| |   ■ Primary prevention: ≥50% reduction of LDL, although this varies based on overall ASCVD risk |
| |   ■ Secondary prevention: LDL ≤70 |
| |   ■ Familial hypercholesterolemia: ≥50% reduction in LDL, ideally LDL <70–100 |
| | ■ While the official AHA guidelines do not yet suggest this, many experts take the perspective of lowering LDL as much as possible, even below 70, in those with high ASCVD risk. |
| | ■ Always titrate statins to the highest tolerated dose and class before considering adjust lipid-lowering therapies. |
| | ■ Learn about alternate lipid-lowering therapies. The two main adjuncts are PCSK9 inhibitors (up to ~60% additional reduction in LDL) and ezetimibe (may lower LDL by an additional 20%). A third-line adjunct is cholestyramine, a bile-acid sequestrant, although it has significant gastrointestinal side effects. |
| **Antidote** | ■ Not applicable |
| **Common Scenarios** | ■ Not applicable |
| **Notes** | ■ Cardiovascular disease risk is correlated to cumulative exposure to LDL-C; additionally, accumulation at a younger age is correlated with a greater risk increase as compared to in an older age, suggesting we should be more aggressively controlling LDL even at a younger age [*J Am Coll Cardiol.* 2020;76(13):1507-1516]. |
| | ■ Pleiotropic effects of drugs may also affect their cardiovascular profile, beyond just the absolute LDL level achieved; this is particularly thought to be the case with statins and contribute to their use as a first-line treatment. |

## MISTAKE: DISCONTINUATION OR LACK OF INITIATION OF STATIN THERAPY IN DIABETICS

| | |
|---|---|
| **Case Example** | A 40-year-old female patient with prediabetes, hyperlipidemia, and hypertension presents for an annual checkup. She has been taking rosuvastatin 20 religiously for the past year after you informed her of an elevated ASCVD risk. However, today she is shocked to learn that she has diabetes (A1c of 6.5%). While in the office, she consults Dr. Google and screams at you for giving her diabetes with the statin. She notes that she will never take a statin again. |

| | |
|---|---|
| **Reasoning Error(s)** | ■ Patient refusal of statin therapy due to the false belief that statins cause diabetes<br>■ Forgetting that statin therapy is indicated in diabetes regardless of LDL<br>■ Lack of knowledge regarding a patient's diabetes status<br>■ Lack of knowledge to counsel patients on the safety of statins in diabetes |
| **How to Avoid the Mistake** | ■ Understand that a common reason patients refuse to take statins is because "statins cause diabetes." This is incorrect. This observation stems from an uninformed analysis of cherry-picked data from the JUPITER trial. All patients who developed diabetes in that trial were patients who had prediabetes and thus very likely to develop diabetes. The average increase in A1c over 2 years was a mere 0.1% and there was a 17% reduction in overall mortality. Notably, there were no new cases of diabetes among patients without major risk factors for diabetes.<br>■ Furthermore, follow-up studies have shown that there is no increase in diabetes in patients who did not have the risk factors for diabetes. In those who had risk factors, even if statins were to cause an increase in diabetes, the overall benefits of statin therapy exceeded the diabetes hazard.<br>■ Gather adequate information to determine ASCVD risk, including diabetes status |
| **Antidote** | ■ Not applicable |
| **Common Scenarios** | ■ Not applicable |
| **Notes** | ■ Though the standard is to start a moderate-intensity statin in a patient with diabetes, you may consider high-intensity statins in the presence of significantly elevated LDL or other risk-enhancing features. Common indications for high-intensity therapy include long-standing diabetes (as evidenced by end-organ manifestations such as albuminuria, retinopathy, and neuropathy) and chronic kidney disease III or greater.<br>■ Data are limited regarding statins in those with diabetes who are age <40 or >75. A discussion of the risks and benefits is recommended, especially in those with long-standing diabetes or the cardiovascular disease risk factors given above. |
| **Further Reading** | ■ In-depth analysis of the JUPITER Trial addressing the signal of increased incidence of diabetes with statin therapy: Ridker PM, et al. Cardiovascular benefits and diabetes risk of statin therapy in primary prevention. *Lancet.* 2012;380(9841):565-571. |

# MISTAKE: WITHHOLDING STATINS IN THE SETTING OF STATIN "INTOLERANCE"

**Case Example**

Your patient in the above example is started on a statin but says that a few days later he felt some joint soreness and myalgias. He also has been working out a bit more after the scare of being started on a new medication for his heart. He wants to know if you think the new medicine could be causing this and if it is worth stopping the statin; after all, he never had this problem before he met you.

**Reasoning Error(s)**

- Thinking that statin intolerance is a class effect rather than a dose or even a nocebo effect
- Lack of understanding regarding statin intolerance and its clinical significance
- Hesitation in trialing lifesaving medications after patients experience adverse events
- Difficulty convincing patients to take statins after experiencing adverse events

**How to Avoid the Mistake**

- While the many of the large-scale statin trials did not show myalgias as a significant difference between statin and placebo, myalgias are an often-reported and well-presumed side effect of statins. Other commonly cited reasons for discontinuation of statins are sleep disturbances, "liver toxicity," and memory issues.
- When a patient presents with muscle symptoms in the setting of statin initiation/uptitration, temporarily stop their statin and administer the Statin-Associated Muscle Symptom Clinical Index (SAMS-CI) to assess if statins could be contributing to the complaint.
- Depending on the degree of elevation of the SAMS score, assess for alternate causes of myalgias, drug interactions, and comorbidities that may be contributing including vitamin D deficiency, hypothyroidism, and renal failure.
- Once symptoms have resolved, work together with the patient on the next step, as patients may be sensitive to suggestions involving statins after perceiving a side effect.
- Consider rechallenging with identical statin and dose (perhaps after discussion of the nocebo effect), lowering the dose, starting an alternative statin, or using alternate-day dosing. Choice of next step is also related to degree of elevation of initial SAMS score.
- If needed, consider alternate lipid-lowering therapy.
- For truly life-changing therapies, always try to find a way to allow the patient to receive maximal benefit.

**Antidote**

- Education regarding nocebo effect, followed by rechallenge
- Change to alternate statin or alternate lipid-lowering agent entirely: Consider pravastatin or pitavastatin as alternate statins given their minimal or lack of metabolism by cytochrome enzymes, thereby thought to induce less myalgias
- Decrease dose
- Alternate-day dosing

**Notes**

- Some have raised questions regarding whether statin-related myalgias is more of a nocebo effect than a true side effect, considering the relative increased reports of muscle complaints compared with those noted in trials.
- Myalgias have a broad differential! Always consider alternative diagnoses of myalgias rather than anchoring on statin-induced muscle complaints.
- Monitor for more severe manifestations of statin injury: Rhabdomyolysis and Immune-mediated necrotizing myopathy are rare but documented side effects of statins that can cause muscular symptoms. They are absolute contraindications to statin reinitiation.
- Bempedoic acid is a recently approved adjunct lipid-lowering medication that works by inhibiting adenosine triphosphate (ATP) citrate lyase, an upstream enzyme to 3-hydroxy-3-methylglutaryl coenzyme A (HMG-CoA) reductase. It may be a first-line consideration as well (and even comes in a single combination pill with ezetimibe). Assess uric acid levels and gout stability before initiation.

**Further Reading**

- Study demonstrating strong evidence for the nocebo effect and ability to restart statins with appropriate counseling regarding the nocebo effect: Wood FA, et al. N-of-1 trial of a statin, placebo, or no treatment to assess side effects. *N Engl J Med.* 2020;383:2182-2184.

## MISTAKE: WITHHOLDING STATINS FOR MILD TRANSAMINITIS

**Case Example**

After much discussion, your patient continues with the statin, and his myalgias resolve. A year later, he goes to see a specialist who happens to be your friend from medical school and who is not as familiar with statin use. Among the labs they send are a routine left function tests (LFTs), which shows alanine transaminase (ALT) and aspartate transaminase (AST) elevations. Concerned and feeling like this is out of their area of expertise, your colleague calls you to ask if the statin should be held.

**Reasoning Error(s)**

- Jumping to attribute LFT abnormalities to statins
- Lack of understanding when to discontinue statins in the setting of LFT abnormalities
- Fear of inducing fulminant drug-induced liver injury

**How to Avoid the Mistake**

- Understand that LFT abnormalities are among the most common laboratory abnormalities that hold a wide differential. Fatty liver (hepatic steatosis) is a common cause of mild transaminitis that is often incorrectly blamed on statins. The incidence of transaminitis attributed to statins in large statin trials such as the Heart Protection Study was essentially zero. In fact, there is some evidence suggesting that statins may improve liver function through pleiotropic effects.
- Understand that statin-induced liver injury usually presents with AST and ALT greater than three times the upper limit of normal. In this case, it is reasonable to hold the statin temporarily.

**Antidote**

- Not applicable

**Notes**
- Do not perform routine monitoring of LFTs while on a statin unless otherwise clinically indicated. It is reasonable to perform a single check before initiating statins and investigate incidentally detected initial elevations as you would any other routinely detected lab abnormality.
- Chronic liver disease, nonalcoholic fatty liver disease (NAFLD), nonalcoholic steatohepatitis (NASH), compensated cirrhosis, and mild-moderate alcohol use are not absolute contraindications to statin therapy, although they may impact the choice of statin (all statins are metabolized by the liver to a certain extent, but rosuvastatin and pravastatin less extensively than others). Decompensated cirrhosis or acute liver failure is a contraindication.
- A post-hoc study of the GREek Atorvastatin and Coronary-heart-disease Evaluation (GREACE) study showed that among patients with mildly abnormal LFTs at baseline (AST or ALT <3 times upper limit of normal) possibly associated with NAFLD, there was a substantial improvement in LFTs among those treated with statins compared with those untreated.
- While the US Food and Drug Administration had originally recommended periodic monitoring of LFTs for patients taking statins, this recommendation was removed in 2012.

**Further Reading**
- Great summary of commonly encountered myths and challenges encountered in statin therapy: Spence JD, et al. Overcoming challenges with statin therapy. *JAHA*. 2016;5:e002497.

## MISTAKE: FORGETTING TO RENALLY DOSE ROSUVASTATIN

**Case Example**
After all that has happened with his statin treatment, you are thankful that your patient continues to see you and continues to take his statin. You continue to treat his diabetes, notice the glomerular filtration rate is slowly decreasing, and refer him to nephrology. "Doc, now that my kidneys aren't working as well as they used to, should I change any of my meds?" You reassure him and note that he is not on any renally dosed medications. A year later, the patient is admitted with severe rhabdomyolysis likely due to elevated rosuvastatin levels.

**Reasoning Error(s)**
- Forgetting that dose adjustments are necessary for rosuvastatin in creatinine clearance (CrCl) <30 because of its predominantly renal clearance
- Thinking all statins are exclusively hepatically cleared
- Lack of thorough medication reconciliation

**How to Avoid the Mistake**
- Although several statins have demonstrated safety in those with chronic kidney injury when dose adjusted, consider using atorvastatin and fluvastatin as first-line statins to avoid dealing with renal dosing adjustments later (and safeguard against providers who may forget).
- Learn the renally cleared statins: rosuvastatin and pravastatin.
- Always perform a thorough medication reconciliation.

**Antidote**
- Decrease rosuvastatin to a maximum of 10 mg daily.

| | |
|---|---|
| **Common Scenarios** | ■ Rosuvastatin<br>■ Pravastatin |
| **Notes** | ■ Watch for statin medication interactions, as most statins (rosuvastatin and pravastatin are notable exceptions) are metabolized by the cytochrome P450 (CYP450) system. For example, many HIV medications are strong inhibitors of the CYP450 system, diltiazem and verapamil are moderate inhibitors, and many antiepileptics are strong inducers. |

## MISTAKE: PRESCRIBING STANDARD DOSES OF ROSUVASTATIN TO ASIAN PATIENTS

| | |
|---|---|
| **Case Example** | A 65-year-old Asian American male with three-vessel coronary artery disease (CAD) presents to you to establish new care. You see that the patient is on only 10 mg of rosuvastatin, and you excitedly increase it to 40 mg without checking a lipid panel. A few days later, the patient is hospitalized with severe rhabdomyolysis. |
| **Reasoning Error(s)** | ■ Not realizing that genetic differences (genetic polymorphisms) may lead to differences in drug metabolism<br>■ Lack of knowledge with prescribing rosuvastatin to patients of Asian descent |
| **How to Avoid the Mistake** | ■ Understand that as a result of CYP genetic polymorphisms, among other factors, rosuvastatin seems to have higher levels of plasma concentration in East Asian populations.<br>■ Initiate at low doses and uptitrate carefully as needed based on LDL level and ASCVD risk. |
| **Antidote** | ■ Not applicable |
| **Common Scenarios** | ■ Not applicable |
| **Notes** | ■ Rosuvastatin in particular should be initiated at a dose of 5 mg in patients of East Asian descent to account for elevated plasma drug levels at higher doses, with increased attention to systemic exposure as you increase the dose.<br>■ Evidence for simvastatin dose differences is conflicting; maintain vigilance when increasing the dose in patients of East Asian descent. |

# Evaluation of Coronary Artery Disease: Exercise Stress Testing

## MISTAKE: WITHHOLDING AN EXERCISE STRESS TEST WHEN UNABLE TO RUN

| | |
|---|---|
| **Case Example** | A 50-year-old male with a prior below-the-knee amputation in the setting of a military injury presents with what seems to be typical angina. During your evaluation, you refer him to a stress test. He looks at you puzzled—"Isn't that the test where I run on a treadmill? I can't do that!" |
| **Reasoning Error(s)** | ■ Lack of knowledge or forgetting the various modes of exercise stress testing available<br>■ Forgetting the prognostic value of evaluating functional status and exercise capacity through stress testing |

| | |
|---|---|
| **How to Avoid the Mistake** | ■ Understand the various types of exercise stress testing: traditional treadmill, bicycle, and hand bicycle.<br>■ Remember that obtaining prognostic information is very useful for future management.<br>■ When faced with an incompatibility, strive to figure out a way to get the complete information you need. |
| **Antidote** | ■ Not applicable |
| **Common Scenarios** | ■ Patients with amputations<br>■ Gait or balance issues<br>■ Severe deconditioning<br>■ Extremes of age |
| **Notes** | ■ Leg cycling is preferred to arm cycling because the size of the muscle groups in the lower extremities more readily allows a person to reach the desired level of exertion.<br>■ Deconditioning, lung disease, or other conditions may preclude a patient from reaching 85% of their maximum predicted heart rate, thereby decreasing the sensitivity of the stress test.<br>■ Bicycle protocols have the benefit of being more portable and yielding clearer electrocardiogram (ECG)/blood pressure (BP) data due to less motion. However, people may be less likely to reach desired heart rate due to deconditioning. |

## MISTAKE: ECG STRESS TESTING IN THE PRESENCE OF BASELINE ECG CHANGES

| | |
|---|---|
| **Case Example** | Before sending him for a stress test, you perform a baseline ECG that shows a left bundle-branch block (LBBB), stable from a similar ECG 1 year earlier. You send him for an ECG stress test but get a call from the cardiologist that the patient had chest pain with exertion, with an ECG showing an LBBB. Thinking that he may have had an ischemic episode, the patient is referred to the emergency department. |
| **Reasoning Error(s)** | ■ Lack of thought as to what you anticipate searching for on the ECG during the stress test and how this may be confounded by preexisting ECG changes<br>■ Lack of a reliable prior ECG |
| **How to Avoid the Mistake** | ■ Perform baseline ECG on patients to triage appropriate testing modality.<br>■ Understand what ECG changes preclude an ECG stress test: LBBB, ventricularly paced rhythms, ST depressions. |
| **Antidote** | ■ Imaging (transthoracic echocardiography [TTE]) or nuclear stress test (single-photon emission computed tomography [SPECT] or positron emission tomography [PET]) |
| **Notes** | ■ Complete right bundle-branch blocks or resting ST depression <1 mm are not absolute contraindications to ECG stress testing because they do not interfere with the detection of ischemia. This is as opposed to ST elevations and LBBB, which can be evidence of ischemia. |

## MISTAKE: EXERCISE STRESS TESTING IN SYMPTOMATIC AORTIC STENOSIS

**Case Example**

During the evaluation of a patient with anginal symptoms, you order TTE, which shows severe aortic stenosis. Concerned about his stable angina that he was reporting to you on your initial interview, you refer him for a stress test. On the treadmill he experiences severe chest pain and has a cardiac arrest.

**Reasoning Error(s)**

- Lack of knowledge or forgetting the absolute contraindications to stress tests
- Not thinking about the pathophysiology of aortic stenosis in relation to stress testing

**How to Avoid the Mistake**

- Understand the absolute contraindications to stress testing (see later).
- Quickly reason through the pathophysiology and its compatibility with the physiology of the clinical action to be undertaken. This will help avoid mistakes in less common scenarios.

**Antidote**

- Not applicable

**Common Scenarios**

- Acute MI, within 2 days
- High-risk unstable angina
- Uncontrolled cardiac arrhythmia with hemodynamic compromise
- Active endocarditis
- Symptomatic severe aortic stenosis
- Decompensated heart failure
- Acute pulmonary embolism, pulmonary infarction, or deep vein thrombosis
- Acute myocarditis or pericarditis
- Acute aortic dissection
- Physical disability that precludes safe and adequate testing
- Resting systolic BP > 200
- Resting diastolic BP >110

**Notes**

- Stress testing in *asymptomatic* aortic stenosis is not contraindicated. In fact, a stress test in asymptomatic aortic stenosis that elicits symptoms on exercise clearly related to aortic stenosis is a Class I indication for aortic valve replacement.

**Further Reading**

- Review article on stress testing in asymptomatic aortic stenosis: Redfors B, et al. Stress testing in asymptomatic aortic stenosis. *Circulation.* 2017;135(20):1956-1976.

## MISTAKE: FORGETTING TO WITHHOLD SPECIFIC MEDICATIONS AND FOODS PRIOR TO STRESS TESTING

**Case Example**

A patient arrives for his 11 a.m. SPECT stress test. In the initial questionnaire, he says he had his usual breakfast including coffee and toast but skipped lunch in preparation for his exercise stress test. He finishes the stress test uneventfully. You interpret the stress test and are pleased to see no evidence of ischemia. However, 2 weeks later, the patient presents to the hospital with crushing chest pain and is soon taken to the cath lab for a high-risk non–ST-segment elevation MI (NSTEMI) (GRACE score 160). Coronary angiogram reveals an 80% lesion of the mid–right coronary artery (RCA).

| | |
|---|---|
| **Reasoning Error(s)** | ■ Lack of understanding regarding the mechanism and physiology of each stress testing modality |
| | ■ Thinking that because a stress test in noninvasive there is no reason to make a patient NPO or change medications |
| **How to Avoid the Mistake** | ■ Remember that holding food for 3 hours prior to a stress test is the only thing that *absolutely* must be done before a stress test of any kind. This is also the only absolute food/medication requirement to participate in an *exercise* stress test; other stress tests have specific requirements as outlined below. |
| | ■ Anticipate problems ahead of time. Prepare patients as if they are going for a vasodilatory pharmacologic stress test even if they are going for an exercise stress test, because there is the possibility that their exercise stress test will be converted into a pharmacologic stress test. Again, these measures are *not absolutely required* for an *exercise* stress test but can save lots of time. |
| | ■ Understand the types of stress tests and their mechanisms in relation to commonly ingested substances: |
| |   ■ Vasodilator stress tests use dipyridamole, adenosine, or regadenoson: |
| |     ■ Methylxanthines, including caffeine-containing compounds and medications (even including some chocolates and ice creams!), absolutely must be held 12 hours prior to a *vasodilator* stress test because they are competitive inhibitors of adenosine. |
| |     ■ Oral dipyridamole is an adenosine analog and therefore should be held at least 48 hours prior to pharmacologic vasodilator stress tests. Not holding oral dipyridamole may still allow for IV dipyridamole use as a vasodilator stress test. |
| |   ■ Synthetic catecholamine stress tests use dobutamine: |
| |     ■ β-Blocker use is a strong relative contraindication to dobutamine stress test given the attenuation in heart rate and inotropic response (thus decreasing the exam sensitivity) but is not an absolute contraindication. |
| **Antidote** | ■ Convert to exercise or dobutamine stress test as needed. |
| **Notes** | ■ Often, it is a good idea to give the stress test lab a call beforehand to ensure that you satisfy all the requirements. |
| | ■ Adenosine-based stress testing uses the principle of coronary steal, where coronary blood flow is directed away from stenosed areas, which are fixed and minimally vasodilatory in response to adenosine. |
| | ■ Continuing antihypertensive medications with antianginal properties (β-blocker [BB], calcium channel blocker [CCB], and nitrates) and angiotensin-converting enzyme inhibitors/angiotensin II receptor blockers will affect stress tests because of the respective medication's impact on heart rate (HR) or BP. Whether to hold such medications for a stress test is an area of debate and mostly decided on a case-by-case basis. An example of when one would be more likely to continue a medication is if the patient is reliant on the BB for their atrial fibrillation; conversely, someone taking amlodipine 5 mg for its mild BP effect likely can hold their medication for a stress test. |

## MISTAKE: NOT RECOGNIZING ABNORMAL BLOOD PRESSURE RESPONSES DURING STRESS TESTING

**Case Example**

A patient's resting BP before the test is 140/85. A few minutes after starting the test, his BP drops to 110/70. You note the drop and continue the stress test. A few moments later, the patient passes out with a cardiac arrest.

**Reasoning Error(s)**

- Assuming that the only signs of ischemia during exercise stress testing are ECG changes
- Lack of attention to vital signs (particularly BP)

**How to Avoid the Mistake**

- Understand the endpoints for exercise stress testing: patient determined (e.g., chest pain, limiting symptoms), provider determined (significant ECG or BP changes), or protocol determined (goal output achieved). Many endpoints do not rely on ECG changes but still may be highly suggestive of significant CAD.
- Pay close attention to the BP during exercise stress testing

**Antidote**

- Not applicable

**Common Scenarios**

- Systolic BP drop >10 mmHg
- Hypertension >~220 mmHg systolic or 100 mm Hg diastolic
- Arrhythmias
- Significant unrelenting angina

**Notes**

- Dehydration or overzealous antihypertensive medication can also cause confounding exercise-induced hypotension.
- Exertional hypotension (exercise systolic BP ≥10 mm Hg below resting BP) or exertional hypertension (systolic >250 or diastolic >115 mm Hg) are indications to stop a stress test and portend future adverse cardiovascular events.

## MISTAKE: STRESS TESTING IN PATIENTS WITH LOW OR HIGH PRETEST PROBABILITY FOR CAD

**Case Example**

A 58-year-old patient with long-standing poorly controlled diabetes, hypertension, a significant smoking history, and peripheral vascular disease presents to your office with complaints that sound quite like typical angina. You refer him to a stress test, which does not demonstrate ischemia. You explain to the patient that despite the negative test, you still believe he has coronary artery disease given his strong comorbidities and the details of his complaint.

**Reasoning Error(s)**

- Not thinking about pretest probabilities and the ideal time to use a test modality, leading to referring all patients with chest pain for stress testing.

**How to Avoid the Mistake**

- Make it a habit to think about when to use a test and what you will do with the information provided by that test prior to ordering it.
- Use stress tests only in intermediate-risk patients, as those are whom a positive and negative test are most likely to change management. If the pretest probability is high, then the patient should usually be referred for a left heart catheterization; if low, even a positive result would be questioned and thus stress testing is not useful.

**Antidote**

- Not applicable

**Common Scenarios**    ■ Not applicable

**Notes**    ■ Bayes theorem of conditional probability is particularly important to remember when interpreting any clinical test. Colloquially, this is often among what people mean when they ask, "Will this test change management?"—they can mean: Am I likely to believe a positive or negative test such that the result would impact my decision making, or will I brush off a result as a false positive or negative?

# Evaluation of Coronary Artery Disease: Myocardial Perfusion Imaging

## MISTAKE: COMMON ARTIFACTS IN MYOCARDIAL PERFUSION IMAGING

**Case Example**    You get a call from the nuclear cardiologist that your 49-year-old patient with typical angina has an inferior heart perfusion defect. Worried about possible ischemia in this critical vascular territory, you request an urgent left heart catheterization, which demonstrates normal and nonoccluded coronary arteries with no segmental wall motional abnormalities.

**Reasoning Error(s)**    ■ Lack of understanding regarding the mechanism of myocardial perfusion imaging
■ Lack of experience with common attenuation artifacts

**How to Avoid the Mistake**
■ Understand the mechanism behind nuclear stress testing, which relies on the relative perfusion to an area compared with surrounding regions.
■ Recognize that perfusion attenuation and/or misdirection can cause the appearance of a relative decrease in perfusion in the absence of ischemia.
■ Note that, rarely, if there is *increased* perfusion to a local area, the surrounding area will appear to have relatively decreased perfusion and, by extension, appear to have coronary artery disease in that territory.
■ Remember common causes of perfusion attenuation:
  ■ Diaphragmatic attenuation: more common in men, attenuation from the left hemidiaphragm may produce an apparent perfusion defect in the inferior segment of the heart.
  ■ Soft tissue attenuation: attenuation from obesity or breasts is very common; the location and severity of the perfusion defect will depend on significance of obesity and/or the size/lay/density/composition of the breasts. Commonly, the anterior or anterolateral wall is affected.
  ■ Liver or bowel attenuation: tracer located in liver or adjacent bowel may erroneously appear as increased perfusion to the inferior wall. This can *hide* native decreased perfusion to the region (overshadow local diseased myocardium) or cause the surrounding areas to appear decreased, and diseased, by comparison.
  ■ Hypertrophic cardiomyopathy: the relative increase in perfusion to the thickened septal myocardium may lead surrounding areas to appear relatively decreased, and therefore erroneously, diseased.
  ■ LBBB: LBBB can present as a septal defect on perfusion imaging. This artifact may be due to decreased diastolic flow from delayed contraction, although the mechanism is not entirely clear.

- There are many methods by which to assess if relative perfusion defects are due to confounding:
  - Acquire images of patient in multiple positions.
  - Use rest and stress images, including both exercise and vasodilator stress.
  - Use ECG image gating.
  - Use attenuation correction algorithms.
- As with all tests, use pretest probability to help inform the interpretation of tests. Do not be scared to take a second look at a result, especially if things do not seem to add up.

**Antidote**
- Not applicable

**Common Scenarios**
- Diaphragmatic attenuation
- Breast attenuation
- Liver/bowel attenuation
- Obesity
- Hypertrophic cardiomyopathy
- LBBB

**Notes**
- None

## MISTAKE: BALANCED ISCHEMIA OR LEFT MAIN STENOSIS AS A FALSE-NEGATIVE PHARMACOLOGIC STRESS TEST

**Reasoning Error(s)**
- Lack of understanding regarding the mechanism of myocardial perfusion imaging
- Not considering the pretest probability of three-vessel disease prior to choosing a nuclear stress test

**How to Avoid the Mistake**
- Understand the mechanism of a nuclear stress test. Nuclear stress tests use a vasodilator (e.g., adenosine) to dilate coronary arteries. Arteries that are healthy and therefore not yet fully dilated will have increased blood flow, whereas stenotic coronary arteries are already maximally dilated and unable to increase blood flow.
- Nuclear stress tests capitalize on this flow difference as a surrogate for perfusion defects (obstructed coronary arteries). Thus, in balanced three-vessel disease or significant proximal left main coronary artery disease, there may be no significant flow difference, providing the appearance of nonobstructive coronary blood flow.
- Use pretest probability to determine the likelihood of three-vessel disease versus no disease at all. Patients with three-vessel disease often have a high pretest probability and should undergo a coronary angiogram rather than a stress test.

**Antidote**
- Not applicable

**Common Scenarios**
- Not applicable

**Notes**
- Interestingly, a study by E. Kostacos et al from the University of Pennsylvania in 2004 demonstrated that only 14% of patients with a false-negative dipyridamole stress test had three-vessel disease, suggesting that the false-negative result was usually not due to balanced ischemia.

# Treatment of Coronary Artery Disease: Pharmacologic
## MISTAKE: FORGETTING TO OPTIMIZE ANTIANGINAL THERAPY

**Case Example**
A patient presents to you with typical angina symptoms. You start him on a BB as part of your treatment plan. He comes back to you a few months later with the great news that his angina is decreased, but he has been having trouble with his asthma—a problem he did not mention to you because he has not really been bothered by it for years. Thinking you are out of options to treat his angina medically, you refer him for revascularization.

**Reasoning Error(s)**
■ Unfamiliarity with the arsenal of medications that can reduce anginal symptoms
■ Misbelief that anginal symptoms represent a problem that can be addressed only with invasive approaches
■ Forgetting to consistently address optimization of antianginal therapy

**How to Avoid the Mistake**
■ Understand the range of medications that help decrease angina: BBs, CCBs, long-acting nitrates, and ranolazine.
  ■ BBs are the first-line treatment for preventing angina via decreasing HR and BP during exercise.
  ■ If BBs are contraindicated or not tolerated, long-acting nondihydropyridine CCBs (verapamil or diltiazem) or long-acting nitrates can be used to prevent angina. Note that CCBs are contraindicated in patients with significant LV dysfunction.
  ■ If symptoms persist despite monotherapy, BBs can be combined with either CCBs or long-acting nitrates.
  ■ Dihydropyridine CCBs are also reasonable choices and may be preferred to non-DHP CCBs in patients with conduction defects.
  ■ Ranolazine can be used as a substitute for BBs if poorly tolerated, ineffective, or contraindicated; it may also be used in refractory angina.
■ Think of antianginal therapy optimization as guideline-directed medical therapy (GDMT) for angina. This may help develop a habit of optimizing antianginal therapy during every patient interaction.

**Antidote**
■ Not applicable

**Common Scenarios**
■ Not applicable

**Notes**
■ Short-acting nitrates (sublingual nitroglycerin or nitroglycerin spray) are the mainstay of acute anginal therapy but are ineffective for day-to-day therapy.
■ Be wary of how long-acting nitrates are scheduled to avoid development of tolerance. Isosorbide mononitrate may be dosed once daily in the morning and isosorbide dinitrate can be dosed once in the morning and again in the early afternoon to allow for a long enough nitrate-free period until the next morning dose.
■ Notably, BBs are contraindicated in vasospastic or variant (Prinzmetal) angina.

■ Ranolazine is metabolized by the CYP3A pathway. Therefore, no more than 500 mg twice daily should be coadministered with diltiazem or verapamil (among other medications). Additionally, ranolazine can significantly increase the plasma concentration of simvastatin.

■ The use of ranolazine use as an antianginal drug is debated, given its side effect profile and questionable efficacy according to some. While there are studies that demonstrate its efficacy (e.g., MARISA, CARISA, ERICA, TERISA), it is not a first-line medication.

## MISTAKE: USING LONG-ACTING NITRATES WITHOUT A NITRATE-FREE INTERVAL

| | |
|---|---|
| **Case Example** | After hearing about the host of medications available to treat angina, you start your patient just discussed on a long-acting nitrate. You get a call saying that he had great control of his angina for a few days, but more recently he feels back to where he was before you started the nitrate. |
| **Reasoning Error(s)** | ■ Forgetting that, unlike most other medications, nitrates lose clinical efficacy with continuous therapy.<br>■ Lack of appropriate scheduling of nitrates to facilitate a nitrate-free interval |
| **How to Avoid the Mistake** | ■ When treating a patient with nitrates, always consider nitrate tolerance.<br>■ Schedule nitrates to include a nitrate-free period to minimize the risk of developing tolerance. |
| **Antidote** | ■ Institute a nitrate-free interval (avoidance of nitrates for 8–12 hours per day).<br> ■ How to arrive at this time window varies by nitrate preparation:<br>  ▪ For oral formulations, rather than a true q8h or q12h schedule, try 8 a.m., 1 p.m., and 6 p.m.; or 8 a.m. and 4 p.m., respectively.<br>  ▪ For transdermal formulations, apply the patch for 12 hours and remove for 12 hours. |
| **Common Scenarios** | ■ Not applicable |
| **Notes** | ■ Although the mechanism of nitrate tolerance is not fully understood, the clinical and hemodynamic implications are well documented, including decreased exercise tolerance and loss of antihypertensive effects with continuous treatment.<br>■ Some data suggest that, while necessary, a nitrate-free interval has significant problems such as inducing rebound ischemia and decreasing the angina threshold during the nitrate-free period. By extension, there is an increased frequency of ischemic episodes during the nitrate-free interval. Therefore, while nitrate-free intervals are the best way to account for nitrate tolerance, it is a far from a perfect solution and accounts for why nitrates are not first-line treatment. |

# Treatment of Coronary Artery Disease: Revascularization

## MISTAKE: REVASCULARIZING ALL STABLE PATIENTS WITH CORONARY ARTERY DISEASE

**Case Example**

A patient presents to you with complaints consistent with stable angina after a coronary angiogram that revealed mild stenosis in a marginal coronary artery branch. Both he and you are concerned that medical therapy would provide insufficient benefit, so you refer him for revascularization. He returns to your clinic sometime later, angry that the interventionalist rejected his case.

**Reasoning Error(s)**

- Long-standing historical teaching that revascularization is superior to medical management of severe CAD
- Well-intentioned thinking that a definitive strategy (revascularization) would be superior to chronic therapy (medical management), which does not bear out in the data

**How to Avoid the Mistake**

- Understand the latest evidence for medical management versus revascularization of stable CAD. The ISCHEMIA trial (*N Engl J Med*, 2020) is a pivotal trial that demonstrated no significant major cardiac death or hospitalization endpoint differences between optimal medical therapy and revascularization in patients with moderate to severe reversible ischemia, including in patients with chronic kidney disease (ISCHEMIA-CKD).
- The more recent REVIVED-BCIS2 trial (N Engl J Med, 2022) trial compared PCI plus OMT to OMT in patients with CAD who were theoretically well suited to benefit from PCI (EF <35%, extensive CAD amenable to PCI, viable myocardium) found no difference in the primary outcome of death from any cause or hospitalization for heart failure at 3.4 years. Longer term outcome data is pending.
- Understand the 2023 ACC/AHA Guideline for the Management of Patients With Chronic Coronary Disease Class I indications for revascularization in chronic coronary disease:
  - CABG plus OMT recommended in significant left main disease with severe LV dysfunction (LV EF ≤35%)
  - Revascularization recommended to improve symptoms with lifestyle-limiting angina despite medical therapy
  - Within those undergoing revascularization, CABG (left internal mammary artery to left anterior descending coronary artery [LAD]) is recommended over percutaneous coronary interventions as a Class I recommendation for those with diabetes and multivessel CAD with involvement of the LAD.
- Patient-centered discussion regarding the risks and benefits of both invasive versus conservative strategies

**Antidote**

- Not applicable

**Common Scenarios**

- Not applicable

**Notes**

- The 2021 and 2023 ACC/AHA/SCAI guidelines have made significant updates to account for recent trials (ISCHEMIA, in particular), which seem to show no significant difference between revascularization and OMT in most cases.
- The STS/AATS-endorsed rebuttal to 2023 ACC/AHA Chronic Coronary Disease Guidelines objects to the 2a/b characterization of CABG for patients with chronic coronary disease and three-vessel CAD in patients without LVEF>35%, and suggest this be upgraded due to its potential survival benefit. Their objection turns on the limitations of the ISCHEMIA trial's structure and its ability to extrapolate to this population.
- ISCHEMIA did demonstrate an improvement in anginal symptoms in patients without chronic kidney disease who underwent revascularization, although this benefit is directly related to the degree of angina before enrollment. This anginal benefit was not demonstrated in the ORBITA (*Lancet*, 2018) trial.
- You can calculate the Society of Thoracic Surgeons risk score to help stratify patients under consideration for CABG.

**Further Reading**

- The landmark ISCHEMIA Trial:
  - Maron DJ, et al. Initial invasive or conservative strategy for stable coronary disease. *N Engl J Med.* 2020;382:1394-1407.
  - The more recent REVIVED-BCIS2 trial and accompanying editorial noting its limitations: *N Engl J Med.* 2022;387:1351-1360 and *N Engl J Med.* 2022;387:1426-1427.
- The ORBITA Trial showed that PCI did not improve exercise times or anginal frequency in patients with stable angina as compared to a sham procedure:
  - Al-Lamee R, et al. Percutaneous Coronary Intervention in Stable Angina (ORBITA): a double-blind, randomised controlled trial. *Lancet.* 2018;391(10115):31-40.
- The FREEDOM Trial showed that CABG is superior to PCI in patients with diabetes and advanced CAD:
- Farkouh ME, et al. Strategies for multivessel revascularization in patients with diabetes. *N Engl J Med.* 2012;367:2375-2384.
- STS/AATS-endorsed rebuttal to 2023 ACC/AHA Chronic Coronary Disease Guidelines: Bakaeen FG, Ruel M, Calhoon JH, Girardi LN, Guyton R, Hui D, et al. STS/AATS-endorsed rebuttal to 2023 ACC/AHA Chronic Coronary Disease Guideline: a missed opportunity to present accurate and comprehensive revascularization recommendations. *J Thorac Cardiovasc Surg.* 2023;166:1115-1118.

## MISTAKE: ALWAYS PERFORMING A CORONARY ANGIOGRAM FOR EVALUATION OF CORONARY ARTERY DISEASE

**Case Example**

A 45-year-old man with hypertension and poorly controlled diabetes presents to you for follow-up after his stress test. The stress test showed no evidence of ischemia. Nevertheless, the patient is concerned about his cardiovascular health. "Why can't I have someone just look inside the arteries, like they do with my colon, to check that everything is OK?" You schedule the patient for a diagnostic left heart catheterization the following week. Unfortunately, the patient passes away from a coronary artery perforation that was discovered late.

| | |
|---|---|
| **Reasoning Error(s)** | ■ Lack of knowledge of the range of diagnostic modalities for evaluating CAD and when each modality is appropriate<br>■ Operator preference over patient-centered decision making |
| **How to Avoid the Mistake** | ■ Always discuss the risks, benefits, and alternatives of each clinical action. This can be particularly important for establishing rapport with patients who have fears and anxieties (whether or not reasonable) regarding certain procedures.<br>■ Consider the pretest probability of finding significant CAD. A very high probability would push you to obtain the definitive angiogram (and potentially allow for intervention at the same time).<br>■ Think about what you will do with the information from a test. For example, the main indication for diagnostic coronary angiography is to identify candidates for revascularization (PCI or coronary artery bypass grafting) and may not be necessary in someone who would not be a candidate.<br>■ Understand the range of tests for evaluating for CAD: coronary angiograms, stress testing, and coronary CT angiogram. |
| **Antidote** | ■ Not applicable |
| **Common Scenarios** | ■ Not applicable |
| **Notes** | ■ Among potential angiogram complications, vascular complications at the insertion site are some of the most common. Other complications include induction of arrythmias during the angiogram, stroke or embolism, and, rarely, perforation.<br>■ Low-contract diagnostic coronary angiograms are possible, usually by specific operators at each institution. |

## MISTAKE: PERFORMING MYOCARDIAL VIABILITY ASSESSMENTS IN ALL PATIENTS WITH UNREVASCULARIZED DISEASE

| | |
|---|---|
| **Case Example** | Your patient with heart failure and a long-standing history of CAD is requesting some kind of surgical intervention. He is frustrated by having to take so many medications every day and feels like there has to be some kind of surgical solution. Before sending him to a surgeon, you pursue myocardial viability assessment imaging. Due to insurance issues, your patient ends up paying for much of the bill himself and is frustrated to hear that the surgeon barely even looked at the study. |
| **Reasoning Error(s)** | ■ Well-intentioned logical thinking that one should know whether there is salvageable myocardium prior to attempted revascularization |
| **How to Avoid the Mistake** | ■ Understand that the viability of myocardium may not adequately discriminate between patients who would derive a mortality benefit from CABG plus OMT compared with OMT alone. In the STICH (Surgical Treatment for Ischemic Heart Failure) trial, the presence of viable myocardium was associated with improvement in left ventricular systolic function; this was irrespective of treatment modality (CABG plus OMT versus OMT alone) and not related to long-term survival. |
| **Antidote** | ■ Not applicable |
| **Common Scenarios** | ■ Not applicable |
| **Notes** | ■ The survival benefit seen in the STICH trial of CABG plus OMT versus OMT did have the trade-off of higher 30-day mortality (4% versus 1%) after CABG, thought to be secondary to surgical complications. |

## CHAPTER 7

# Acute Coronary Syndromes

Balakrishnan Pillai

Mistake: Overlooking New Murmurs in Late-Presenting Myocardial Infarction

Mistake: Suppressing Post–Myocardial Infarction Arrhythmias With Antiarrhythmic Drugs

**Post–Acute Coronary Syndromes Care: Secondary Prevention and Guideline-Directed Medical Therapy**

Mistake: Lack of β-Blocker Post–Myocardial Infarction

Mistake: Overlooking Cardiac Rehabilitation on Discharge

Mistake: Lack of Counseling and Resources on Lifestyle Modifications

Mistake: Not Screening for Depression Post–Acute Coronary Syndromes

# Diagnostics: History

## MISTAKE: NOT RECOGNIZING ACUTE CORONARY SYNDROMES IN THE ABSENCE OF CHEST PAIN

**Case Example**

A 68-year-old male with a history of hyperlipidemia and hypertension presented to his primary care physician (PCP)'s office as a same day visit after he developed left sided neck and arm pain while shoveling snow. The pain started while he was shoveling but continued to worsen so he presented to his PCP. He was diagnosed with muscular strain and sent home with acetaminophen, ibuprofen, and a lidocaine patch. That evening his pain continued to worsen and he presented to the nearest ED, where a 12-lead ECG showed 2-mm ST-segment elevations in leads II, III, and aVF with deep Q waves in those same leads. Coronary angiography showed a 100% mid–right coronary artery (RCA) lesion.

**Reasoning Error(s)**

- Lack of knowledge or experience with atypical presentations of acute coronary syndromes (ACS)
- Not holding a higher suspicion for atypical presentations of ACS in select patients
- Not asking explicitly regarding both chest pain and chest pressure
- Lack of a differential diagnosis, even for seemingly common and straightforward presentations
- Not using pretest probabilities to inform differentials
- Skipping low-cost, low-effort diagnostics that may significantly change management to save time or avoid inconvenience or because the probability of ACS is deemed "low"

**How to Avoid the Mistake**

- Be sure to consider the adage "chest pain is more than pain in the chest" as stated in the 2021 American Heart Association Chest Pain guidelines. Approximately 30% of ACS is thought to present without chest pain. Hold higher suspicion for atypical ACS in older patients, females, and persons with diabetes.
- Remember the atypical and/or associated symptoms of ACS: atypical location of pain (neck, jaw, shoulder, back, arm, and epigastric), shortness of breath, nausea/vomiting, diaphoresis, and significant acute-onset fatigue. Other history that may be "ischemic equivalents" are syncope (due to ventricular tachycardia [VT]), palpitations, and new heart failure symptoms (recent myocardial infarction [MI] versus flash pulmonary edema).

- Realize that patients may answer your questions very literally. Thus, it is essential to ask about chest pressure and/or chest discomfort rather than asking about only chest pain. You would be surprised at how many patients who deny chest pain have chest pressure or other discomfort. Notably, all three forms of chest symptoms (i.e., pain, pressure, vague discomfort) possess similar sensitivities and specificities (~70% and ~40%, respectively).
- Always form a differential diagnosis guided by pretest probabilities. In an older patient with several cardiac risk factors, as in our example, the patient always has ACS unless proven otherwise. Keep in mind do-not-miss diagnoses.
- Remember that the electrocardiogram (ECG) is a very low-cost and low-effort maneuver that can quickly provide key diagnostic information. There may be various signs concerning for ACS beyond ST elevations, although a non–ST-segment elevation myocardial infarction (NSTEMI) may present with a completely normal ECG. All patients for whom ACS is even a slim consideration require an ECG within 10 minutes of presentation.

**Antidote**

- Not applicable

**Note(s)**

- A common misconception is that abdominal or chest pain that resolves with an antacid (H2-blocker, proton pump inhibitor [PPI], Maalox [aluminum hydroxide and magnesium hydroxide suspension]) rules out ACS. This is absolutely not true, and ACS must still be ruled out with due diligence and workup.
- Nonaspirin nonsteroidal anti-inflammatory drugs (NSAIDs) have been associated with increased risk of major adverse cardiac events (MACE) in individuals at elevated risk for CAD. NSAIDs all inhibit cyclooxygenase enzymes 1 and 2 (COX-1/-2) to some degree due to a relative increase in thromboxane levels, where thromboxane has prothrombotic, platelet-activating effects. Aspirin at low doses (81 mg) is an irreversible inhibitor of COX-1 (much more than COX-2), which allows for its unique effects on inhibiting platelet aggregation. The cardiovascular risks are even greater with COX-2 selective inhibitors such as celecoxib.

## MISTAKE: BRUSHING OFF SYMPTOMS CONSISTENT WITH ACUTE CORONARY SYNDROMES IN PSYCHIATRICALLY OR COGNITIVELY CHALLENGED PATIENTS

**Case Example**

A 54-year-old undomiciled male with a history of schizoaffective disorder presented to the ED complaining of chest pain. He has been to the emergency department (ED) six times in the past 2 months with similar complaints and had been discharged with PCP follow-up with the diagnosis of musculoskeletal versus psychogenic pain. On this occurrence, the pain woke him from sleep and felt like a squeezing weight on his chest. His current medications are lithium and olanzapine. He smokes a pack of cigarettes a day and has done so for 20 years. In the emergency department, he is agitated and diaphoretic, yelling out in pain. He is given IV haloperidol and on reassessment he is calm. He is discharged soon thereafter with another diagnosis of musculoskeletal versus psychogenic pain.

| | |
|---|---|
| **Reasoning Error(s)** | ■ Implicit bias toward psychiatric and/or cognitive conditions that lowers a physician's pretest probability of "real" symptoms (in this case, ACS) |
| | ■ Recency bias leading this emergency physician to anchor on the diagnosis of psychogenic chest pain |
| | ■ Overlooking increased risk for ACS with use of atypical antipsychotics |
| **How to Avoid the Mistake** | ■ Do not allow psychiatric and/or cognitive conditions to alter pretest probabilities. All patients, including those with mental illness, merit the same basic ACS workup regardless of their comorbidities. |
| | ■ Form your own assessment based on your own history and objective data first. Reading notes from prior visits and other clinicians can significantly bias you. Compare your assessment to those of supporting documents and reconcile differences. |
| | ■ Recognize that atypical antipsychotic use (i.e., olanzapine, quetiapine, clozapine, risperidone) are a risk factor for cardiovascular disease as they can cause obesity, type 2 diabetes, dyslipidemia, and the metabolic syndrome. |
| **Antidote** | ■ Not applicable |
| **Common Scenarios** | ■ Psychiatric illness (e.g., schizophrenia, depression) |
| | ■ Cognitive illness (e.g., dementia) |
| | ■ Patients who visit the ED frequently |
| **Note(s)** | ■ Patients with schizophrenia are at higher risk for tobacco use disorder, which is a strong risk factor for ACS. |

## MISTAKE: OVERLOOKING ACUTE CORONARY SYNDROMES MASQUERADING AS DIABETIC KETOACIDOSIS

| | |
|---|---|
| **Case Example** | A 45-year-old male with a history of hyperlipidemia, hypertension, and type 1 diabetes presented to his PCP's office as a same day visit complaining of weakness and frequent urination. His PCP obtained a urinalysis, which was positive for glucose and ketones, and he was sent to the ED for further diagnosis and management. In the ED, the patient was diagnosed with diabetic ketoacidosis (DKA) and was resuscitated with fluids and started on an insulin infusion. After a few hours, on assessment by the admitting team, the patient was complaining of shortness of breath. Vital signs at that time were significant for an oxygen saturation of 90% on room air, auscultation of the chest revealed crackles bilaterally, and anteroposterior chest radiography showed bilateral infiltrates consistent with pulmonary edema. A 12-lead ECG showed 2-mm ST- segment elevations in leads V5, V6, I, and aVL with developing Q waves in those same leads. The patient was given aspirin and rushed to the cardiac catheterization laboratory, where coronary angiography showed a 100% mid-left circumflex (LCx) lesion. |
| **Reasoning Error(s)** | ■ Anchoring on the diagnosis of DKA without considering triggers or complications |
| | ■ Lack of experience with ACS in the setting of DKA |
| | ■ Not revisiting and reorganizing a differential diagnosis throughout a patient's visit |
| | ■ Lack of close monitoring with appropriate reactions to a changing clinical scenario |

| | |
|---|---|
| **How to Avoid the Mistake** | ■ Constantly reassess a clinical scenario as it evolves. You should never be "bored" and consider a case mundane if you continue to keep abreast of clinical developments. Differential diagnoses should be reconstructed as the case evolves. |
| | ■ Always consider underlying triggers of DKA when managing patients. Know that ischemia is a trigger, and it can also be a complication. As DKA causes significant volume depletion, coronary blood flow may be significantly decreased resulting in ischemia especially in the setting of preexisting stenoses. |
| **Antidote** | ■ Not applicable |
| **Common Scenarios** | ■ DKA |
| | ■ Pneumonia |
| | ■ Sepsis |
| **Note(s)** | ■ Approximately 5–10% of patients hospitalized with pneumonia have evidence of an MI in-hospital. The risk of MI continues to be elevated even after discharge. |
| | ■ Acute infection can lead to type 1 MI via various mechanisms such as activating inflammatory cells within atherosclerotic plaques to facilitate rupture and increasing prothrombotic potential. |

## MISTAKE: IMPROPER DIFFERENTIATION OF TYPE 1 VERSUS TYPE 2 MYOCARDIAL INFARCTION

| | |
|---|---|
| **Case Example** | A 55-year-old female with a history of hyperlipidemia, hypertension, and breast cancer was recovering after a double mastectomy on postop day 2. She noted chest pain that morning; she described it as starting 10 minutes ago and as squeezing and substernal, a "fist to the chest." The intern promptly obtained a 12-lead ECG, which showed diffuse ST-segment depressions in the inferior and lateral leads. She ordered troponins, gave full-dose aspirin, and started a heparin drip. However, the bedside nurse noted that the patient's right-sided breast drain output had been putting out a significant amount of blood overnight, much more than before, and much more than the left-sided drain. As the intern went to examine the drain, he noted bright red blood that was visibly accumulating in the right drain. The patient's hemoglobin result from the morning is 5 g/dL down from 7 g/dL immediately postoperatively (baseline 10 g/dL). STAT troponin levels returned at 2.1 ng/dL (upper limit of normal 0.017 ng/dL). |
| **Reasoning Error(s)** | ■ Inadequate history to differentiate between plaque rupture and demand |
| | ■ Equating tropinemia associated with chest pain as pathognomonic of plaque rupture |
| **How to Avoid the Mistake** | ■ Obtain a thorough history yourself. Focus on causes of demand (the reasons are infinite) and fully characterize the chest pain (e.g., worse with exertion and better with rest). The distinction between type 1 and type 2 MI is purely based on the history. |
| | ■ Remember that even if a patient has typical chest pain, this may be due to supply/demand mismatch and in not necessarily a plaque rupture event. In other words, all anginal pain means is that there is a significant oxygen-demand mismatch, only some of which is due to a hemodynamically significant coronary stenosis. |

| | |
|---|---|
| **Antidote** | ■ Not applicable |
| **Common Scenarios** | ■ Severe anemia (usually acute) |
| | ■ Sepsis |
| | ■ Hyperthyroidism |
| | ■ Acute severe illness (e.g., acute decompensated heart failure) |
| | ■ Hypertensive emergency |
| **Note(s)** | ■ A type 2 MI event is not the same as nonischemic myocardial injury. Nonischemic myocardial injury is defined by biomarker evidence of cardiomyocyte damage (i.e., elevated troponin) without evidence of ischemia (e.g., myocarditis). A type 2 MI event is one that meets the fourth universal definition of MI by including a rise and fall of cardiac biomarkers in conjunction with evidence of cardiac ischemia such as anginal chest pain or the equivalent, ECG evidence of ischemia, or imaging evidence of wall motion abnormalities. Patients with type 2 MI often have underlying coronary artery disease (CAD), and a future ischemic evaluation is warranted (usually when the current situation/ stress has resolved). |
| | ■ A type 2 MI is frequently thrown around even in the setting of no obvious reason for increased demand. Remember that there must be an etiology to the increased demand. |

## Diagnostics: Physical Exam

### MISTAKE: INACTION ON NEW MURMURS OR GALLOPS IN ACUTE CORONARY SYNDROMES

| | |
|---|---|
| **Case Example** | An 80-year-old male with a history of hyperlipidemia, hypertension, and three-vessel coronary artery bypass graft surgery (CABG) performed 15 years earlier presented to the ED via emergency medical services (EMS) with a complaint of new chest pain. This was the first time he has had chest pain since his operation 15 years earlier. His pain was worse when he was moving but was present at rest and relieved with nitroglycerin. He was given aspirin in the field and takes a baby aspirin and high-intensity statin daily. ECG on presentation showed sinus rhythm with nonspecific ST-segment and T-wave changes. His first troponin was negative. The admitting team physician examined the patient and noted stable vital signs and a patient who is well appearing and chest pain free after two nitroglycerin tablets. His cardiovascular exam was significant for warm and well-perfused extremities, a soft 2/6 mid-systolic murmur at the apex, no rubs, no gallops, and a nondisplaced point of maximal impulse (PMI). Most notable are bibasilar rales, although the patient's oxygen saturation is 100% on room air and denies dyspnea. You reassure the patient and note that a new troponin level will be checked in 3 hours. At 30 minutes later, the patient is found in acute respiratory distress requiring escalation to bilevel positive airway pressure (BiPAP), and a STAT troponin is elevated at 4.2 ng/dL. A bedside transthoracic echocardiogram (TTE) reveals a flail posterior mitral leaflet. |

| | |
|---|---|
| **Reasoning Error(s)** | ■ Expectation of a significant and/or obvious change in the physical exam<br>■ Lack of knowledge on patient's prior physical exam baseline<br>■ Inaction on an uncertainty (e.g., unclear baseline exam) |
| **How to Avoid the Mistake** | ■ Understand that most patients with ACS have normal physical exams. Signs of mechanical complications of ACS may be obvious (e.g., new hypotension, significant rales, cold extremities) or subtle (e.g., soft new murmur). In particular, ischemic mitral regurgitation due to papillary muscle rupture displays a widely variable new murmur that may be prominent or nonexistent (when severe due to the lack of a pressure gradient between the left atrium [LA] and left ventricle [LV]).<br>■ Obtain a description of a patient's baseline physical exam to help differentiate old from new exam findings. This may involve carefully searching the electronic medical record (including through connections to outside records) or calling outside hospitals/providers for collateral.<br>■ If unable to be certain regarding a patient's baseline exam (or any other aspect such as history), and the information is critical to patient care, act to obtain the necessary information. This may include expediting a workup at your own institution (in the case above, a transesophageal echocardiogram [TEE]). |
| **Antidote** | ■ Emergent bedside TTE |
| **Common Scenarios** | ■ Ischemic mitral regurgitation<br>■ Ischemic ventricular septal defect<br>■ Cardiogenic shock |
| **Note(s)** | ■ Remember that the absence of abnormal findings (i.e., a normal physical exam) does not rule out ACS. Most patients with ACS do not have obvious new physical exam findings, and the presence of new findings such as rales usually indicates more severe myocardial dysfunction from ACS. Severe ischemic mitral regurgitation may present without a murmur. |

## MISTAKE: NOT CHECKING FOR A LOW-OUTPUT STATE IN PATIENTS WITH ACUTE CORONARY SYNDROMES

| | |
|---|---|
| **Case Example** | A 72-year-old male with a history of hyperlipidemia, hypertension, type 2 diabetes, and coronary artery disease status post three-vessel CABG 10 years ago presented to the ED. He was quite confused at home and very sleepy, hard to arouse out of bed this morning. In the ED, his vital signs were significant for blood pressure of 84/66, pulse of 120/min, respirations of 18/min, and $SpO_2$ of 94% on room air. The admitting team ordered fluid resuscitation and sent a workup for sepsis. When the admitting team examined the patient, they noted cool extremities and put a blanket on the patient. A few hours later the patient's initial labs come back significant for creatinine 1.6 (baseline 0.8), and troponin of 4.0 ng/dL (upper limit of normal 0.017 ng/dL). A 12-lead ECG was then obtained, which showed 2-mm ST-segment elevations in leads II, III, and aVF with deep Q waves in those same leads. The patient proceeded to go into VF arrest; although return of spontaneous circulation (ROSC) was achieved, he was transitioned to comfort focused care the next day per his prior wishes. |

**Reasoning Error(s)**
- Overlooking cool extremities subjectively ("it is cool but should be okay," low index of suspicion) as a marker of poor perfusion
- False reassurance by the patient of prior cool extremities
- Lack of understanding on how to assess perfusion state
- Not considering all etiologies of shock in a hypotensive patient

**How to Avoid the Mistake**
- Understand that cool extremities are often overlooked subjectively with a low index of suspicion, though this should never be the case without objective evidence for a well-perfused state. Furthermore, remember that there is little point in performing an exam maneuver if the information will not be used or acted upon.
- Realize that many patients have cool extremities, particularly the distal appendages such as toes, feet, fingers, and hands. While difficult to attribute the coolness to poor baseline circulation versus a new hypoperfused state, it is important to check the temperature of the legs up to the knees in all patients. A patient in cardiogenic shock will usually have not only cold feet but also cold shins and even a cold knee. Furthermore, cool is different from icy cold, which is a red flag sign of hypoperfusion.
- Incorporate additional markers of perfusion into your overall assessment: pulse pressure, tachycardia (including relative tachycardia from baseline), mentation, and end-organ markers (e.g., creatinine, liver function tests, urine output, lactic acidosis).
- Refrain from jumping to the most common etiology of shock (septic shock). Meticulously consider all etiologies for each patient in shock even if septic shock is the most common, or you will miss the other types of shock.

**Antidote**
- Not applicable

**Common Scenarios**
- Not applicable

**Note(s)**
- The varying degrees of congestion and hypoperfusion in ACS were expertly categorized by Forrester et al and briefly summarized in Table 7.1.
- Cardiogenic shock is an emergent indication for angiography in non–ST-elevation acute coronary syndromes (NSTE-ACS) and patients presenting with low output states should be immediately triaged as such.
- Many patients who are hypotensive may be fluid responsive, but administering fluids to a patient in cardiogenic shock could be detrimental.
- Early revascularization and mechanical circulatory support are the best ways to manage cardiogenic shock due to acute ischemia.
- Examples of potentially reversible causes of cardiogenic shock include acute MI, acute valvular regurgitation (aortic or mitral), fulminant acute myocarditis, malignant arrhythmia (VT or VF), progression of primary cardiomyopathy, severe heart failure with reduced ejection fraction, and low output state.
- Remember that all patients presenting with chest pain or other potential cardiac issues (including cardiogenic shock) should receive a 12-lead ECG within 10 minutes of presentation.

TABLE 7.1 ■ **Forrester Hemodynamic Profiles**

| | |
|---|---|
| Cardiac index >2.2 L/min/m² <br> PCWP <18 mmHg <br> Forrester Class I (normal) | Cardiac index >2.2 L/min/m² <br> PCWP >18 mmHg <br> Forrester Class II (pulmonary edema) |
| Cardiac index <2.2 L/min/m² <br> PCWP <18 mmHg <br> Forrester Class III (low output state) | Cardiac index <2.2 L/min/m² <br> PWCP >18 mmHg <br> Forrester Class IV (true cardiogenic shock) |

# Diagnostics: ECG (refer to Chapter 3)

## MISTAKE: RULING OUT ISCHEMIA BASED ON A NORMAL ECG

**Case Example**

A 68-year-old male with a history of hyperlipidemia and hypertension presented to his PCP's office as a same day visit after he developed squeezing chest discomfort. The pain started while he was walking out to his car but continued to worsen, so he presented to his PCP's office two blocks away. An ECG was obtained in office and showed normal sinus rhythm. He was diagnosed with muscular strain and sent home with Tylenol (acetaminophen), ibuprofen, and a lidocaine patch. That evening his pain continued to worsen and he presented to the nearest ED, where a 12-lead ECG showed 1-mm, horizontal ST-segment depressions in diffuse leads with ST elevation in aVR. Troponin was 3.05 ng/dL (normal <0.017 ng/dL).

**Reasoning Error(s)**

- Assuming that a normal ECG rules out ischemia
- Not considering the relationship between ECG changes and time course of ischemia
- Thinking that an ECG during ischemia always demonstrates obvious signs of ischemia

**How to Avoid the Mistake**

- Treat ECGs as medical tests with a fixed sensitivity and specificity, but keep in mind that they have limits just like all medical tests. The ECG is like a "biopsy of time" wherein you catch a glimpse of the electrical activity of the heart. This fact can be very powerful and lead to the diagnosis of acute myocardial ischemia and MI; however, it is also limited and can miss the phenomenon of myocardial ischemia.
- The most powerful ECGs are the ones obtained *during* the event in question (chest pain, palpitations, syncope, etc.). However, keep in mind that most ECG changes evolve over time and may not be prominent (nonspecific or subtle) early in the course of ischemia. Trend ECGs in patients suspected of ACS.

**Antidote**

- Serial ECGs

**Common Scenarios**

- Not applicable

**Note(s)**

- The ischemic cascade represents the time sequence of events (Fig. 7.1) at the cellular and macroscopic level that occur after myocardial ischemia. Theoretically, an ECG obtained during an episode of chest pain should show changes, but the issue is that the changes may not be diagnostic (e.g., may be a nonspecific T-wave change or a subtle ST elevation that does not meet criteria), particularly earlier in the course of ischemia.

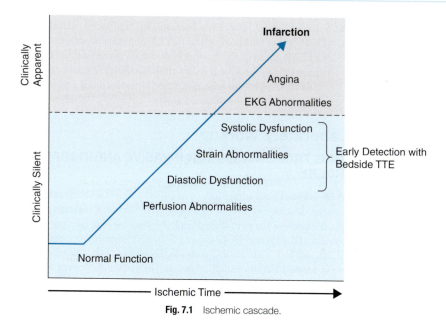

**Fig. 7.1** Ischemic cascade.

## MISTAKE: OVERLOOKING DIFFUSE ST DEPRESSIONS

**Case Example**  A 70-year-old female with a history of type 2 diabetes and tobacco use disorder presented to the ED with epigastric discomfort and hiccups. Vital signs were normal on presentation, and physical exam was within normal limits. An ECG was obtained and demonstrated global ST depressions with ST elevation in aVR. Initial troponin value was 4.04 ng/dL (normal <0.017 ng/dL). The patient was admitted to the cardiology floor with the diagnosis of NSTEMI and was medically managed. Coronary angiogram the following day showed a 70% left main coronary artery lesion.

**Reasoning Error(s)**
- Lack of knowledge on diffuse ST depressions as a presentation consistent with ischemia
- Lack of proper reconciliation (clinical inaction) of an unusual clinical finding

**How to Avoid the Mistake**
- Understand that diffuse ST depressions (particularly when accompanied by ST elevation in aVR) are highly concerning for significant CAD leading to "global" ischemia (left main, proximal LAD, or multivessel disease).
- High-risk findings on surface ECG should warrant, at the least, early consultation with the interventional cardiology team. Do not choose inaction on clinical findings that you do not fully understand with confidence.

**Antidote**
- Clarify all questionable ECG findings with the interventional team or other colleagues

**Common Scenarios**  ■ Not applicable

| | |
|---|---|
| **Note(s)** | ■ Some institutions prefer not loading with dual antiplatelet therapy (DAPT) (i.e., withholding the P2Y12 inhibitor) in patients with NSTEMI, particularly those at high risk of multivessel CAD that may require CABG, because it delays time to CABG (a washout period is required). Check with your institution's interventional and cardiothoracic teams on the institutional policy. |

# Diagnostics: Laboratory Workup

## MISTAKE: CHECKING TROPONINS AFTER INVASIVE ANGIOGRAPHY OR CARDIAC SURGERY

| | |
|---|---|
| **Case Example** | A 68-year-old male with a history of hyperlipidemia and hypertension presented to the ED after he developed left-sided neck and arm pain while shoveling snow. The pain started while he was shoveling but continued to worsen, and a 12-lead ECG showed 2-mm ST-segment elevations in leads II, III, and aVF with small Q waves in those same leads. Coronary angiography showed a 100% mid-RCA lesion. The patient underwent successful suction thrombectomy followed by a single drug-eluting stent placement. He was then admitted to the cardiac care unit for further management. The next morning on prerounds, the patient was asymptomatic and well, with no chest pain, and was ambulating about the unit without dyspnea. The junior resident had ordered a troponin level for that morning because he was in the habit of trending troponins for all ACS events. The troponin level continued to rise from 10.04 ng/dL (normal <0.017 ng/dL) to 15.39 ng/dL. The resident was worried and obtained an ECG, which showed resolution of ST elevation from prior. Concerned, she brought it up to the fellow. |
| **Reasoning Error(s)** | ■ Unnecessary laboratory investigation was performed, which sparked further worry and testing.<br>■ Forgetting that invasive coronary angiography will increase troponins due to subclinical distal embolization of atherosclerotic plaques (e.g., while passing a wire over a plaque)<br>■ Not understanding the time kinetics of various cardiac biomarkers<br>■ Forgetting to think of what will be done with newly obtained clinical information |
| **How to Avoid the Mistake** | ■ It is not commonplace to check troponin levels after coronary intervention or cardiac surgery as they are presumed to be positive either from residual elevation from the initial event or from myocardial injury from instrumentation or transient coronary occlusions intraprocedurally. In the absence of symptoms or hemodynamic instability, do not screen for reinfarction after reperfusion.<br>■ Troponins have slow kinetics and will be positive for days following an acute ischemic event (ACS). This is less true of high-sensitivity troponins, which nearly mimic creatine kinase (CK)-MB. If suspicion is high for reinfarction, standard troponins will be of little value and testing should include either high-sensitivity troponins and/or CK-MB.<br>■ Always think about how new clinical information changes management. How will you interpret and use the new information? |
| **Antidote** | ■ Not applicable |

**Common Scenarios** ■ Not applicable

**Note(s)** ■ Troponin I is more specific for myocardial injury compared to troponin T. Noncardiac causes of troponin elevation include chronic kidney disease, sepsis (i.e., demand), muscle damage, and stroke.

■ An elevated troponin without a rise and fall (i.e., a troponin that is always elevated at baseline, such as in the setting of CKD) is known as chronic myocardial injury.

## MISTAKE: CHECKING CREATINE KINASE–MB TO DIAGNOSE MYOCARDIAL INFARCTION

**Case Example**    A 43-year-old male with no significant past medical history presented to the ED complaining of chest pain. This pain was new for him and started earlier that day. He described it as a substernal squeezing that occurred as he was walking up the stairs in his home, it went away after a few minutes when he rested at the top. The patient's 12-lead ECG showed evidence of left ventricular hypertrophy with downsloping ST depressions in the lateral leads and T-wave inversions in these same leads. The admitting intern is concerned about ACS, gives the patient aspirin, and orders a CK-MB with thoughts that troponin may not be positive yet due to the timing of his symptoms.

**Reasoning Error(s)** ■ Thinking that CK-MB is value in diagnosis of new MI because it may be detectable earlier than standard troponins

■ Old-school practice patterns

**How to Avoid the Mistake** ■ Unless attempting to diagnose reinfarction in a patient with confirmed ACS or quantifying size of infarction, refrain from ordering CK-MB. CK-MB is less sensitive and less specific than cardiac troponin and has been replaced as the recommended biomarker to use in diagnosis of ACS. CK-MB use for initial diagnosis of ACS wastes money and time and can lead to errors and delays in treatment.

■ Although classic troponin may not be positive initially for a patient with ACS, as it takes time to be detectable, high-sensitivity troponin assays are reducing this time to approximately 2–3 hours. The decision to treat as ACS in this case could be made based on the clinical presentation and the ECG findings—as even in the absence of biomarker positivity this patient meets the definition of NSTE-ACS, specifically unstable angina at this point (since biomarkers have not yet resulted).

■ Continue to stay updated on recent advances.

**Antidote** ■ Not applicable

**Common Scenarios** ■ Not applicable

**Note(s)** ■ The biomarker of choice to prove myocardial injury, and in the setting of myocardial ischemia/MI, is cardiac troponin. The specific assay (troponin T, troponin I) will vary per institution, but there is a trend toward high-sensitivity troponins nationwide to expedite the ACS rule-out process.

■ Order CK-MB only for diagnosing reinfarction, as the kinetics of CK-MB show a rise and fall over the course of 48–72 hours of the index infarction. This allows for diagnosis of reinfarction, as other biomarkers (troponins) remain positive for days after infarction.

# Diagnostics: Stress Testing (refer to Chapter 6)

## MISTAKE: RULING OUT ACUTE CORONARY SYNDROMES BASED ON A RECENT NORMAL STRESS TEST

**Case Example**

A 68-year-old male with a history of hyperlipidemia and hypertension presented to the ED after he developed left-sided neck and arm pain while walking home from the gym. The pain started while he was walking but continued to worsen; he then experienced a "soreness" in his chest. The ED provider looked through his chart and saw a negative exercise stress echocardiogram from 3 years prior and held off on ordering an ECG as a result-opting to treat with acetaminophen and a lidocaine patch for musculoskeletal pain. At change of shift, a 12-lead ECG was obtained that showed 2-mm ST-segment elevations in leads II, III, and aVF with small Q waves in those same leads. Coronary angiography showed a 100% mid-RCA lesion. The patient underwent successful suction thrombectomy followed by a single drug-eluting stent placement. Follow-up echocardiogram showed an ejection fraction of 30%.

**Reasoning Error(s)**

- Lack of understanding regarding the pathophysiology of ACS
- Lack of knowledge regarding the sensitivity and specificity of various stress tests (i.e., thinking that negative stress tests rule out ischemia/ACS)
- Not factoring in clinical context

**How to Avoid the Mistake**

- ACS pathophysiology is one of plaque rupture and thrombus formation, which can occur with hemodynamically insignificant soft plaques that can be physiologically silent on stress testing (all modalities except coronary CT angiography [CTA] provide a binary depiction of ischemia or not, which leads to ignorance of nonobstructive lesions) and missed. Hence, a negative stress test in the past does not absolutely rule out the possibility of ACS.
- Take stress test results into context as one piece of data. A negative stress test in the recent past (specifically a negative coronary CTA within 2 years or negative stress test within 1 year) makes ischemic heart disease a less likely phenomenon to explain a current presentation but does not rule it out. Clinical context should be the single most important factor guiding your decisions.
- The sensitivity of stress testing is ~70% on ECG stress testing, 80% on echocardiographic stress testing, 85%–90% on nuclear stress testing, and 90%–93% with CTA. Thus, a convincing clinical presentation should usually override recent stress testing results.

**Antidote**

- Not applicable

**Common Scenarios**

- Not applicable

**Note(s)**

- There are many factors that go in to the "warranty" of a stress test or coronary evaluation to gauge future events such as angiographic (or CT) appearance of lesion, mode of stress (exercise versus pharmacologic), age, known coronary disease or first diagnosis, and so forth.
- In general, a negative myocardial perfusion scan, coronary CTA, or stress echocardiogram is associated with a risk of MI/death of <1% per year for ~2–3 years.
- In general, a completely negative coronary angiogram is associated with a low risk of MI/death for ~3–5 years.

# Therapeutics: Medical Management

## MISTAKE: FAILURE TO ADMINISTER ASPIRIN EARLY IN ACUTE CORONARY SYNDROMES

**Case Example**

A 43-year-old male with no significant past medical history presented to the emergency department complaining of chest pain. The patient's 12-lead ECG shows evidence of horizontal ST-depressions in the lateral leads and T-wave inversions in these same leads. Initial troponin was 3.08 ng/dL (normal <0.017 ng/dL). The admitting intern diagnosed the patient with a type I MI and wished to proceed with an early invasive strategy of reperfusion. They immediately told the nurse to administer aspirin and start a heparin infusion. After awaiting an hour for the pharmacy to verify and prepare the bag of heparin, aspirin was administered at the same time.

**Reasoning Error(s)**
- Lack of understanding the evidence behind aspirin in ACS
- Not thinking about timeliness of administering aspirin
- Lack of insight or oversight of logistics that delay essential medications

**How to Avoid the Mistake**
- Understand that aspirin reduces mortality by 20% versus placebo, with no significant increase in intracranial or gastrointestinal bleeding, based on the landmark ISIS-2 trial, which cemented its role in the treatment of ACS.
- Once the diagnosis of ACS has been made, there should be no delay (unless true aspirin allergy) in giving chewable, non–enteric-coated aspirin 162–325 mg once, followed by 81 mg daily.
- Shoulder responsibility for ensuring that essential orders are carried out in a timely fashion. Check-in with team members such as nursing to ensure that there are no logistical barriers. If barriers arise, help overcome them so patients may receive care expeditiously.

**Antidote**
- Not applicable

**Common Scenarios**
- Not applicable

**Note(s)**
- Although anticoagulant medication is recommended in the treatment of ACS *in addition to antiplatelet agents*, this should not take precedence over antiplatelet agents, especially aspirin. In fact, unfractionated heparin infusion *alone* was shown not to have a mortality benefit in patients with unstable CAD.
- Additionally, subcutaneous enoxaparin at 1 mg/kg every 12 hours has more evidence (Class IA recommendation) than unfractionated heparin infusion (Class IB). Part of the reason for this has been postulated as the erratic pharmacokinetics of unfractionated heparin versus the reliable anticoagulation of enoxaparin.

**Further Reading**
- The practice-changing ISIS-2 trial that demonstrated mortality reduction in ACS with aspirin: ISIS-2 Collaborative Group. Randomised trial of intravenous streptokinase, oral aspirin, both, or neither among 17 187 cases of suspected acute myocardial infarction: ISIS-2. *Lancet.* 1988;332(8607):349-360.

## MISTAKE: NOT PROVIDING A HIGH-INTENSITY STATIN IMMEDIATELY ON DIAGNOSIS OF ACUTE CORONARY SYNDROMES

**Case Example**

A 67-year-old female with a past medical history of hypertension and tobacco use disorder presented to the emergency department complaining of chest pain. The patient's 12-lead ECG shows evidence of symmetric T-wave inversions in the inferior and lateral leads. Initial troponin was 1.08 ng/dL (normal <0.017 ng/dL) The admitting intern diagnosed the patient with a type 1 MI and began appropriate medical management with aspirin, ticagrelor, enoxaparin, and metoprolol with nitroglycerin as needed. The patient had resolution of her chest pain with these interventions. The intern signed the patient out to the night team with an echocardiogram, lipid panel, and hemoglobin A1c pending.

**Reasoning Error(s)**
- Thinking that the decision to initiate a statin in a patient experiencing ACS depends on lipid levels and/or ASCVD risk scores
- Lack of knowledge regarding the benefit of statins in ACS
- Thinking that statins provide long-term rather than short-term benefit (as in the setting of ACS)

**How to Avoid the Mistake**
- A high-intensity statin should be started for secondary prevention for all patients with clinical atherosclerotic cardiovascular disease, of which ACS is a subcategory. Lipid levels and ASCVD risk scores do not apply here because the patient is experiencing ASCVD (no need to predict it!).
- Understand that high-intensity statin therapy has been shown in a randomized controlled trial (MIRACL) to reduce the risk of death and recurrent ischemic events when started early after ACS diagnosis (within 24–96 hours of hospital admission). This phenomenon of high-intensity statins that protects against the once high rate of recurrent ischemia and death in the early period after ACS diagnosis appears to be unrelated to its lipid-lowering effects (possibly explained by pleiotropic antiinflammatory effects).

**Antidote**
- Not applicable

**Common Scenarios**
- Not applicable

**Note(s)**
- High-intensity statin options are atorvastatin 40/80 mg and rosuvastatin 20/40 mg.
- As noted in Chapter 6, rosuvastatin is renally cleared and should be administered cautiously up to a maximum dose of 10 mg in GFR <30. Our preference is to choose atorvastatin for patients with significant CKD because dose adjustment is often overlooked and cumbersome.

**Further Reading**
- The MIRACL study: Schwartz GG, et al. Effects of atorvastatin on early recurrent ischemic events in acute coronary syndromes—the MIRACL study: a randomized controlled trial. *JAMA.* 2001;285(13):1711-1718.

## MISTAKE: NOT PROVIDING P2Y12 INHIBITORS FOR DELAYED REVASCULARIZATION

**Case Example**

A 70-year-old female with a history of depression, type 2 diabetes, hyperlipidemia, and tobacco use disorder presented to the ED with nausea and dyspnea. Vital signs were normal on presentation, and physical exam was within normal limits. An ECG was obtained and showed sinus rhythm with nonspecific ST/T-wave changes. The patient was given aspirin and admitted to cardiology. Her first troponin level was 3.04 ng/dL (normal <0.017 ng/dL). The patient received medical management with aspirin, heparin, metoprolol tartrate, and rosuvastatin, with plans for an early invasive approach and coronary angiogram scheduled for the next day.

**Reasoning Error(s)**
- Fear of increased bleeding during revascularization
- Fear of delaying potential CABG

**How to Avoid the Mistake**
- Realize that the decision to delay CABG after receiving DAPT is not only institution dependent but also surgeon dependent. Usually, surgeons require the P2Y12 inhibitor to be held 2–5 days prior to CABG. Unless coronary anatomy is going to be quickly determined (via angiogram with intent for reperfusion), DAPT should be given up front for maximal medical management of ACS and decisions about CABG may be made down the line.
- Understand that DAPT with either clopidogrel or ticagrelor plus low-dose aspirin should be given by the medical team upon diagnosis of ACS unless the patient is definitely going for angiography within 24 hours. In that case, reperfusion therapy with primary PCI and definition of coronary anatomy by angiography will take temporal precedence, or indications for CABG will be defined.

**Antidote**
- Administer DAPT if delay is anticipated.

**Common Scenarios**
- Logistical delays (e.g., catheterization delayed until after the weekend)
- Likely CABG candidate

**Note(s)**
- The 600-mg clopidogrel load has quicker onset of action and more predictable pharmacokinetics. The 600-mg load is standard for ACS, but a 300-mg load can be used in patients >75 years old or those with high bleed risk.
- Ticagrelor is preferred to clopidogrel in terms of DAPT choice; however may not be covered by as many insurance carriers and may be cost-prohibitive for some patients.
- DAPT with prasugrel and low-dose aspirin should be used only in select cases (i.e., when PCI is planned and the patient has low bleed risk with no contraindications) and never in patients who are not undergoing planned PCI.
- In ACS, the PLATO trial showed ticagrelor (given as 180-mg load then 90 mg twice a day) with aspirin significantly reduced the risk of death from vascular causes, MI, or stroke without an increase in major bleeding but with an increase in non–procedure-related bleeding compared to clopidogrel and aspirin.

- In ACS, the TRITON-TIMI-38 trial showed that in patients scheduled to undergo coronary intervention, prasugrel (given as 60-mg load followed by 10 mg daily) with aspirin reduced rates of MI, revascularization, and in-stent thrombosis with a significant increase in bleeding complications (fatal and nonfatal) compared to clopidogrel with aspirin, with no difference in overall mortality.
- Clouding the picture, the ISAR-REACT 5 study showed that in patients undergoing coronary intervention for ACS, prasugrel with aspirin reduced rates of death, MI, or stroke with no significant difference in incidence of bleeding when compared to ticagrelor with aspirin.

## MISTAKE: LACK OF DUAL ANTIPLATELET THERAPY AFTER ACUTE CORONARY SYNDROMES IRRESPECTIVE OF REPERFUSION STRATEGY

**Case Example**

A 70-year-old female with a history of depression, type 2 diabetes, hyperlipidemia, and tobacco use disorder presented to the emergency department with nausea and dyspnea. Vital signs were normal on presentation, and physical exam was within normal limits. An ECG was obtained and showed sinus rhythm with nonspecific ST-T wave changes. The patient was given aspirin and admitted to cardiology. Her first troponin level was 3.04 ng/dL (normal <0.017 ng/dL). The patient received medical management with aspirin, ticagrelor, heparin, metoprolol tartrate, and rosuvastatin, with plans for an early invasive approach and coronary angiogram scheduled for the next day. She underwent coronary angiography and received a single drug-eluting stent to a mid-left circumflex artery lesion. She was asymptomatic the following day and felt well with stable vital signs. The intern was about to discharge her with 90 days of DAPT.

**Reasoning Error(s)**

- Confusing DAPT after ACS with DAPT after stenting only (not in the setting of ACS)
- Not understanding the data for DAPT after ACS
- Difficulty balancing bleeding risk with ischemic risk

**How to Avoid the Mistake**

- Remember that regardless of treatment approach for ACS (reperfusion with primary PCI or medical management alone), DAPT should be provided for up to 12 months in patients without contraindications. This is an IB recommendation by the American Heart Association. Indeed, patients with ACS represent a subset of patients with clinical ASCVD who are at high risk of MACE; therefore, it is crucial to reduce this risk, especially in the immediate time surrounding an event (such as ACS).
- The choice of DAPT, and the ultimate length of DAPT, after ACS has to consider the patient's bleeding risk, the patient's coronary anatomy, and the type (PCI or CABG) of revascularization strategy (if any). For example, in high bleed risk situations post-ACS, there are IIA recommendations for stopping the 81-mg aspirin component after 1–3 months of DAPT and IIB recommendations for stopping the P2Y12 inhibitor component after 6 months of DAPT. Always consult with your interventional team.
- Do not confuse the duration of DAPT after ACS with that after a stent alone. The duration of DAPT post-ACS is 12 months, which is much longer than one would prescribe DAPT for a DES alone (without associated ACS). This belies the underlying high-risk phenotype of patients who have ACS.

| | |
|---|---|
| **Antidote** | ■ Not applicable |
| **Common Scenarios** | ■ Not applicable |
| **Note(s)** | ■ In general, DAPT with prasugrel has the highest bleeding risk, followed by ticagrelor, followed by clopidogrel. The degree of reduction in MACE is in the reverse order. |
| **Further Reading** | ■ The PLATO and ISAR-REACT 5 studies are the original studies that suggested superiority of ticagrelor (compared with clopidogrel) and prasugrel (compared with ticagrelor) after ACS.<br>　　■ Wallentin L, et al. Ticagrelor versus clopidogrel in patients with acute coronary syndromes. *N Engl J Med.* 2009;361:1045-1057.<br>　　■ Schupke S, et al. Ticagrelor or prasugrel in patients with acute coronary syndromes. *N Engl J Med.* 2019;381:1524-1534. |

## MISTAKE: FORGETTING UNIQUE CONTRAINDICATIONS TO PRASUGREL

| | |
|---|---|
| **Case Example** | A 77-year-old female with a history of depression, type 3 diabetes, hyperlipidemia, prior cerebrovascular accident (CVA), and tobacco use disorder presented to the ED with nausea and dyspnea. Vital signs were normal on presentation. and physical exam was within normal limits. An ECG was obtained and showed sinus rhythm with ST depressions in the inferior leads. The patient was given aspirin and prasugrel and admitted to cardiology. Her first troponin level was 3.04 ng/dL (normal <0.017 ng/dL). The patient elected to receive medical management with aspirin, prasugrel heparin, metoprolol tartrate, and rosuvastatin. |
| **Reasoning Error(s)** | ■ Lack of knowledge regarding the contraindications to prasugrel<br>■ Patchy understanding of the evidence behind prasugrel use in ACS |
| **How to Avoid the Mistake** | ■ Remember that prasugrel is contraindicated in patients above the age of 75, with a history of CVA (due to increased risk of ICH), or with weight <60 kg. One way to better remember these contraindications is to remember prasugrel as the antiplatelet agent with the highest risk of bleeding.<br>■ Understand that bleeding risk is highest with prasugrel then ticagrelor then clopidogrel. Carefully discuss with the patient the benefit of a small superiority in MACE reduction versus an increase in bleeding risk.<br>■ Only prasugrel as choice of DAPT with aspirin order if the patient is *definitely* going to receive PCI *and* the patient is low risk for bleeding. Prasugrel as choice of DAPT was not studied in patients who were not going for scheduled angiogram with intent for revascularization. This is typically only known by the proceduralist, and hence prasugrel upfront (especially for NSTE-ACS) is discouraged.<br>■ Prasugrel is uniquely used, with aspirin, for ACS management (particularly in STEMI) in patients *undergoing PCI* with *low bleed risk* who are *<75 years of age with no history of CVA/TIA and weight >60 kg*. If there is any doubt regarding these factors, then one should avoid the use of prasugrel. |

| | |
|---|---|
| **Antidote** | ■ Not applicable |
| **Common Scenarios** | ■ Not applicable |
| **Note(s)** | ■ Prasugrel is not the P2Y12 inhibitor of choice for NSTE-ACS due to there being a larger range of revascularization options, the prescribing team not knowing for certain that a stent will be placed, and there being higher risks compared with clopidogrel and ticagrelor in terms of fatal bleeding |
| | ■ ISAR-REACT 5 did cast some doubt in terms of prasugrel bleeding risk versus ticagrelor, implying that it did not increase the risk of bleeding significantly but did reduce thrombotic complications. This study does not change the above-mentioned contraindications and caveats to its use in ACS. |
| **Further Reading** | ■ The TRITON-TIMI-38 study: Wiviott SD, et al. Prasugrel versus clopidogrel in patients with acute coronary syndromes. *N Engl J Med.* 2007;357:2001-2015. |

## MISTAKE: CONTINUING HEPARIN AFTER SUCCESSFUL REVASCULARIZATION

| | |
|---|---|
| **Case Example** | A 70-year-old female with a history of depression, type 2 diabetes, hyperlipidemia, and tobacco use disorder presented to the ED with nausea and dyspnea. Vital signs were normal on presentation, and physical exam was within normal limits. An ECG was obtained and showed sinus rhythm with ST depressions in the lateral leads. The patient was given aspirin and admitted to cardiology. Her first troponin level was 1.04 ng/dL (normal <0.017 ng/dL). The patient received medical management with aspirin, ticagrelor, heparin infusion, metoprolol tartrate, and rosuvastatin, with plans for an early invasive approach and coronary angiogram scheduled for the next day. She underwent coronary angiography and received a single drug-eluting stent to a mid-left circumflex artery lesion. She was asymptomatic the following day and feeling well with stable vital signs but continued on heparin to round out the medical management of NSTEMI. |
| **Reasoning Error(s)** | ■ Lack of understanding the role of heparin in ACS |
| | ■ Not considering the risks of a common medication such as heparin |
| **How to Avoid the Mistake** | ■ Understand that the role of anticoagulation with heparin in ACS is to reduce hemostatic effects that may facilitate expansion of existing thromboses or development of new thromboses. When added to aspirin (but not with heparin alone), heparin significantly reduces mortality and complications from myocardial infarction. |
| | ■ Remember that once a plaque is stabilized (e.g., with stent placement), there is no role for heparin as the plaque is definitively stabilized, obviating the need for further medical efforts at stabilization. Stop heparin for whichever comes first: 48 hours of therapeutic heparin therapy or definitive revascularization (e.g., with a stent). |
| | ■ Always consider contraindications and side effects, even for routine medications such as supplemental oxygen and acetaminophen. Heparin is a common medication in the treatment of ACS that possesses significant bleeding risk and should be used for only the shortest necessary duration. |

| | |
|---|---|
| **Antidote** | ■ Stop heparin when no longer indicated |
| **Common Scenarios** | ■ Not applicable |
| **Note(s)** | ■ If heparin needs to be continued for another indication, there is a delay based on the access site for angiogram. Specifically, restarting any heparin product must wait until the coronary angiogram access site is stable after the sheath has been pulled. |

## MISTAKE: ROUTINE AND/OR PROLONGED TRIPLE THERAPY

| | |
|---|---|
| **Case Example** | A 75-year-old male with a history of diabetes, atrial fibrillation on apixaban, and hypertension presented to the ED complaining of chest pain. He described it as a substernal squeezing that got worse when he thought about his divorce; it went away after a few minutes with no particular intervention, but these episodes increased in frequency throughout the day. The patient's 12-lead ECG showed 2.3-mm ST elevations in V2-4; the patient was given aspirin and taken to the catheterization laboratory, where a stent was placed for a 100% proximal left anterior descending artery lesion, with successful reperfusion. He was given a load of 600 mg clopidogrel on the table and a bolus of heparin as well. Postprocedurally he was asymptomatic, and his echocardiogram showed an ejection fraction of 45%. He was started on optimal therapies and planned to discharge on 1 year of DAPT, metoprolol, rosuvastatin, and lisinopril, in addition to his preexisting medications. |
| **Reasoning Error(s)** | ■ Lack of considering cumulative bleeding risk from DAPT and anticoagulation<br>■ Lack of knowledge of evidence for alternatives to triple therapy<br>■ Only considering ischemic risk rather than balancing ischemic and bleeding risk |
| **How to Avoid the Mistake** | ■ Understand that, unsurprisingly, the bleeding risk with DAPT plus anticoagulation (known as triple therapy) is very high. In general, this is reserved for patients who have no increased bleeding risk and very high ischemic risk (e.g., a lot of myocardium at risk with a stent to the proximal left anterior descending artery).<br>■ Learn the evidence behind triple therapy. Because atrial fibrillation is a common comorbidity in patients with ACS, the optimal balance of DAPT and anticoagulation has been extensively studied using atrial fibrillation as a model disease. Most recently, the AUGUSTUS trial demonstrated that the addition of aspirin to apixaban and a P2Y12 inhibitor increased bleeding risk significantly without a clear reduction in thrombotic events.<br>■ Triple therapy is almost never indicated for *prolonged* periods; however, for the immediate peri-stent period it may be indicated. This period is determined by the operator who placed the stent usually but may vary from 1 week to 1 month, as guided by the thrombotic and bleeding risk. After this period, aspirin is usually omitted, and the patient continues on P2Y12 inhibitor with anticoagulation (DOAC preferred over warfarin, unless contraindications). |
| **Antidote** | ■ Deescalate triple therapy as soon as possible. |

**Common Scenarios**　■　Not applicable

**Note(s)**
■ DAPT is prescribed to reduce the probability of in-stent thrombosis. The risk of in-stent thrombosis is higher in drug-eluting stents than bare metal stents due to the drugs that prevent smooth muscle proliferation also slowing reendothelialization. Thus, DAPT duration is longer for drug-eluting stents than for bare metal stents. DAPT is always indicated immediately after a coronary stent placement.

**Further Reading**
■ The AUGUSTUS trial answered many questions regarding triple therapy: Lopes RD, et al. Antithrombotic therapy after acute coronary syndrome or PCI in atrial fibrillation. *N Engl J Med.* 2019;380:509-1524.

## MISTAKE: NITRATES FOR INFERIOR ST-SEGMENT ELEVATION MYOCARDIAL INFARCTION (NOT NON–ST-SEGMENT ELEVATION MYOCARDIAL INFARCTION) WITHOUT ASSESSING FOR RV INFARCTION

**Case Example**
A 50-year-old female with a history of depression, type 2 diabetes, hyperlipidemia, and tobacco use disorder presented to the ED with nausea and dyspnea. Vital signs were normal on presentation, and physical exam was within normal limits. An ECG was obtained and showed 1 mm ST-elevations in leads II, III, and aVF with 1-mm ST depressions in leads I and aVL. After notifying the catheterization laboratory, the intern ordered aspirin, atorvastatin, and nitroglycerin given her discomfort. Following these interventions, she lost consciousness and her blood pressure was 70/40 with heart rate of 120. The cardiology fellow started a fluid bolus and placed the patient in Trendelenburg position with improvement in vital signs to blood pressure of 90/60 and heart rate of 95.

**Reasoning Error(s)**
■ Forgetting that an inferior STEMI may involve right ventricular (RV) involvement
■ Lack of knowledge on how to check for RV infarction
■ Not understanding the physiology associated with RV infarction

**How to Avoid the Mistake**
■ All patients with inferior STEMIs should have a right-sided ECG obtained in order to rule out RV infarction. A right-sided ECG is obtained by moving the precordial leads V3-6 to their mirror image positions on the right side of the chest, while leaving leads V1-2 in place. In this new arrangement, the old V2 becomes V1R and the old V1 becomes V2R, while V3-6 become V3R-6R.
■ Bedside echocardiography is also very useful in determining if the RV has been involved by inferior STEMI (can be as simple as gross loss of contractility), ideally in the apical four-chamber or RV inflow/outflow views as these can technically allow for more advanced quantitative measurements if the operator is experienced in them.
■ Learn the interplay in physiology behind RV infarction and nitroglycerin. An RV infarction leads to a preload-dependent state, which benefits from IV fluids and may cause profound hypotension with preload-lowering agents such as nitrates and high-dose morphine.

| | |
|---|---|
| **Antidote** | ■ IV fluids |
| | ■ Trendelenburg position |
| **Common Scenarios** | ■ Not applicable |
| **Note(s)** | ■ Nitrates are used for NSTEMI as long as the patient is not hypotensive and has not had a phosphodiesterase inhibitor (e.g., sildenafil) recently. Notably, an NSTEMI with ST depressions that are in the inferior leads (II, III, aVF) does not necessarily localize to the inferior myocardium as in a STEMI (i.e., you cannot localize ST depressions). Thus, an "inferior" pattern NSTEMI is not a contraindication to nitrates. |
| | ■ Nitroglycerin is contraindicated in patients with significant pulmonary hypertension on advanced medical therapies such as riociguat, epoprostenol, and iloprost, since they share the cGMP pathway for vasodilation and profound hypotension may result. |

## MISTAKE: UNDERTREATING PAIN IN ACUTE CORONARY SYNDROMES

| | |
|---|---|
| **Case Example** | A 59-year-old male with a history of type 2 diabetes and BPH presented to the ED complaining of chest pain. This pain was new for him and started that evening. He described it as a substernal squeezing that went away after a few minutes when he rested. The patient was chest pain free in the ED and with stable vital signs, and a normal physical exam. The patient's 12-lead ECG shows voltage criteria for left ventricular hypertrophy and symmetric terminal T-wave inversions in V2-4. The admitting intern was concerned about Wellen syndrome, give the patient aspirin, and called interventional cardiology. While the intern was on the phone with the catheterization laboratory, the patient developed recurrence of his chest pain and diaphoresis and was in visible distress. His vital signs were significant at that time for blood pressure of 180/110 and heart rate of 110. ECG now showed 2-mm ST elevations in V2-5 with depressions in II and III. The intern was afraid to give pain medications for risk of hypotension. |
| **Reasoning Error(s)** | ■ Not knowing when to treat anginal pain with opioids |
| | ■ Incorrect association of hypotension with opioid use in ACS |
| | ■ Lack of knowledge of when opioids are contraindicated in ACS |
| **How to Avoid the Mistake** | ■ Treat angina with antianginals if the patient has no other contraindications. If the patient is not already hypotensive, antianginals are relatively safe. Opioids are not first-line antianginals; however, they are effective should nitroglycerin and beta blockers fail while awaiting urgent angiography. |
| | ■ If a patient is obviously hypotensive with systolic BP <90, most antianginals will be relatively contraindicated, as will most opioids due to sympatholytic effects. Anginal pain is extremely distressing and warrants prompt treatment with antianginal medications, however, and usually patients will have BP room to tolerate these (nitrates, β-blockers, calcium channel blockers if β-blockers contraindicated). |
| | ■ Use the localization of ST elevations (or right-sided ECG or echocardiogram; see prior case) to reassure against RV infarction. Once that is done—and medication reconciliation is negative for any phosphodiesterase inhibitors—nitrates may be used with close clinical monitoring. If refractory to as-needed nitroglycerin, a nitroglycerin infusion is an effective antianginal for up to 24 hours. |

| | |
|---|---|
| **Antidote** | ■ Not applicable |
| **Common Scenarios** | ■ Not applicable |
| **Note(s)** | ■ Similar preload-dependent conditions in which nitrates are contraindicated include HOCM and severe aortic stenosis. |

## MISTAKE: PROVIDING 100% SUPPLEMENTAL OXYGEN TO ALL PATIENTS IN ACUTE CORONARY SYNDROMES

| | |
|---|---|
| **Case Example** | An 80-year-old male with a history of type 2 diabetes and COPD presented to the ED complaining of chest pain. This pain was new for him and started that morning. He described it as crushing pain in the center of his chest. The patient was chest pain free in the ED with stable vital signs, and a normal physical exam. The patient's 12-lead ECG showed voltage criteria for left ventricular hypertrophy and nonspecific ST/T-wave changes. The initial troponin was 1.07 ng/dL (normal <0.017 ng/dL). The patient was started on aspirin, ticagrelor, metoprolol, and atorvastatin and given enoxaparin as a subcutaneous injection. The nurse puts on supplemental oxygen citing the "MONABASH" dictum. |
| **Reasoning Error(s)** | ■ Lack of knowledge on when oxygen is indicated in ACS<br>■ Following an outdated mnemonic used to teach the basics of ACS management |
| **How to Avoid the Mistake** | ■ Remember that supplemental oxygen is a drug with side effects just like any other and specific indications. It should not be reflexively started and is indicated only in patients with new hypoxemia with $SpO_2$ under 90% or respiratory distress (may help with comfort).<br>■ As medical trainees transition from medical school to residency and beyond, they should prioritize verifying and/or relearning key aspects of medical management taught in medical school because many early teachings are oversimplified. Always strive to keep up to date with new medical advances and evidence. |
| **Antidote** | ■ Remove supplemental oxygen if not indicated |
| **Common Scenarios** | ■ Not applicable |
| **Note(s)** | ■ Supplemental oxygen may increase coronary vascular resistance. |

## Therapeutics: Reperfusion Strategies

## MISTAKE: ASSUMING ALL ACUTE CORONARY SYNDROMES REQUIRE URGENT ANGIOGRAPHY

| | |
|---|---|
| **Case Example** | A 61-year-old male with a history of diabetes and hypertension presented to the ED complaining of chest pain. He described it as a substernal pressure that has worsened over the past 2 hours. The patient's 12-lead ECG showed 1.0-mm ST depressions in the inferior leads, and the patient was started on optimal medical management with aspirin, ticagrelor, enoxaparin subcutaneously, metoprolol tartrate, rosuvastatin, with as-needed nitroglycerin. Following these interventions, the patient was pain free, with stable vital signs, and with normal physical exam. The initial troponin level was 1.04 ng/dL (normal <0.0017 ng/dL). Given the "heart attack,", you insist to no success that interventional cardiology rush this patient to the cath lab. |

| | |
|---|---|
| **Reasoning Error(s)** | ■ Lack of knowledge on the indications for immediate coronary angiography, urgent coronary angiography, early coronary angiography, and delayed coronary angiography in terms of reperfusions strategies in ACS<br><br>■ Discomfort with the role of maximal medical management for ACS |
| **How to Avoid the Mistake** | ■ Understand that some patients benefit more from early reperfusion than others. A number of trials have been conducted to determine the patients who will benefit the most from reperfusion in ACS and the timing of reperfusion strategies (PCI with stenting vs CABG).<br><br>   ■ All patients with STEMI should receive revascularization of the culprit lesion, with primary PCI, within 90 minutes of medical contact at a PCI-capable facility (Class IA) or within 120 minutes of medical contact at a PCI incapable facility assuming a ≤30-minute transfer time to a PCI-capable center (Class IB).<br><br>   ■ Patients with NSTE-ACS (unstable angina and NSTEMI) should receive revascularization based on their risk and coronary anatomy—this may result in PCI with stenting or CABG.<br><br>      ■ If uncontrolled ischemic pain, hemodynamic instability, electrical instability (ventricular arrhythmias), or acute heart failure/cardiogenic shock, the patient should go urgently for coronary angiogram (Class IA).<br><br>      ■ If the patient has elevated TIMI or GRACE scores predictive of major adverse clinical cardiac events or has a positive troponin (especially if rising rapidly), early coronary angiography should be pursued (within 24 hours) (Class IB).<br><br>      ■ If the patient is not at high risk for events and is initially stabilized, it is reasonable to pursue a delayed coronary angiogram (25–72 hours) (Class IIA-B)<br><br>      ■ If the patient is at a lower risk for clinical events, and is initially stabilized, it is reasonable to pursue an ischemia-driven approach and defer invasive angiography pending results of noninvasive testing or recurrent ischemic symptoms (Class IIB-B).<br><br>      ■ Revascularization should not be pursued if the patient has extensive comorbidities and risks outweigh benefits. |
| **Antidote** | ■ Not applicable |
| **Common Scenarios** | ■ Not applicable |
| **Note(s)** | ■ A GRACE score >140 is generally the threshold for elevated-risk patients necessitating early angiography. A GRACE score <109 is generally the threshold for low-risk patients that can be managed with an ischemia-driven approach if troponin negative. |

## MISTAKE: DELAYING OR AVOIDING CORONARY ANGIOGRAPHY IN CHRONIC KIDNEY DISEASE AND/OR ACUTE KIDNEY INJURY

**Case Example**

A 67-year-old male with a history of diabetes, hypertension, and chronic kidney disease (CKD) IIIb presented to the ED complaining of 3 hours of crushing substernal chest pain. The patient's 12-lead ECG showed 1.2-mm ST depressions diffusely with ST elevations in aVR. The initial troponin level was 1.3 ng/dL (normal <0.017 ng/dL). The patient was given aspirin and started on optimal therapies for NSTEMI. The patient's troponin level continued to increase with the next result being 10 ng/dL, and the next set of vital signs showed a blood pressure of 95/65 with exam notable for cool extremities and some general sleepiness. The admitting team was hesitant to call for an angiogram for fear of precipitating acute kidney injury (AKI) on CKD.

**Reasoning Error(s)**

- Not realizing that coronary angiograms can be performed with low-dose contrast
- Inability to properly weigh risks and benefits
- Lack of patient-centered decision-making
- Lack of knowledge on maneuvers to decrease risk of contrast nephropathy

**How to Avoid the Mistake**

- In stage II and III CKD, an early invasive strategy is reasonable in patients who require it for management of NSTE-ACS (Class IIA-B). There is a trend toward reduced mortality and reinfarction in patients with ACS and CKD who receive revascularization and a reduction in recurrent hospitalization.
- The CKD population is a unique one that is both at risk for complications from ACS and at risk for treatment-related complications, and the risk and benefit should be individualized in each patient.
- Few select operators at most large medical institutions are able to perform coronary work with lower doses of contrast. Reach out to the cath lab at your institution to learn more about who qualifies for these procedures and who performs them.
- In patients with high-risk ACS (e.g., patient with impending cardiogenic shock in the case example), the theoretical risk of kidney damage does not outweigh the risks of developing cardiogenic shock (which will guarantee kidney damage) and/or mechanical complications of ACS. Always weigh risks and benefits carefully in discussion with the patient, who may prioritize certain risks and benefits differently from traditional medical providers.
- When possible (i.e., allowed by comorbidities), consider hydrating patients with 0.5–1 L of IV fluids prior to contrast exposure. Other potential associations with reduced risk of contrast-induced nephropathy are a radial artery approach and pretreatment with a high-intensity statin.

**Antidote**

- Angiogram when clinically necessary

**Common Scenarios**

- Not applicable

**Note(s)**

- The creatinine begins to rise within 24 hours in contrast-induced nephropathy and typically produces an FeNa that mimics prerenal injury (<2%). The kidneys usually recover within 3–7 days of contrast exposure.

## MISTAKE: LACK OF SALVAGE PERCUTANEOUS CORONARY INTERVENTION AFTER FIBRINOLYSIS FOR ST-SEGMENT ELEVATION MYOCARDIAL INFARCTION

**Case Example**

A 60-year-old male with a history of diabetes and hypertension presented to the ED complaining of 3 hours of chest pain. It started that evening and was maximal intensity after about an hour, feeling like a crushing pressure. The patient's 12-lead ECG showed 2.3-mm ST elevations in V2-4, and the patient was given aspirin and clopidogrel. The hospital to which he presented was 2 hours from the nearest PCI-capable facility and had only fibrinolytic capabilities. He underwent fibrinolysis yet had persistent typical angina. He received 48 hours of unfractionated heparin infusion. He was started on optimal therapies and planned to discharge on 1 year of DAPT, metoprolol, rosuvastatin, and lisinopril, in addition to his preexisting medications.

**Reasoning Error(s)**
- Not understanding salve (or "rescue") PCI
- Thinking that fibrinolysis is definitive
- Not aware of steps after fibrinolytic therapy

**How to Avoid the Mistake**
- Understand that management does not stop after fibrinolytic therapy, regardless of whether successful. Revascularization after fibrinolytic therapy is known as salvage or rescue PCI. The term is most often used in the setting of incomplete reperfusion from fibrinolytic therapy.
- After fibrinolysis, the patient should be transferred to a PCI-capable facility for angiography and PCI of the culprit lesion should be done as soon as possible (noting only that salvage PCI should not be done within 3 hours of fibrinolytic therapy). The following are more detailed guideline indications:
  - Immediate transfer if the patient is in cardiogenic shock or heart failure (Class IB)
  - Urgent transfer if the patient has evidence of failed reperfusion or continued ischemia (Class IIA-B)
  - Within 3–24 hours after successful fibrinolysis (Class IIA-B)
  - Greater than 24 hours after successful fibrinolysis (Class IIB-B)

**Antidote**
- Not applicable

**Common Scenarios**
- Failed fibrinolysis
- Successful fibrinolysis without subsequent transfer to PCI-capable center

**Note(s)**
- DAPT should be given in patients who receive fibrinolysis. However, only clopidogrel has been studied specifically in this regard.
- Anticoagulation should be given to patients who receive fibrinolytic therapy, up to 8 days or until revascularization.
- A late-presenting STEMI is defined as >12 hours after symptom onset.

## MISTAKE: USING FIBRINOLYTICS IN NON–ST-ELEVATION ACUTE CORONARY SYNDROMES

**Case Example**

A 65-year-old female with a history of diabetes and hypertension presented to the ED complaining of 3 hours of chest pain. The pain started that morning and was a vice-like pressure around her chest. The patient's 12-lead ECG showed 1.0-mm ST depressions in V5 and V6, and the patient was given aspirin and clopidogrel. Initial troponin was 3.03 ng/dL (normal <0.0017 ng/dL). The hospital to which she presented was 2 hours from the nearest PCI-capable facility and had only fibrinolytic capabilities. The admitting team gives fibrinolytic therapy prior to transfer to a PCI-capable facility for further management.

**Reasoning Error(s)**

- Lack of understanding indications for fibrinolytic therapy
- Not reasoning through the pathophysiology of NSTE-ACS
- Associating fibrinolysis with "buzz" scenarios such as a PCI-incapable center

**How to Avoid the Mistake**

- Understand that STEMI (or STEMI-equivalent posterior infarct pattern) is the only ECG criterion that would allow for fibrinolytic therapy for ACS. Fibrinolysis is useful only as second-line therapy when PCI is not available, AND it is not logistically feasible to perform PCI within 120 minutes of medical contact. It is best to administer fibrinolysis within 30 minutes of medical contact, if it is to be used.
- Remember that because NSTE-ACS does not represent a total acute occlusion, there is almost always time to transfer the patient to a PCI-capable center. Furthermore, NSTE-ACS may also be managed medically. Fibrinolysis in patients with ST depressions and not a true posterior MI has not been shown to improve mortality or MACE (TIMI IIIb Trial).
- Even though fibrinolysis is most commonly used in areas without access to PCI, that itself is not the key indication for fibrinolytic therapy. STEMI must be present.

**Antidote**

- Not applicable

**Common Scenarios**

- Unstable angina
- NSTEMI

**Note(s)**

- Fibrinolytic therapy includes agents such as tissue plasminogen activator (tPA), streptokinase, and urokinase.

# Therapeutics: Revascularization Strategies

## MISTAKE: INCOMPLETE REVASCULARIZATION OF NONCULPRIT LESIONS IN ST-SEGMENT ELEVATION MYOCARDIAL INFARCTION

**Case Example**

A 65-year-old male with a history of hypertension, dyslipidemia, occasional tobacco use, and BPH presented to the ED complaining of 1 hour of crushing substernal chest pressure. The patient's 12-lead ECG showed 2.3-mm ST elevations in V2-4, and the patient is given aspirin and taken to the catheterization laboratory where a 100% proximal left anterior descending artery lesion is stented with successful reperfusion. A 70% RCA lesion was also noted, which was not intervened upon at the time of primary PCI. He was given a load of 600 mg clopidogrel on the table and a bolus of heparin as well. Postprocedurally, he was asymptomatic, and his echocardiogram showed an ejection fraction of 45%. He was started on optimal therapies and planned to discharge on 1 year of DAPT, metoprolol, rosuvastatin, and lisinopril, in addition to his preexisting medications.

**Reasoning Error(s)**
- Lack of knowledge regarding complete revascularization in STEMI
- Incomplete understanding of data regarding complete revascularization in STEMI

**How to Avoid the Mistake**
- Understand that prior data on revascularization of nonculprit lesions in STEMI had conflicting data. However, this is thought largely due to the nonrandomized nature of the studies. Smaller randomized trials prior to COMPLETE demonstrated a benefit of complete revascularization.
- Understand that in 2019 the COMPLETE trial showed that in patients with STEMI and multivessel disease, complete revascularization significantly reduced cardiovascular death, MI, or ischemia-driven revascularization. Thus, our preference (and at minimum, a consideration of yours) is that STEMI patients undergo complete PCI.

**Antidote**
- Consider discussing complete revascularization with the interventional team.

**Common Scenarios**
- Not applicable

**Note(s)**
- Perhaps unsurprisingly, up to half of patients presenting with STEMI are found with multivessel coronary artery disease.

**Further Reading**
- While yet to be incorporated into guidelines, the COMPLETE trial is worth reading about: Mehta SR, et al. Complete revascularization with multivessel PCI for myocardial infarction. *N Engl J Med*. 2019;381(15):1411-1421.

## MISTAKE: LACK OF CONSIDERATION FOR CORONARY ARTERY BYPASS GRAFTING IN ACUTE CORONARY SYNDROMES (NONSTABLE ISCHEMIC DISEASE)

**Case Example**    A 75-year-old male with a history of diabetes, dyslipidemia, gout, and hypertension presented to the ED complaining of 3 hours of substernal discomfort associated with nausea. The patient's 12-lead ECG showed 1.5-mm ST segment depressions in the inferior and lateral leads, and the patient was given aspirin and ticagrelor loads. He was started on enoxaparin subcutaneously and was given metoprolol and nitroglycerin as needed. With these interventions, his chest pain resolved. His initial troponin was 2.04 ng/dL (normal <0.017 ng/dL) and peaked at 5 ng/dL. His transthoracic echocardiogram showed an ejection fraction of 35%. Once medically stabilized as above, he went for coronary angiogram as part of an early invasive strategy. Angiogram showed 70% stenoses in the RCA, left anterior descending artery, and left circumflex arteries. The interventional team reported these results to the primary team. The primary team asked them to move forward with multivessel PCI.

**Reasoning Error(s)**    ■ Lack of knowledge regarding indications for CABG
                    ■ Not knowing the evidence between PCI and CABG

**How to Avoid the Mistake**    ■ Understand the big picture. Revascularization consists of either PCI with stenting or CABG. The indications for revascularization in coronary artery disease depend on whether the patient is presenting with ACS or chronic stable angina or heart failure due to ischemic heart disease. The patients who benefit most from revascularization have few comorbidities (low surgical risk), a large area of myocardium at risk, and a reduced ejection fraction.

■ Learn the indications that favor CABG over PCI. Multivessel disease, left main disease, reduced ejection fracture, anatomic complexity of lesions with high SYNTAX score, and diabetes all favor CABG as revascularization for symptom reduction and mortality benefit.

■ Conversely, anatomically amenable lesions, single- or dual-vessel disease, and surgical comorbidity favor PCI over CABG as revascularization for symptom reduction and reduction of mortality, MI, and urgent revascularization depending on the indication (ACS versus chronic CAD).

**Antidote**    ■ Not applicable

**Common Scenarios**    ■ Not applicable

| | |
|---|---|
| **Note(s)** | ■ The SYNTAX score is an angiographically derived score that quantifies difficulty of PCI. It considers coronary anatomy, lesion complexity and distribution, and vessel characteristics. It does not account for prior revascularization (PCI or CABG). |
| | ■ In ACS with STEMI, the preferred revascularization approach is culprit artery PCI as soon as possible with emergency CABG of culprit lesion being performed only if PCI is not feasible, has failed, or in the setting of mechanical complications of STEMI. Once the culprit artery has been addressed, the nonculprit lesions can be revascularized via staged PCI or elective CABG depending on the anatomy. |
| | ■ In chronic stable angina/stable ischemic heart disease, CABG is the favored revascularization approach for patients with left main coronary artery disease or a reduced ejection fraction (with benefit correlating with degree of reduction in ejection fraction). This strategy confers a mortality benefit (as well as addresses symptoms) over medical therapy alone and has fairly strong data supporting its use. CABG may be reasonable for three vessel disease (with normal ejection fraction and no left main disease) but the benefits are less as compared to the group with left main disease or a reduced ejection fraction (when compared to optimal medical therapy alone). |

## Post-ACS Care: Complications

### MISTAKE: NOT RECOGNIZING POSTANGIOGRAPHY COMPLICATIONS

| | |
|---|---|
| **Case Example** | A 65-year-old male with a history of hypertension, dyslipidemia, occasional tobacco use, and BPH presented to the ED complaining of 1 hour of crushing substernal chest pressure. The patient's 12-lead ECG showed 2-mm ST elevations in V1-4, and the patient was given aspirin and taken to the catheterization laboratory, where right femoral access was obtained due to failed radial access. A 100% proximal left anterior descending artery lesion was stented with successful reperfusion. Postprocedurally that evening, he was noted to be newly hypotensive to 80s/40s and appeared sleepy with pinpoint pupils. He was noted to have flank ecchymoses bilaterally but otherwise his exam was normal. The overnight intern ordered fluids, held the patient's nitroglycerin, and discontinued all opioids as he thought the patient was "snowed." The morning labs were notable for a hemoglobin of 4.5 g/dL (was 10 g/dL the day prior). CT abdomen and pelvis with contrast showed a large retroperitoneal hematoma with active extravasation. |
| **Reasoning Error(s)** | ■ Lack of knowledge regarding common postangiography complications |
| | ■ Thinking that complications are rare and unlikely |
| | ■ Premature closure (only considering a "routine" differential and forgetting to consider procedural complications) |
| **How to Avoid the Mistake** | ■ Following femoral access, the complications in Table 7.2 should be high on the differential diagnosis. A positive diagnostic workup for any of the above complications should prompt a vascular surgery consult STAT. |
| | ■ Realize that postangiography complications are possible even if rare nowadays (generally 1% for the most common complications). Always examine the access site upon return from the catheterization laboratory and the following day. |
| | ■ Always keep a broad differential, ensuring to include postprocedural complications. |

TABLE 7.2 ■ **Common Complications of Coronary Angiography**

| Finding | Diagnostic Consideration | First Diagnostic Action |
| --- | --- | --- |
| Groin pain/mass | Pseudoaneurysm/hematoma | Direct compression ultrasonography |
| Hypotension, abdominal or back pain | Retroperitoneal hematoma | CT abdomen/pelvis with contrast |
| Access side leg pain | Arterial dissection/clot | CT angiogram of lower extremity |

**Antidote** ■ Not applicable

**Common Scenarios** ■ Not applicable

**Note(s)** ■ Following radial access, one should be aware of the expanding hematoma, which is common and will be directly visualized. This requires direct manual compression for a minimum of 20 minutes but is less life threatening than retroperitoneal hematoma precisely because this is a compressible space.

■ Another notable post coronary angiogram complication when stents are placed is stent thrombosis. This is a true medical emergency and presents as a STEMI with ST elevations in the region of myocardium supplied by the newly stented artery. The risk of this is highest in the first month following stent placement as this is the time when endothelialization is occurring. DAPT is provided to reduce this risk but does not reduce it to zero always; this phenomenon should be on your radar in the patient with postangiogram chest pain.

## MISTAKE: OVERLOOKING NEW MURMURS IN LATE-PRESENTING MYOCARDIAL INFARCTION

**Case Example**     A 65-year-old male with a history of hypertension, dyslipidemia, and heavy tobacco use of two packs per day presented to the ED complaining of dyspnea. The dyspnea started yesterday, and he has not been able to walk around his home without feeling short of breath. He noted that 2 days prior to presentation he had a severe bout of indigestion that lasted almost the entire day and went away when he went to bed. Vital signs were stable, and exam was unremarkable. The patient's 12-lead ECG showed deep Q waves in V2-4 with symmetric and deep T-wave inversions in those same leads. The patient was given aspirin, and his initial troponin was 40 ng/dL (normal <0.017 ng/dL). He was taken to the catheterization laboratory, where a 100% mid left anterior descending artery lesion was stented, with sluggish filling. He was taken to the cardiac care unit, and a resting echocardiogram showed anterolateral hypokinesis with an ejection fraction of 30%. The next morning the patient was acutely dyspneic and hypoxemic to 88% on room air. Physical exam was notable for a faint holosystolic murmur at the apex. A STAT chest radiograph showed pulmonary edema. The primary resident ordered Lasix for decongestion.

| | |
|---|---|
| **Reasoning Error(s)** | ■ Thinking that late-presenting ACS patients are out of the window for mechanical complications |
| | ■ Lack of knowledge on mechanical complications of ACS, risk factors, and their timeline |
| | ■ Cursory physical exam in a late-presenting patient (mentality of "nothing on exam will change management because the presentation is so late") |
| **How to Avoid the Mistake** | ■ Understand that mechanical complications generally occur within the first week of the index event and are more common in patients who wait a long time prior to reperfusion, are older, female, and taking antiinflammatory medications. |
| | ■ Acute mitral regurgitation due to papillary muscle rupture occurs between days 3 and 5 postinfarct and presents as acute heart failure with pulmonary edema and hypoxemia. As there is rapid equalization of left atrial and left ventricular pressures with acute mitral regurgitation, the classic holosystolic murmur may be absent or faint on exam. |
| | ■ Acute ventricular septal defect occurs between days 3 and 5 postinfarction and presents as a harsh holosystolic murmur and ensuing shock. |
| | ■ Ventricular free wall rupture occurs approximately 7 days postinfarction and presents as chest pain and rapidly progresses to cardiac arrest. |
| | ■ Postinfarction pericarditis may occur acutely as an extension of myocardial inflammation or approximately weeks (or months) later as an autoimmune phenomenon (Dressler syndrome). This presents as classic pericarditis chest pain, but stent thrombosis should always be ruled out clinically. |
| | ■ Always perform a thorough physical exam. Even if a patient presents late, they are still at risk for the consequences of unrevascularized disease and extensive disease. In fact, post-MI complications are usually seen in late-presenting patients because there is more damage from longer time without revascularization! |
| **Antidote** | ■ STAT echo |
| | ■ STAT surgical consultation |
| **Common Scenarios** | ■ Acute mitral regurgitation |
| | ■ Acute ventricular septal defect |
| | ■ Ventricular free wall rupture |
| | ■ Postinfarction pericarditis |
| **Note(s)** | ■ All mechanical complications with rupture of a portion of the myocardium carry a high mortality and are medically temporized with afterload reduction, diuresis, and IABP placement but often require emergent surgery. The patients typically have poor prognoses. |
| | ■ Acute mitral regurgitation may occur at the time of the ACS event due to restriction of the posterior mitral leaflet in association with inferolateral wall motion abnormalities secondary to left ventricular dysfunction as a manifestation of acute ischemia. This is treated with reperfusion therapy and is a functional mitral regurgitation as opposed to papillary muscle rupture as above. |
| | ■ Postinfarction pericarditis is treated with high-dose aspirin and colchicine, but not NSAIDs or steroids, which increase the rate of mechanical complications as mentioned above. |

## MISTAKE: SUPPRESSING POST–MYOCARDIAL INFARCTION ARRHYTHMIAS WITH ANTIARRHYTHMIC DRUGS

| | |
|---|---|
| **Case Example** | A 75-year-old male with a history of diabetes, hyperlipidemia, and hypertension presented to the ED complaining of chest pain. The patient's 12-lead ECG showed 2.5-mm ST elevations in V1-4. In the cath lab, a 100% proximal left anterior descending artery lesion was successfully stented. He was given a loading dose of 600 mg clopidogrel on the table and a bolus of heparin as well. Postprocedurally he was asymptomatic, and his echocardiogram showed an ejection fraction of 45%. He was started on DAPT, metoprolol, rosuvastatin, and lisinopril, in addition to his preexisting medications. The next day he was noted to have a wide-complex rhythm at 87 beats per minute; the patient was asymptomatic and hemodynamically stable. The cross-cover resident reflexively orders lidocaine and amiodarone for suppression of VT. |
| **Reasoning Error(s)** | ■ Well-intentioned, logical thinking that arrhythmia suppression post-MI improves mortality<br>■ Lack of knowledge regarding empiric outcomes data with post-MI arrhythmia suppression |
| **How to Avoid the Mistake** | ■ Understand the data for post-MI arrhythmia suppression. In the CAST trials, an increase in mortality was seen in post-MI patients treated with Class 1C antiarrhythmics.<br>■ Understand that the best way to prevent lethal ventricular arrhythmias is to optimize volume status, perfusion, and electrolyte imbalances and treat any associated heart failure or shock.<br>■ VT and VF that are not hemodynamically tolerated are addressed via ACLS protocol with defibrillation and antiarrhythmic drug therapy. There is no role for routine antiarrhythmic suppression/prophylaxis against these rhythms although starting a β-blocker within 24 hours of presentation reduces the incidence of VF. |
| **Antidote** | ■ Not applicable |
| **Common Scenarios** | ■ Monomorphic VT |
| **Note(s)** | ■ AIVR, NSVT, and VPCs are expected postreperfusion and require no specific therapies.<br>■ β-Blockers should be started within 24 hours unless contraindicated based on heart failure, hypotension, shock, etc., which have the added benefit of reducing risk for VF.<br>■ Ventricular rhythms (VT and VF) are commonly ischemic in nature and are the number one causes of out-of-hospital cardiac arrest due to ACS. |

# Post–Acute Coronary Syndromes Care: Secondary Prevention and Guideline-Directed Medical Therapy

## MISTAKE: LACK OF β-BLOCKER POST–MYOCARDIAL INFARCTION

**Case Example**

A 75-year-old male with a history of diabetes, hyperlipidemia, and hypertension presented to the ED complaining of chest pain. The patient's 12-lead ECG showed 2.5-mm ST elevations in V1-4, and the patient was given aspirin and taken to the catheterization laboratory, where stenting was performed for a 100% proximal left anterior descending artery lesion with successful reperfusion. He was given a loading dose of 600 mg clopidogrel on the table and a bolus of heparin as well. Postprocedurally, he was asymptomatic, and his echocardiogram showed an ejection fraction of 45%. He was started on DAPT, rosuvastatin, and lisinopril, in addition to his preexisting medications, with a plan for discharge.

**Reasoning Error(s)**

- Lack of knowledge regarding role of β-blockers in the management of ACS
- Association of β-blockers with heart failure as the principal indication

**How to Avoid the Mistake**

- Understand that β-blockers have been extensively studied in ACS, both STEMI and NSTE-ACS, and there is a Class IA recommendation to start β-blockers within 24 hours of presentation for an ACS event.
- β-Blockers reduce not only rate of major adverse cardiovascular events post-ACS but also mortality. This has been studied even in the modern PCI era and holds true regardless of ejection fraction.
- If the ejection fraction on post-ACS echocardiogram is ≤40%, then one of the three mortality-reducing β-blockers (carvedilol, metoprolol succinate, or bisoprolol) should be used specifically for that population. Barring this, any β-blocker would be sufficient.

**Antidote**

- Not applicable

**Common Scenarios**

- Not applicable

**Note(s)**

- A commonly used regimen is metoprolol tartrate 12.5 mg every 6 hours PO, with transition to metoprolol succinate on discharge.
- A "β-blocked" state is achieved at a heart rate of 60 beats per minute at rest; this is not always achieved during the index hospitalization and should not be the goal immediately as adequate titration takes time to do safely. A massive dose of β-blocker upfront increases the risk of side effects, hemodynamic intolerance, and decreases adherence in the long term.
- The primary reasons not to start a β-blocker are cardiogenic shock or high risk for cardiogenic shock (low cardiac output states), acute heart failure, prolonged PR interval >0.24 second, high-grade AV block, symptomatic bradycardia, or active bronchospasm.

# MISTAKE: OVERLOOKING CARDIAC REHABILITATION ON DISCHARGE

**Case Example**

A 50-year-old male with a history of tobacco use, hyperlipidemia, and hypertension presented to the ED complaining of chest pain. The patient's 12-lead ECG showed 2.5-mm ST elevations in V1-4, and the patient was given aspirin and taken to the catheterization laboratory where stenting was performed for a 100% proximal left anterior descending artery lesion with successful reperfusion. Postprocedurally he was asymptomatic, and his echocardiogram showed an ejection fraction of 45%. He was started on DAPT, metoprolol, rosuvastatin, and lisinopril, in addition to his preexisting medications. The next day he was set for discharge after being cleared by physical and occupational therapy. The patient was worried that he would never be able to run again.

**Reasoning Error(s)**
- Lack of awareness of the existence of cardiac rehabilitation programs
- Not understanding what cardiac rehabilitation entails

**How to Avoid the Mistake**
- Understand that ACS events are psychologically stressful for patients and frequently they are left coping with their mortality in ways they never had before. Ischemic heart disease is a limitation for physical activity when there is ongoing/inducible ischemia, and patients fear this frequently.
- Learn that cardiac rehabilitation is a supervised exercise program that allows for safely increasing the maximal heart rate during exercise (under close monitoring), optimal risk factor modification, and improved outcomes for secondary prevention. Referral to a cardiac rehabilitation program is a core performance measure following ACS.

**Antidote**
- Not applicable

**Common Scenarios**
- Not applicable

**Note(s)**
- Patients should be told that, in addition to postangiogram precautions at the access site, they should modify their physical activity after an ACS event. They can resume symptom-limited walking/leisure activity almost immediately, aerobic exercise 1–2 weeks after successful revascularization, and resistance training 2–4 weeks after aerobic training has been initiated and tolerated. A cardiac rehabilitation program supervises and ensures this progression.
- However, if the patient is left without revascularization after ACS, additional physical restrictions apply due to concern for ongoing ischemia (and potential infarction) being provoked by activity.
- Overall, exercise is beneficial and should be recommended to all, especially post ACS, for reducing symptoms, weight loss, improving insulin sensitivity and glucose tolerance, and improving functional capacity.

## MISTAKE: LACK OF COUNSELING AND RESOURCES ON LIFESTYLE MODIFICATIONS

**Case Example**

A 75-year-old male with a history of diabetes, hyperlipidemia, tobacco use, and hypertension presented to the ED complaining of chest pain. The patient's 12-lead ECG showed 2.5-mm ST elevations in V1-4. The patient was given aspirin and taken to the catheterization laboratory, where stenting was performed for a 100% proximal left anterior descending artery lesion with successful reperfusion. He was started on DAPT, metoprolol, rosuvastatin, and lisinopril, in addition to his preexisting medications. The next day he was asymptomatic and was eager to leave the hospital. On his way home that evening, the primary resident saw the patient smoking a cigarette two blocks from the hospital.

**Reasoning Error(s)**
- Only focusing on medical interventions
- Reliance on PCP for counseling on lifestyle

**How to Avoid the Mistake**
- Understand that all patients who smoke should be counseled for smoking cessation at every opportunity and provided options and support to help them quit, such as pharmacotherapy or support groups. Other lifestyle modifications include diet and exercise. Remember that risk factor modification is essential to preventing recurrent ACS (e.g., discontinuing smoking can reduce MACE by up to 40%).
- Remember that lifestyle modification is a challenge for all patients. They benefit from frequent reinforcement. Furthermore, less-compliant patients benefit from frequent reassessment on whether they are amenable to considering lifestyle changes. Last, PCPs are often inundated with so many tasks and considerations that such counseling likely do not happen often enough—it is your responsibility to ensure your patients receive appropriate education and counseling.

**Antidote**
- Inquire about tobacco use in all ACS patients and, if positive, counsel to quit and provide resources. Nicotine replacement therapy works well in the hospital and can be continued easily on discharge. Close PCP follow-up after engaging with this topic decreases loss to follow-up in patients and increases adherence.
- Varenicline no longer holds the black-box warning regarding suicidality and is a very effective medication for smoking cessation; bupropion can also be considered.

**Common Scenarios**
- Not applicable

**Note(s)**
- Tobacco use is dwindling in the US, but it is still an extremely potent modifiable risk factor for clinical ASCVD.

## MISTAKE: NOT SCREENING FOR DEPRESSION POST–ACUTE CORONARY SYNDROMES

**Case Example**

A 50-year-old male with a history of tobacco use, hyperlipidemia, and hypertension presented to the ED complaining of chest pain. The patient's 12-lead ECG showed 2.5-mm ST elevations in V1-4. The patient was given aspirin and taken to the catheterization laboratory, where stenting was performed for a 100% proximal left anterior descending artery lesion with successful reperfusion. Postprocedurally he was asymptomatic, and his echocardiogram showed an ejection fraction of 45%. He was started on optimal therapies of DAPT, metoprolol, rosuvastatin, and lisinopril, in addition to his preexisting medications. The next day he was set for discharge. However, the patient was in tears and was worried that he would never be able to run again.

**Reasoning Error(s)**

- Exclusive focus on cardiology for ACS care
- Lack of knowledge regarding the link between ACS and depression

**How to Avoid the Mistake**

- Understand that a holistic approach is needed to patient care in any specialty. Depression is a common comorbidity of patients who experience major life-changing events such as ACS. In otherwise healthy or young patients, ACS events can be especially psychologically traumatic. Approximately 20% of patients experience signs or symptoms of depression after their first heart attack.

**Antidote**

- Consider referral to a psychiatrist and/or therapist

**Common Scenarios**

- Not applicable

**Note(s)**

- ACS events commonly cause severe health anxiety, depressive mood (and can potentially precipitate a major depressive episode), and an enhanced perception of bodily processes.

## CHAPTER 8

# Heart Failure

Bliss J. Chang

## CHAPTER OUTLINE

Mistake: Dismissal of FeNa as a Valuable Test for Guiding Diuresis in Heart Failure

Mistake: Increasing Diuretic Dosage Rather than Frequency in Nonrefractory Diuresis

Mistake: Blind Favor of Bolus Diuresis Over Drip Diuresis

Mistake: Forgetting to Bolus When Initiating Drip Diuresis

Mistake: Using Thiazides in Moderate to Severe Hyponatremia

Mistake: Not Screening for Diuresis-Antagonistic Medications

Mistake: Delay in Redosing Diuretics in Resistant or Refractory Diuresis

Mistake: Diuresing to Documented "Dry Weight" Rather Than Clinical Judgment

Mistake: Frequent Manual Potassium Repletion During Diuresis

Mistake: Acetazolamide to Correct Metabolic Alkalosis Without Checking Potassium

Mistake: Lack of Consideration for Nasal Intermittent Positive-Pressure Ventilation in All Patients With Acute Decompensated Heart Failure

Mistake: Use of Nasal Intermittent Positive-Pressure Ventilation in Acute Decompensated Heart Failure With Soft Blood Pressures

Mistake: Use of Ineffective or Evidence-Lacking Strategies for Diuresis

**Treatment: Guideline-Directed Medical Therapy**

Mistake: Limited GDMT Therapy in the Setting of Soft Blood Pressures

Mistake: Forgetting to Actively Uptitrate GDMT to Target Doses

Mistake: Deferring GDMT Initiation/Uptitration to the Outpatient Setting

Mistake: Holding All GDMT During Acute Decompensated Heart Failure

Mistake: Discontinuing GDMT in Recovered HFrEF

Mistake: Holding or Withdrawing ACEIs/ARBs for Increasing Creatinine After Initiation

Mistake: Not Trialing an ARB After ACEI Angioedema

Mistake: Not Using or Discontinuing Low-Dose ACEI/ARB Therapy in CKD/ESRD

Mistake: Maintaining ACEIs/ARBs Instead of ARNIs

Mistake: Transitioning to ARNIs From ACEIs Without a Washout Period

Mistake: Liberal Vasodilator Use in Severe Aortic Stenosis

Mistake: Prescribing Metoprolol in the Setting of Hypotension

Mistake: Rapid Uptitration of β-Blocker Dosing (Particularly in New Heart Failure)

Mistake: Withholding β-Blockers in Bronchospastic Disease

Mistake: Treating Cocaine as an Absolute Contraindication to β-Blocker Therapy

Mistake: Withholding ACEIs/ARBs/ARNIs and/or Spironolactone for Mild Hyperkalemia

Mistake: Prescribing SGLT2 Inhibitors to Patients With Frequent UTIs

Mistake: Forgetting to Consider Hydralazine/Nitrates, Ivabradine, or ICD Therapy for GDMT

Mistake: Lack of Patient-Centered Consideration for a LifeVest for Severe Ischemic HFrEF During GDMT Optimization

Mistake: Forgetting Aerobic Exercise Prescriptions in HFrEF and HFpEF

Mistake: Not Considering GDMT for HFpEF

**Treatment: Vasopressors and Inotropes**

Mistake: Use of β-Blockers While on Catecholaminergic Pressors or Inotropes

Mistake: Liberal Use or Incorrect Choice of Inotropes in Patients With Arrhythmic Substrate and/or Ischemia

Mistake: Aggressive Weaning or Sudden Discontinuation of Inotropes

Mistake: High-Dose Phenylephrine in Afterload-Sensitive Diseases

Mistake: Using Dobutamine or Norepinephrine in Hypotension in the Setting of Left Ventricular Outflow Tract Obstruction

# Diagnosis: Symptoms

## MISTAKE: RULING OUT ACUTE DECOMPENSATED HEART FAILURE BASED ON ABSENCE OF COMMON SYMPTOMS OR EXAM FINDINGS

**Case Example**

A 63-year-old female with heart failure (HF) with reduced ejection fraction (HFrEF) (EF = 30%), chronic obstructive pulmonary disease (COPD), venous insufficiency, and severe peripheral artery disease (PAD) status post popliteal stent presents with worsening shortness of breath (SOB). He denies orthopnea and consistently sleeps using a single pillow. He also denies awakening early at night gasping for air and weight gain. On exam, he has no edema on the left leg but 2+ edema up to the right knee. There is no obvious jugular vein distention (JVD) at 60 and 45 degrees. While awaiting further testing, you incorrectly conclude, based on the lack of corroborating symptoms such as orthopnea (remembering that orthopnea and paroxysmal nocturnal dyspnea [PND] are some of the most specific symptoms of HF) and the lack of obvious leg edema (attributing the right leg edema to venous insufficiency), that the SOB is more likely secondary to another common etiology such as pneumonia or progression of COPD.

**Reasoning Error(s)**

- Forgetting that symptoms and exam findings are either specific or sensitive for HF but not both. For example, the specificity of orthopnea is 77%, whereas its sensitivity (i.e., ability to rule out HF) is 50%. Conversely, the specificity of worsening dyspnea on exertion is 34%, whereas its sensitivity is 84%.
- Misunderstanding how to correctly perform the physical exam (e.g., equating edema as only that of the lower extremities rather than gravity dependent, or an inability to visualize JVD due to a high angle of the head of the bed). Refer to page 164.
- Attributing a key symptom or exam finding to an alternate existing diagnosis. For example, attributing unilateral leg edema to venous insufficiency rather than (1) leaving open the possibility of an atypical (asymmetric) presentation of leg edema or (2) considering that the visible leg edema is excess fluid superimposed upon baseline edema from venous insufficiency (or other cause, such as leg edema due to calcium channel blockers).

**How to Avoid the Mistake**

- Understand the diagnostic accuracy of common symptoms and exam findings.
- Hone history-taking and physical exam techniques to optimize quality of data.
- Avoid anchoring: stay flexible with interpretation of key data and revisit assumptions or determinations that you have made if the story is not fitting.
- Always obtain information on a patient's baseline prior medical presentations.
- Diagnose based on the summation of all data available: history, physical exam, laboratory testing, and imaging. Revise your differential diagnosis as you gain new information.

**Antidote**

- Not applicable

**Common Scenarios**

- Lack of orthopnea: Inquire about not only the number of pillows used but also whether they sleep in a chair or recliner. Some patients may use one pillow but sleep in a recliner!
- Lack of exertional dyspnea: Patients may experience a gradual decline in exercise tolerance that is less noticeable. For example, patients may not believe their ability to walk has decreased but perhaps they are aware that they can no longer golf as many rounds. Assess for worsening exercise tolerance in a manner relevant to the patient's lifestyle.
- Lack of weight gain: HF is a cachectic disease and over time patients will lose weight not attributable to fluid balance. Pay close attention to the date of the last recorded dry weight—the more recent the weight, the more likely to be accurate. Furthermore, there is no guarantee that the last recorded dry weight was the patient's true dry weight (e.g., some clinicians may discharge before fully reaching a dry weight with plans to diurese more in the outpatient setting).
- Lack of leg edema: Edema is gravity dependent. For example, in bedbound patients, the most gravity-dependent point is the sacrum; thus, patients may appear to have little leg edema but have copious hidden sacral edema. Furthermore, in very obese patients, volume may hide well, and you may not easily visualize pitting edema.

**Note(s)**

- The two most specific symptoms for HF (elevated left-side pressures) are paroxysmal nocturnal dyspnea and orthopnea.
- The most sensitive symptom for HF is dyspnea on exertion.
- The two most specific exam findings for HF are an S3 (ventricular) gallop and jugular venous distention.
- The absence of lower extremity edema on exam is only 50% sensitive for HF.
- Bendopnea (shortness of breath when bending forward, such as to tie shoelaces) is a symptomologic cousin of orthopnea that carries prognostic significance, particularly of an increased risk of HF admission within 3 months.

**Further Reading**

- Excellent overview of the diagnostic accuracy of various symptoms, exam findings, and laboratory testing for HF: Wang CS, et al. The rational clinical examination: does this patient in the emergency department have congestive heart failure? *JAMA.* 2005;294(15):1944-1956.

## MISTAKE: RULING OUT ACUTE DECOMPENSATED HEART FAILURE BASED ON PRESENCE OF UNCOMMON AND UNFAMILIAR SYMPTOMS OR EXAM FINDINGS

**Case Example**  An 82-year-old male with ischemic cardiomyopathy (EF = 15%), hypertension (HTN), and hyperlipidemia (HLD) presents with worsening SOB. The patient also endorses sleeping on multiple pillows in a recliner and awakens in the middle of the night frequently gasping for air. His legs have become visibly swollen and he complains of a distended abdomen. He also notes significant right upper quadrant pain and early satiety, wincing when you attempt a hepatojugular reflux test. Given multiple prior presentations of decompensated HF and the clear picture of volume overload, you are almost convinced that this is another HF exacerbation. However, the abdominal pain and distended abdomen throw you off and you attempt to search for Occam's razor, eventually incorrectly setting on decompensated liver failure as higher on the differential prior to seeing lab results.

**Reasoning Error(s)**
- Overreliance on classic and common presentations with decreased awareness and/or comfort of atypical presentations of common diseases
- Lack of knowledge of less common HF symptoms
- Failure to think through how an atypical symptom may align with the pathophysiology of HF

**How to Avoid the Mistake**
- Realize that the most common cases you see are common presentations of common diseases and that the next most common are atypical presentations of a common disease.
- Consider how uncommon or unfamiliar symptoms may manifest given the most likely pathophysiology at play—for example, right upper quadrant abdominal pain may manifest from severe venous congestion and early satiety from gut edema.
- Consider keeping a diary or a list of unusual patient presentations for future reference.

**Antidote**
- Not applicable

**Common Scenarios**
- Severe venous congestion: abdominal pain (especially right upper quadrant)
- Gut edema: early satiety, nausea/vomiting, diarrhea
- Pulmonary congestion: coughing
- Inadequate cardiac output: confusion, altered mental status, lethargy, chest pain, decreased urine output
- Genetic/nonischemic cardiomyopathy: young age

**Note(s)**
- Patients with New York Heart Association (NYHA) Class IV HF seem to experience more atypical signs and symptoms.

## MISTAKE: FORGETTING TO SCREEN FOR DEPRESSION IN PATIENTS WITH HEART FAILURE

| | |
|---|---|
| **Case Example** | A 72-year-old male with HFrEF (EF = 15%) is admitted to your service for decompensated HF for the seventh time in 4 months. The patient's length of stay is usually quite short, as he often leaves against medical advice, citing an inability to tolerate the strict salt and fluid restrictions. However, you persuade him to stay the entire hospitalization this time. The day of discharge, he complains of significant fatigue even though his volume exam appears baseline. You tell the patient that with his EF, he will always feel some fatigue, and that he appears much better than when he presented. He re-presents 3 days later with subjective SOB, fatigue, and only mild lower extremity edema. |
| **Reasoning Error(s)** | ■ Focusing too much on one's own medical specialty<br>■ Bias against psychiatry as less of a "real" medical problem<br>■ Lack of awareness about the prevalence of major depression among HF patients |
| **How to Avoid the Mistake** | ■ Approach patient care with a holistic mindset regardless of chosen specialty.<br>■ Understand that patients with HF commonly experience depression, from as low as 8% in NYHA Class I HF to as much as 40% in NYHA Class IV. |
| **Antidote** | ■ Not applicable |
| **Common Scenarios** | ■ Not applicable |
| **Note(s)** | ■ Depression is an extremely important comorbidity to treat in HF patients. It has been linked to worse symptom management and more frequent hospitalizations. |

# Diagnosis: Physical Exam

## MISTAKE: BEING FALSELY REASSURED OF ADEQUATE CARDIAC OUTPUT BASED ON NORMAL SYSTOLIC BLOOD PRESSURE

| | |
|---|---|
| **Case Example** | The nurse urgently pages you about a patient who has acutely become hypoxic. Walking into the patient's room, you see a blood pressure of 115/98 and breathe a sigh of relief that the systolic blood pressure is robust. However, on a bedside Swan, the estimated cardiac output is shown to be 1.8 (normal >2.2). |
| **Reasoning Error(s)** | ■ Assuming an unwavering direct relationship between systemic blood pressure and perfusion<br>■ Lack of reference to a patient's individual baseline blood pressures<br>■ Cursory glance at the blood pressure without considering the diastolic or pulse pressure |

| | |
|---|---|
| **How to Avoid the Mistake** | ■ Understand that hypoperfusion may occur in both systemic hypotension and normotension; that systemic hypotension does not necessarily result in hypoperfusion. |
| | ■ Assess the pulse pressure (systolic minus diastolic) for each patient. A sustained pulse pressure of <25 mmHg is a sign of decreased cardiac output. |
| | ■ Integrate multiple data sources (history, vitals, exam, labs) to determine perfusion state. |
| **Antidote** | ■ Not applicable |
| **Common Scenarios** | ■ Normal systolic blood pressure with a low pulse pressure |
| | ■ Normal pulse pressure in the setting of severe aortic regurgitation |
| **Note(s)** | ■ Nonhypotensive cardiogenic shock appears to predominantly occur in patients with large anterior wall infarctions or those with baseline uncontrolled HTN. That is, it is more likely in patients with a more robust intrinsic vasoconstrictor response (leading to higher systemic vascular resistance). In other words, since BP = CO × SVR, blood pressure (BP) may appear normal in the setting of low cardiac output (CO) if systemic vascular resistance (SVR) is elevated due to neurohormonal activation in HF (e.g., sympathetic and renin-aldosterone system activation). |
| | ■ The alternation of weak and strong pulses, known as pulsus alternans, is a sign of severe left ventricular (LV) dysfunction. The mechanism is thought secondary to an increased preload in the setting of poor cardiac output, leading to a larger cardiac output and hence stronger following beat. |
| **Further Reading** | ■ SHOCK Trial first describing nonhypotensive cardiogenic shock: Menon V, et al. Acute myocardial infarction complicated by systemic hypoperfusion without hypotension. *Am J Med*. 2000;108(5):374-380. |

## MISTAKE: MISIDENTIFICATION OR INABILITY TO VISUALIZE THE JUGULAR VENOUS PULSE

| | |
|---|---|
| **Case Example** | You search the right neck of a patient for the jugular venous pulse (JVP), beginning near the clavicles and searching for anything pulsating. You are unable to identify a pulsation and thus note "No JVP." |
| **Reasoning Error(s)** | ■ Lack of knowledge of correct landmarks for JVP assessment |
| | ■ Improper setup for visualization (head of the bed, neck positioning, lighting, external wiring, etc.) |
| | ■ Lack of knowledge regarding how JVP reacts to changes in position |

**How to Avoid the Mistake**

- Understand the correct anatomic landmarks for identifying JVP (Fig. 8.1). The key landmark is the sternoclavicular muscle heads that flank the internal jugular vein. These are better exposed when the patient turns their head. The clavicle forms the inferior border of the triangular region. Note that the external jugular vein lies lateral to the clavicular head of the sternoclavicular muscle.
- Take a systematic approach, starting with identifying landmarks each time. Avoid the temptation to jump to looking for any fluttering vasculature.
- If unsure whether carotid or JVP, gently place a finger on the vessel—an internal jugular pulse disappears, whereas a carotid pulse does not.
- Ensure visualization of two quick flutters of the vessel per heartbeat.
- When unable to visualize the JVP, attempt adjusting the angle of the head of the bed. As the angle becomes more upright, the vertical top of the venous column decreases (the actual JVP does not change but rather the JVP becomes more or less visible). In patients with very high right-sided pressures, the JVP may not be visible at 45 (or even 60) degrees; conversely, patients with very low right-sided pressures may need to be at a substantially low angle (e.g., 20 degrees) to visualize the JVP.
- Attempt increasing the JVP temporarily with the hepatojugular reflux maneuver: press firmly on the mid-abdomen (avoid pressing in the right upper quadrant in patients with significant congestive hepatopathy as it can be quite painful) for at least 10 seconds, checking to see if your hypothesized JVP rises.
- Remember that the angle of the bed/neck/head does not matter for measuring the JVP as long as you can see the top of the venous column. Measure the vertical ($y$-axis) height of the IJ vein, which does not change with head position. The neck adjustment may be needed to *see* the top of the column, if the value is quite high or low, but does not affect the actual numerical value of the JVP (a common misconception).

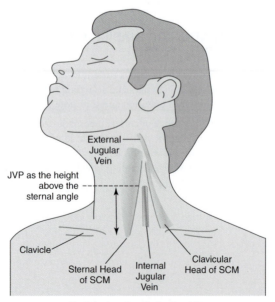

**Fig. 8.1**   Landmarks for the JVP.

| | |
|---|---|
| **Antidote** | ■ Not applicable |
| **Common Scenarios** | ■ Inability to identify any semblance of a JVP |
| | ■ Mistaking the carotid artery for the JVP |
| | ■ Mistaking the external jugular vein for the JVP |
| **Note(s)** | ■ Always note the approximate angle of the bed when reporting a JVP. This is to help others better identify the JVP rather than because the true JVP value changes (it does not change as noted above). |
| | ■ Per data from the SOLVD (Studies of Left Ventricular Dysfunction) Trial, the most specific physical exam signs of HF exacerbation are the presence of JVD and an S3 gallop. |
| | ■ S3 corresponds to left atrial pressures >20 mmHg and LV end-diastolic pressure (LVEDP) >15 mmHg |
| | ■ You may ultrasound the internal jugular vein using a linear probe to confirm your visualize estimation. At the JVD, ultrasound should reveal spontaneous collapse of the vein. |
| **Further Reading** | Bickley LS, et al. *Bates' Guide to Physical Examination and History-taking.* Wolters Kluwer; 2017:10.4. |

## MISTAKE: EQUATING THE JUGULAR VENOUS PULSE WITH VOLUME STATUS

| | |
|---|---|
| **Case Example** | You assess the JVP of a patient with HFrEF (30%) and severe tricuspid regurgitation who is admitted to you for possible HF exacerbation. You visualize the JVP elevated to the mid-neck at 45 degrees and, despite a clear chest radiograph and no obvious edema, decide that the patient is significantly volume overloaded and proceed to diurese aggressively. Two hours later, the patient's blood pressure falls precipitously. |
| **Reasoning Error(s)** | ■ Thinking of JVP as synonymous with volume |
| | ■ Forgetting to consider causes of elevated right-sided heart pressures beyond volume |
| | ■ Incomplete access to information regarding a patient's comorbidities that may falsely elevate the JVP |
| **How to Avoid the Mistake** | ■ Remember that the JVP is a simply a marker of venous (right-sided) pressures, specifically in the right atrium. It is thus altered by anything that increases right-sided heart pressures, including increased intravascular volume but also conditions such as tricuspid regurgitation and pulmonary HTN. |
| | ■ Always ask yourself what all the possible contributors to a patient's JVP are rather than equating JVP as a synonym for volume. Consider nonvolume causes of elevated right-sided heart pressures. |
| | ■ In patients with uncommon diseases (e.g., constrictive pericarditis), reason through the pathophysiology to determine if it induces increased right-sided pressures. |
| | ■ Perform a thorough physical exam to elicit potential signs (e.g., murmur of tricuspid regurgitation) that point toward a potential confounder of JVD interpretation. |

| | |
|---|---|
| **Antidote** | ■ If overdiuresed, replenish intravascular volume (i.e., a certain degree of increased intravascular volume is necessary for the patient to maintain enough driving pressures to prevent hemodynamic collapse in the setting of significant right-sided pressures).<br>■ If possible, temporarily hold agents and interventions that significantly decrease preload (diuretics, nitrates, invasive ventilation).<br>  ■ Although certain agents such as angiotensin-converting enzyme inhibitors (ACEIs), angiotensin II receptor blockers (ARBs), β-blockers (BBs), and calcium channel blockers (CCBs) may decrease preload slightly, they have a minor effect compared with the above. |
| **Common Scenarios** | ■ Moderate-severe tricuspid regurgitation<br>■ Moderate-severe pulmonary HTN<br>■ Submassive or massive pulmonary embolism<br>■ Right ventricular dysfunction (right-sided HF, cor pulmonale)<br>■ Tamponade<br>■ Constrictive pericarditis |
| **Note(s)** | ■ While the JVP in the setting of increased right-sided heart pressures is not reliable as a binary indicator of volume status, you may be able to trend changes in the JVP with interventions (e.g., diuresis). |

## MISTAKE: IMPROPER EXAM TECHNIQUES: ASSESSMENT OF EDEMA, HEPATOJUGULAR REFLUX, S3

| | |
|---|---|
| **Case Example** | You assess the legs of a patient for edema by placing your fingers on their leg at a random point then pressing gently for a half-second. You find no edema and proceed to the next part of your exam. |
| **Reasoning Error(s)** | ■ Insufficient knowledge or experience with proper exam technique<br>■ "See one, do one" approach to learning without verification through official sources |
| **How to Avoid the Mistake** | ■ Edema: Press firmly, ideally against a bony prominence such as the tibia, for a minimum of 3–5 seconds. Quick and gentle pressing is ineffective for eliciting nonsevere pitting edema. Note that edema is gravity dependent—patients who have been bedbound may have significant sacral edema rather than lower extremity edema. Large amounts of subcutaneous tissue can also hide visible pitting edema.<br>■ Hepatojugular reflux: Press firmly with steady pressure to the upper abdomen for at least 10 seconds. Avoid pressing for merely a few seconds. Also avoid pressing in the right upper quadrant if a patient has significant known congestive hepatopathy as it may be very painful.<br>■ JVP: refer to page 164.<br>■ S3: Use the bell, positioning the patient in left lateral decubitus if able. First identify the S1 and S2 only—tune out all other sounds. Then think "right after S2, right after S2, right after S2" to hone your ears on the S3 (a quick dull sound). Do not be afraid to ask the patient to hold their breath if you cannot hear well. |
| **Antidote** | ■ Verify all fundamental concepts and techniques through an independent learning source.<br>■ Ask experts to observe and provide feedback on your exam technique. |

| | |
|---|---|
| **Common Scenarios** | ■ Edema |
| | ■ Hepatojugular reflux |
| | ■ JVP |
| | ■ S3 |
| **Note(s)** | ■ Depending on the study, as much as half of what trainees learn in fellowship from their peers may have at least a small inaccuracy. |
| **Further Reading** | Bickley, LS et al. *Bates' Guide to Physical Examination and History-taking.* Wolters Kluwer; 2017:10.4, 10.9. |

## MISTAKE: RULING OUT CARDIOGENIC SHOCK BASED ON WARM EXTREMITIES

| | |
|---|---|
| **Case Example** | A 57-year-old male with HFrEF (EF = 10%) presents with altered mental status and increased dyspnea. On your exam, you first assess his feet for warmth and discover that his feet are warm. Reassured, you triage the patient to the floor after which the patient's labs results demonstrate marked transaminitis and acute kidney injury, along with decreased urine output suggesting cardiogenic shock. |
| **Reasoning Error(s)** | ■ Equating an absolute relationship of warm extremities with good perfusion |
| | ■ Incorrectly concluding warm extremities based on use of gloves that decrease temperature sensitivity |
| **How to Avoid the Mistake** | ■ Understand that warm extremities alone do not rule out cardiogenic shock. |
| | ■ When possible, avoid using gloves during temperature assessment. Always compare multiple locations and on both sides. |
| | ■ When assessing for extremity warmth, assess for temperature of not only the feet but also the legs and knees—the more proximal the coldness, the more likely a patient is in shock. |
| | ■ Many people have cold hands and feet, and there is a difference between cool and icy! |
| **Antidote** | ■ Not applicable |
| **Common Scenarios** | ■ Ruling out shock based on warm extremities |
| | ■ Ruling in shock based on cold extremities |
| **Note(s)** | ■ How do you define cardiogenic shock? In the SHOCK Trial, it was defined as meeting the following three criteria:<br>　■ Blood pressure criteria |
| | ■ SBP <90 mmHg for >30 minutes OR vasopressor support to maintain SBP >90 mmHg<br>　■ Evidence of end-organ damage as defined by UOP <30 mL/h or cool extremities<br>　■ Hemodynamic criteria |
| | ■ CI <2.2 AND |
| | ■ PCWP >15 mmHg |
| **Further Reading** | ■ Original paper describing the 2 × 2 hemodynamic profiles of HF: Nohria A, et al. Clinical assessment identifies hemodynamic profiles that predict outcomes in patients admitted with heart failure. *JACC.* 2003;41(10):1797-1804. |

## MISTAKE: RULING OUT DECOMPENSATED HEART FAILURE BASED ON WHEEZING

**Case Example**

You are caring for a patient with both COPD and HFrEF. On lung auscultation, you hear prominent wheezing. The volume exam is difficult due to habitus. The patient does not have a prominent history of COPD exacerbations and does not endorse an increase in his sputum production or an increase in sputum purulence. You equate wheezing with COPD exacerbation and start the patient on steroids for a COPD exacerbation and hold off on diuresis. After 5 days of steroids, the patient continues to have a wheeze and has now become visibly volume overloaded.

**Reasoning Error(s)**

- Equating wheezing as synonymous with COPD/asthma (obstructive lung disease)
- Not considering the additional causes of wheezing (such as volume overload)
- Lack of experience seeing patients with common conditions present atypically

**How to Avoid the Mistake**

- Incorporate multiple pieces of data to determine the most likely etiology.
- Reason through the pathophysiology of how wheezing occurs and what pathologic processes can culminate in the same physiology to cause wheezing.
- Cardiac wheezes are most common at nighttime due to recumbency.

**Antidote**

- Not applicable

**Common Scenarios**

- COPD
- Asthma
- HF decompensation (cardiac asthma)

**Note(s)**

- While not all wheezes are caused by COPD or asthma, all wheezes are ultimately due to obstructive physiology.
- Cardiac wheeze is caused by bronchial hyperreactivity secondary to the accumulation of unaccustomed fluid in the bronchioles, triggering J-receptors.

# Diagnosis: Laboratory Testing

## MISTAKE: RULING OUT ACUTE HEART FAILURE BASED ON FALSELY LOW BNP/NT-proBNP

**Case Example**

An obese (BMI 74) female with HF with mid-range EF (HFmrEF) (EF = 45%) presents with worsening dyspnea. Your volume exam is limited due to body habitus. You obtain a B-type natriuretic peptide (BNP) and N-terminal pro-BNP (NT-proBNP) level (183 ng/L) and conclude that patient is unlikely to be volume overloaded, ultimately favoring a standalone COPD exacerbation. Later, the patient receives an echocardiogram that demonstrates markedly elevated right-sided pressures as well as a newly reduced EF.

| Reasoning Error(s) | ■ Forgetting to consider causes of falsely low BNP/NT-proBNP levels |
|---|---|
| | ■ Lack of knowledge of the most common causes of a falsely low BNP/NT-proBNP level |
| | ■ Incomplete access to information regarding a patient's comorbidities that may lower the BNP or NT-proBNP levels |
| | ■ Incomplete understanding of the physiology behind BNP or NT-proBNP elevation |
| |    ■ Levels rise primarily as the LV stretches due to either volume or pressure; hence conditions such as mitral regurgitation that result in HF symptoms without compromising the stretch of the LV may result in lower than expected BNP or NT-proBNP levels. |
| How to Avoid the Mistake | ■ Use multiple pieces of data (labs, exam) to determine volume status and likelihood of decompensated HF. |
| | ■ Always consider the top two causes (obesity, acute HF) of a falsely low BNP/NT-proBNP. |
| | ■ Always compare BNP/NT-proBNP levels to baseline. |
| | ■ Understand the physiology of BNP and NT-proBNP levels. |
| Antidote | ■ Begin diuresis and document patient's BNP during decompensation for future reference. |
| Common Scenarios | ■ Obesity (most common) |
| | ■ Flash pulmonary edema |
| | ■ Structural causes prior to the LV |
| |    ■ Acute or early HF |
| |    ■ Mitral stenosis/regurgitation |
| |    ■ Constrictive pericarditis |
| Note(s) | ■ HF is a syndrome of symptoms that may result from a variety of mechanisms (i.e., ventricular, valvular, pericardial, electrical). |
| | ■ Natriuretic peptides also hold prognostic significance—higher levels are associated with worse outcomes and greater mortality. |
| | ■ While the BNP is usually normal in constrictive pericarditis, it is often elevated in restrictive cardiomyopathies because the myocardium is involved. |

## MISTAKE: RULING-IN ACUTE HEART FAILURE BASED ON FALSELY ELEVATED BNP/NT-proBNP

| Case Example | A 92-year-old male with HFrEF (EF = 35%) presents with increasing SOB. The volume exam is not convincing for volume overload, though the lung exam is limited by cooperation. You obtain an NT-proBNP of 1453 ng/L and start aggressive diuresis. The next morning, patient is oligouric and his creatinine has doubled. |
|---|---|
| Reasoning Error(s) | ■ Forgetting to consider common causes of falsely elevated BNP/NT-proBNP |
| | ■ Lack of knowledge regarding age-adjusted cutoffs for NT-proBNP levels used to rule-in HF |

**How to Avoid the Mistake**
- Use multiple pieces of data (labs, exam) to determine volume status and likelihood of decompensated HF.
- Always consider the top two causes (elderly, renal failure) of a falsely elevated NT-proBNP
  - <50 years: >450 ng/L
  - 50–75 years: >900 ng/L
  - >75 years: >1800 ng/L
- Always compare BNP/NT-proBNP levels to baseline.
- Understand the physiology of BNP/NT-proBNP levels.

**Antidote**
- Give back intravascular volume.

**Common Scenarios**
- Increased age
- Renal failure
- Sustained severe HTN (e.g., SBP >180 mm Hg)
- Massive pulmonary embolism
- High cardiac output states
  - Sepsis
  - Severe anemia (usually Hb <8)
  - Hypothyroidism
  - Cirrhosis

**Note(s)**
- There is no good correlation between the degree of BNP elevation and degree of hypervolemia (some patients will always have extremely elevated levels).
- An age-independent NT-proBNP cutoff of <300 ng/L excludes decompensated HF with 94% sensitivity.

**Further Reading**
- Article investigating age-adjusted NT-proBNP cutoffs for ruling-in HF: Januzzi J, et al. N-terminal pro-B-type natriuretic peptide in the emergency department: the ICON-RELOADED Study. *JACC.* 2018;71(11):1191-1200.

## MISTAKE: MISATTRIBUTION OF ABNORMAL LIVER FUNCTION TESTS IN ACUTE DECOMPENSATED HEART FAILURE

**Case Example**
A 49-year-old female with biventricular nonischemic cardiomyopathy (EF = 25%) and severe functional tricuspid regurgitation is admitted for acute decompensated HF. Basic labs reveal an indirect hyperbilirubinemia to 2.2 and mildly elevated aspartate transaminase, alanine transaminase, and alkaline phosphatase. The patient denies any abdominal pain and has no history of prior liver/biliary pathology. You instinctively order a right upper quadrant ultrasound to workup possible pathologies such as chole-cystitis or choledocholithiasis.

**Reasoning Error(s)**
- Lack of knowledge regarding congestive hepatopathy
- Only associating congestive hepatopathy with right-sided HF.
- Reflex interpretation of abnormal liver function tests (LFTs) as due to liver/biliary pathology

| | |
|---|---|
| **How to Avoid the Mistake** | ■ Identify comorbidities that may increase the likelihood of congestive hepatopathy. |
| | ■ Understand that left-sided HF can lead to severe venous congestion that transmits to the liver as in right-sided HF. |
| | ■ Congestive hepatopathy may result in significant right upper quadrant abdominal pain which, when in conjunction with abnormal LFTs, may present a diagnostic dilemma. In these cases, history is especially useful—does the patient have a history of biliary/liver disease? What is their likelihood of having a separate pathology at the same time as acute decompensated HF? What are the ramifications of a tincture of time and diuresis prior to further workup of the LFTs? |
| **Antidote** | ■ Not applicable |
| **Common Scenarios** | ■ Right-sided HF, including as a consequence of: |
| | ■ Left-sided HF (most common cause) |
| | ■ Severe tricuspid regurgitation |
| | ■ Severe pulmonary HTN |
| | ■ Severe mitral stenosis |
| | ■ Constrictive pericarditis |
| **Note(s)** | ■ Severe tricuspid regurgitation is an especially common culprit of hepatic congestion given the significant transduction of right ventricular pressures into the hepatic vasculature. |
| | ■ The LFTs of >2600 patients with chronic HF were characterized in the CHARM study, of which the main goal was to assess the mortality benefit of ARBs in HFrEF. About 10% of patients shared abnormal LFTs, and hyperbilirubinemia was the strongest predictor among liver function tests of mortality and morbidity from HF. |

## MISTAKE: EXCLUDING CARDIAC AMYLOID BASED ON NORMAL ECG VOLTAGE

| | |
|---|---|
| **Case Example** | A routine TTE demonstrates a 1.6-cm interventricular septum and LV posterior wall. Examining an ECG, you notice that the voltages are normal in all leads. Given the lack of low voltage, you dismiss the possibility of cardiac amyloidosis. |
| **Reasoning Error(s)** | ■ Focusing on a low-voltage ECG as the defining feature on ECG for cardiac amyloid |
| | ■ Searching for low voltage in all leads rather than in one set (precordial or limb) |
| | ■ Lack of knowledge regarding the low sensitivity of a low-voltage ECG for cardiac amyloid |
| | ■ Forgetting to consider that low-voltage ECG is likely a late manifestation of cardiac amyloid |

**How to Avoid the Mistake**
- Analyze whether voltages are decreased out of proportion to the hypertrophy rather than searching exclusively for a low-voltage ECG. For example, normal voltage for a 1.6-cm LV wall is abnormally normal.
- Realize that low voltage need not be present in all leads. Low voltage in either the precordial or limb leads may signal amyloid.
- Rule out other causes of low voltages such as obese habitus and severe lung disease.

**Antidote**
- Not applicable

**Common Scenarios**
- Not applicable

**Note(s)**
- Approximately 50% of AL and 25% of TTR cardiac amyloidosis cases are associated with a low-voltage ECG, depending on the criteria used to define low voltage.
- The most common criteria for a low-voltage ECG are <10 mV in the precordial leads and <5 mV in the limb leads.
- Small studies suggest that ECG voltages are likely normal in early cardiac amyloid.

## MISTAKE: EXCLUDING CARDIAC AMYLOID BASED ON NORMAL SPEP/UPEP

**Case Example**
A 62-year-old female with prior HTN presents to your clinic for shortness of breath and is found on TTE to have a preserved EF and markedly thick walls (interventricular septum [IVS] 1.7, left ventricular posterior wall [LVPW] 1.5). You send off serum and urine protein electrophoresis (SPEP and UPEP, respectively), which both return normal. You are reassured and agree to see the patient in follow-up, but she becomes lost to follow-up. Years later, the patient re-presents as an admission for decompensated HF, at which point a biopsy is taken, revealing transthyretin (TTR) cardiac amyloidosis.

**Reasoning Error(s)**
- Lack of knowledge on the sensitivity of SPEP/UPEP for AL amyloid
- Forgetting to consider TTR amyloid (which does not affect SPEP/UPEP)

**How to Avoid the Mistake**
- Initiate workup for TTR amyloid based on clinical suspicion, regardless of SPEP/UPEP.
- Maintain a high degree of clinical suspicion for cardiac amyloidosis.
  - Bilateral carpal tunnel syndrome
  - Autonomic dysfunction: resolution of prior HTN or new orthostasis
  - New increased LV wall thickness in a patient without known HTN

**Antidote**
- Not applicable

**Common Scenarios**
- AL (primary) amyloidosis
- TTR amyloidosis

**Note(s)**
- TTR amyloid is significantly underdiagnosed. For example, a 2015 study demonstrated 13% of patients with HFpEF cases were secondary to TTR. A 2017 study from Columbia University demonstrated that 16% of patients with severe aortic stenosis had TTR cardiac amyloidosis.
- TTR is associated with low-flow low-gradient aortic stenosis.

## MISTAKE: DISCHARGING PATIENTS WITHOUT A DRY WEIGHT AND DRY BNP/NT-proBNP

**Case Example**

You successfully treat a patient with decompensated HF. Despite a prior standing dry weight of 74 kg, you continued to diurese significantly based on your clinical judgment. You happily discharge the patient. The patient is then readmitted the following month for decompensated HF, and the next team sees the old dry weight of 74 kg and uses that as a target for diuresis. The new team stops diuresing once that goal is reached and discharges the patient, only to have her re-present a few days later.

**Reasoning Error(s)**
- Forgetting to effectively transition care across healthcare settings
- Lack of thought toward how one can best help future teams care for the patient and prevent readmission

**How to Avoid the Mistake**
- Understand that providing an effective transition of care facilitates improved care for the patient in the future in other healthcare settings with different providers.
- Think about the key pieces of data that would help future providers care for the patient. For instance, a dry weight and dry NTproBNP level should always be recorded upon discharge. This is particularly important in heart failure which is a long-term cachexia-inducing disease which means that the true dry weight of a patient may decrease over time.
- Consider using a discharge checklist to ensure patients are fully ready for discharge. This may include recording relevant diagnostic data as well as ensuring appropriate therapeutic care such as optimizing GDMT. Many cardiac institutes use such checklists to ensure standardized and top notch care.

**Antidote**
- Not applicable

**Common Scenarios**
- Not applicable

**Note(s)**
- Though a patient may be unable to stand (e.g. due to limited mobility or deconditioning) for a weight measurement, an optimized bed weight may be better than not recording a weight. Optimizing the bed weight includes consistently taking off extra weight such as pillows, blankets, devices, and anything else that would overestimate the patient's dry weight. It is important to always note the content (standing or not) of the recorded weight.

# Diagnosis: Swan-Ganz Catheter

## MISTAKE: ROUTINE USE OF SWAN-GANZ CATHETER IN ACUTE DECOMPENSATED HEART FAILURE

**Case Example**

A 74-year-old female ith HFrEF (EF = 15%) is admitted to your service with acute decompensated HF.

**Reasoning Error(s)**
- Reassurance from the mere presence of objective data (increased comfort using numerical data compared to careful clinical assessment)
- Forgetting that every intervention is associated with risks

| | |
|---|---|
| **How to Avoid the Mistake** | ■ Avoid routine use of Swan-Ganz catheters (SGCs) and carefully ask yourself the benefit of using one (what information could I obtain with the SGC that would significantly change management?). |
| | ■ Understand the data behind clinical practice to decrease bias of good intention (well-reasoned logic that does not bear out empirically). |
| | ■ Always consider risks, even with seemingly common procedures. |
| **Antidote** | ■ Not applicable |
| **Common Scenarios** | ■ Not applicable |
| **Note(s)** | ■ Per the ESCAPE Trial, there was no reduction in overall mortality, hospitalization days, and symptomatic improvement with the use of SGCs versus clinical judgment. However, there was an increased rate of adverse events with SGC use. |
| | ■ In the ESCAPE Trial, orthopnea of two or more pillows was associated with PCWP >= 30 mmHg |
| **Further Reading** | ■ The ESCAPE Trial: Binanay C, et al. Evaluation study of congestive heart failure and pulmonary artery catheterization effectiveness: the ESCAPE Trial. *JAMA*. 2005;294(13):1625-1633. |

## MISTAKE: APPROXIMATING WEDGE PRESSURE VIA THE PULMONARY ARTERY DIASTOLIC PRESSURE IN PULMONARY HYPERTENSION

| | |
|---|---|
| **Case Example** | A 52-year-old female with HFrEF (15%), COPD, and severe group III pulmonary HTN is admitted to the ICU for cardiogenic shock and a SGC is soon placed. You glance at the patient's monitor, notice that the PA diastolic pressure is 28 mmHg, and assume that the patient has a significantly elevated PCWP but is surprised to find on right heart catheterization a PCWP of 10 mmHg. |
| **Reasoning Error(s)** | ■ Forgetting to consider confounding factors that influence the PA diastolic pressure |
| | ■ Lack of knowledge regarding the patient's comorbidities |
| **How to Avoid the Mistake** | ■ Establish crude estimates of how the PA diastolic pressure correlates to the PCWP in each individual patient. |
| | ■ Be aware that the PA diastolic pressure may overestimate the PCWP in patients with significant pulmonary HTN (not group II). |
| **Antidote** | ■ Not applicable |
| **Common Scenarios** | ■ Pulmonary HTN (all classes except group II) |
| **Note(s)** | ■ In general, the PA diastolic pressure correlates with the PCWP but always |
| | ■ The gold standard for measuring pressures within the heart is a right heart catheterization. |
| | ■ The transpulmonary gradient (TPG) is a useful marker of whether a patient possesses intrinsic disease of the pulmonary arteries. TPG = PCWP – mean PAP. TPG >12 indicates intrinsic disease suggesting that the pulmonary HTN is not due to class II (left-sided HF). |

## MISTAKE: OBTAINING A WEDGE PRESSURE DURING INSPIRATION ON AN INTUBATED PATIENT

**Case Example**

You are called to the bedside to measure the PCWP on an intubated patient in cardiogenic shock. As a first-year fellow, you astutely remember that PCWP should be obtained at end-expiration to minimize the influence of intrathoracic pressure swings. Given that the intrathoracic pressure swings are reversed in positive pressure ventilation, you confidently obtain the PCWP at maximal inspiration. Your attending solemnly pats you on the back.

**Reasoning Error(s)**

- Lack of understanding regarding the impact of the respiratory cycle on intrathoracic pressures and hence PCWP
- Confusing the goal point for measuring PCWP as the most negative intrathoracic pressure rather than neutral (ambient) pressure

**How to Avoid the Mistake**

- The simple rule is, no matter what type of respiratory support, PCWP should always be measured at end-expiration.
- Understand the normal respiratory cycle's impact on PCWP. During inspiration, the intrathoracic pressure decreases and conversely it increases during expiration. The ideal measurement of PCWP would be when the intrathoracic pressure is closest to zero, that is, there is equalization of pressure inside the lungs with the outside world (no air movement). This is in end-expiration.
- In positive-pressure ventilation, the lowest intrathoracic pressure continues to occur during end-expiration. The difference is that the end-expiratory pressure is non-zero, since there is a constant pressure maintained to keep the alveoli open.

**Antidote**

- Not applicable

**Common Scenarios**

- Positive-pressure ventilation
  - High-flow nasal cannula
  - Continuous positive airway pressure (CPAP)
  - Bilevel positive airway pressure (BiPAP)
  - Mechanical ventilation

**Note(s)**

- One proposed method of eliminating the effect of positive pressure ventilation on PCWP has been use of an expiratory hold maneuver.
- Remember that positive end-expiratory pressure (PEEP) increases right ventricular afterload, which may transiently dilate the right ventricle into the LV (ventricular interdependence), leading to a higher than true PCWP.

**Further Reading**

- "Expiratory hold" approach to measuring PCWP in intubated patients: Yang W, et al. "Expiratory holding" approach in measuring end-expiratory pulmonary artery wedge pressure for mechanically ventilated patients. *Patient Prefer Adherence*. 2013;7:1041-1045.

# Diagnosis: Imaging

## MISTAKE: USING INFERIOR VENA CAVA COLLAPSIBILITY AS A PROXY FOR VOLUME STATUS WITHOUT CONSIDERING CONFOUNDING FACTORS

**Case Example**

A TTE report on a newly intubated patient reports a distended IVC that collapses <5 0%. In light of a difficult volume exam, you decide to diurese the patient aggressively while awaiting chest imaging and other lab results. Three hours later, the patient's blood pressure drops significantly requiring brief pressor support.

**Reasoning Error(s)**

- Not taking into consideration the impact of various confounders when interpreting IVC size and collapsibility, positive pressure, on intrathoracic pressures, and IVC size
- Not considering confounding sources of elevated right-sided pressures
- Determining volume status based on a single data source (IVC collapsibility) or overly weighing one data point

**How to Avoid the Mistake**

- Consider confounding factors when interpreting IVC size and collapsibility, such as positive pressure ventilation and structural issues leading to elevated right-sided heart pressures.
    - Take into consideration respiratory support settings when measuring the IVC.
    - Understand that high PEEP may increase right atrial pressure and hence increase IVC size.
- If applicable, decrease PEEP temporarily to obtain a higher fidelity IVC measurement.
- Determine volume status based on multiple data sources.

**Antidote**

- Give back intravascular volume if overdiuresed.

**Common Scenarios**

- Positive-pressure ventilation
    - Mechanical ventilation (intubation)
    - High-pressure BiPAP
- Elevated right-sided heart pressures
    - Pulmonary HTN
    - Tricuspid regurgitation/stenosis
    - Right ventricular failure
    - Massive PE

**Note(s)**

- Remember to request a sniff or gentle cough when measuring the IVC collapsibility in a patient without positive pressure.

## MISTAKE: EQUATING NEWLY DISCOVERED REDUCED EJECTION FRACTION WITH RECENT-ONSET HEART FAILURE

**Case Example**

A 52-year-old male presents with worsening exercise tolerance and undergoes a TTE that shows LV end-diastolic diameter (LVEDD) 6.1 cm, IVS 1.1 cm, LV posterior wall 1.1 cm, LVEF by Simpson's biplane method 27%, severe left atrial enlargement, moderate functional mitral regurgitation, and a noncollapsible inferior vena cava. You become especially worried that the patient may have had a recent infarct (perhaps silent) that led to this newly reduced EF.

| Reasoning Error(s) | ■ Focusing exclusively on the new discovery of a decreased EF<br>■ Lack of knowledge on using structural information from a TTE to interpret chronicity of reduced EF |
|---|---|
| How to Avoid the Mistake | ■ Take into consideration all the information provided by a TTE rather than the EF in isolation.<br>■ Analyze the LVEDD. The natural history of systolic dysfunction is for the LV to dilate. A true recent reduction in EF would be unlikely to demonstrate structural changes such as a dilated LV or significantly enlarged left atrium.<br>■ Analyze the mitral valve for evidence of regurgitation secondary to a dilated LV cavity, known as functional (or secondary) mitral regurgitation, that would suggest a more chronic reduction in EF. This occurs due to the pulling apart of the mitral leaflet and malcoaptation as the mitral annuli are pulled farther away from each other due to compensatory dilation of the LV. |
| Antidote | ■ Not applicable |
| Common Scenarios | ■ Not applicable |
| Note(s) | ■ Cardiomyopathies that are rarely associated with evidence of significant structural changes reflecting long-term disease include stress (Takotsubo's), giant cell, viral, peri/postpartum, and single-incident toxin-induced (e.g., cocaine). Note that all these causes result in very acute presentations of HF that does not provide the cavity enough time to dilate. |

## MISTAKE: RULING OUT HEART FAILURE BASED ON A NORMAL EJECTION FRACTION

| Case Example | An 85-year-old female with no known past medical history is evaluated for progressive dyspnea. TTE demonstrates LVEDD 4.7, IVS 1.1, LVPW 1.0, LVEF 65%, moderate left atrial enlargement, and a heavily calcified mitral valve without mitral stenosis. You conclude that the patient does not have HF and proceed to evaluating other causes of progressive dyspnea. |
|---|---|
| Reasoning Error(s) | ■ Not considering HF with preserved EF (HFpEF/diastolic dysfunction)<br>■ Ruling out HFpEF despite no mention of a patient's diastolic function on the TTE report<br>■ Lack of evaluation of a patient's diastolic function when reading a TTE<br>■ Failing to consider risk factors for diastolic dysfunction |
| How to Avoid the Mistake | ■ Consider both types of HF: systolic and diastolic dysfunction.<br>■ Always evaluate diastolic function when able on TTE.<br>■ Do not rule out HFpEF based on a lack of information on diastology. Rather, state that HFpEF cannot be ruled out without further information.<br>■ Consider risk factors for HFpEF (increasing age, obesity, female gender, HTN). |
| Antidote | ■ Not applicable |
| Common Scenarios | ■ Not applicable |

| | |
|---|---|
| **Note(s)** | ▪ As our population has aged alongside vastly improved revascularization techniques, HFpEF has grown to account for the majority (slightly >50%) of HF cases now.<br>▪ The presence of LV hypertrophy (LVH) does not automatically mean a patient has HFpEF as it is possible to have LVH without diastolic dysfunction.<br>▪ It is possible to have concomitant diastolic dysfunction with systolic HF (HFrEF). |

# Treatment: General

## MISTAKE: TREATING HEART FAILURE DECOMPENSATION WITHOUT TREATING THE TRIGGER(S)

| | |
|---|---|
| **Case Example** | A patient presents with acute decompensated HF after binge eating Chinese food. You diurese the patient over 2 days and subsequently discharge her home. The patient comes back a week later with another exacerbation, proclaiming that the Chinese food was "delicious!" |
| **Reasoning Error(s)** | ▪ Focusing exclusively on treating the acute scenario<br>▪ Forgetting to consider the underlying cause or trigger<br>▪ Lack of familiarity with the most common causes of HF exacerbation |
| **How to Avoid the Mistake** | ▪ Always consider the underlying cause/trigger. Remember, preventing future occurrences is just as important as treating the acute scenario at hand!<br>▪ For the most common causes of HF exacerbation, think through the mnemonic FAILURE:<br>   ▪ *F*orgot medications<br>   ▪ *A*rrhythmias<br>   ▪ *I*nfection/*I*schemia/*I*nfarction<br>   ▪ *L*ifestyle changes (e.g., too much salt or fluid intake)<br>   ▪ *U*remia<br>   ▪ *R*enal failure<br>   ▪ *E*mbolism (i.e., PE) |
| **Antidote** | ▪ Not applicable |
| **Common Scenarios** | ▪ Not applicable |
| **Note(s)** | ▪ The most common causes of HF exacerbation are medication nonadherence and inappropriate lifestyle.<br>▪ The number of HF hospitalizations is prognostic of a patient's morbidity and mortality. |

## MISTAKE: AVOIDANCE OF DIHYDROPYRIDINE CALCIUM CHANNEL BLOCKERS FOR HYPERTENSION IN HFpEF

| | |
|---|---|
| **Case Example** | A patient with uncontrolled HTN, HFpEF (EF = 65%), and CKD IV is admitted to the ICU for hypertensive emergency. Despite max-dose nitroprusside drip, the patient's blood pressure hardly budges, with continued floaters in both visual fields. A nicardipine drip is suggested for easy titration, but you decide against it given the patient's HFpEF. Continued management with pushes of labetalol becomes increasingly difficult to manage and offer little blood pressure control. |

| | |
|---|---|
| **Reasoning Error(s)** | ■ Inference of adverse effects of dihydropyridine CCBs in HFpEF given the strong recommendation to avoid all CCBs in HfrEF |
| | ■ Well-intentioned reasoning without understanding the evidence |
| | ■ Failure to differentiate HF into preserved and reduced EF |
| **How to Avoid the Mistake** | ■ Always strive to understand the evidence rather than rely solely on well-intentioned logic. |
| | ■ Avoid inferring among distinct medical entities. |
| | ■ Understand the difference in management between HfpEF and HfrEF. |
| **Antidote** | ■ Not applicable |
| **Common Scenarios** | ■ Amlodipine |
| | ■ Nifedipine |
| | ■ Nicardipine |
| **Note(s)** | ■ Nondihydropyridine CCBs also appear to be safe and well tolerated in HFpEF (excluding amyloidosis), but preference is given to DHP CCBs because they have less cardiac effects (e.g., negative inotropy and chronotropy). |
| | ■ Second-generation CCBs such as amlodipine appear to be safe in HFrEF but are still discouraged given lack of any additional benefits (e.g., mortality) and numerous alternate agents with blood pressure–lowering effects that provide secondary benefits. |

## MISTAKE: LIBERAL USE OF ATRIOVENTRICULAR NODAL BLOCKERS IN CARDIAC AMYLOIDOSIS

| | |
|---|---|
| **Case Example** | A patient with TTR cardiomyopathy (EF = 55%) presents for a routine checkup and is found with new-onset atrial fibrillation. The patient is hemodynamically stable with a rate of 108 bpm. You decide to start the patient on a β-blocker to help with rate control. The next day, you receive an alert that the patient was hospitalized for profound hypotension and heart block. |
| **Reasoning Error(s)** | ■ Lack of knowledge regarding poor tolerance of certain medications in cardiac amyloidosis |
| | ■ Well-intentioned use with thought to potential benefit with medications in question despite risk of intolerance; "worth challenging" |
| **How to Avoid the Mistake** | ■ Understand that the amyloid fibrils bind very avidly to certain medications, such as calcium channel blockers and digoxin, causing increased effectiveness. The medications are not absolutely contraindicated but rather there should be a clear risk-benefit discussion. |
| | ■ Understand that cardiac output in cardiac amyloidosis is significantly dependent on heart rate given a fixed and low stroke volume. |
| | ■ Challenge patients with medications in a controlled setting (e.g., inpatient). |
| **Antidote** | ■ Discontinuation of intolerant medications |
| | ■ No evidence to support the use of therapies in overdose of these medications, such as lipid emulsion therapy |

| | |
|---|---|
| **Common Scenarios** | ■ β-Blockers |
| | ■ Calcium channel blockers |
| | ■ Digoxin |
| | ■ Amiodarone (increased risk of heart block) |
| **Note(s)** | ■ Unsurprisingly, patients with more advanced cardiac amyloidosis demonstrate greater intolerance to medications such as β-blockers. |
| **Further Reading** | ■ Interesting new study on potential mortality benefit in TTR amyloid patients with exposure to β-blockers. Given the lack of robust data in this area and potentially significant benefit, this is an area worth following closely over the next few years: Barge-Caballero G, et al. Beta-blocker exposure and survival in patients with transthyretin amyloid cardiomyopathy. *Mayo Clin Proc.* 2021;97(2):261-273. |

## Treatment: Diuresis

### MISTAKE: DIURESING WITH STANDARD NET-NEGATIVE GOALS (OR LACK OF A GOAL) IN PRELOAD-DEPENDENT STATES

| | |
|---|---|
| **Case Example** | A patient with severe aortic stenosis is admitted to you for HF exacerbation. You diurese aggressively with Lasix (furosemide) for a net negative 2 L/day. The next day, the patient's blood pressure falls drastically with an extremely narrow pulse pressure. At morbidity and mortality conference, you are told that the patient likely had hemodynamic collapse from taking off volume too quickly, leading to inadequate preload and hence cardiac output. |
| **Reasoning Error(s)** | ■ Not considering the presence of a preload-dependent physiology |
| | ■ Forgetting to consider the synergistic effect of multiple preload-dependent pathologies |
| | ■ Memorizing buzz words such as "aortic stenosis" as associations for preload dependence without understanding the physiology and applicability of this concept to other preload-dependent states. |
| | ■ Lack of recognition that the diuresis goal is not a fixed and/or memorized value |
| | ■ Lack of recognition that diuresis goals can be spread over time, including shorter intervals, rather than over the course of an entire day |
| **How to Avoid the Mistake** | ■ Consider preload every time you diurese. |
| | ■ If preload dependent, diurese gently (lower net negative goal such as 0.25–1.0 L/day or equivalent hourly rate). |
| | ■ Diurese more frequently as needed: start slow and uptitrate as needed. |
| **Antidote** | ■ Give back intravascular volume (e.g., lactated Ringer's, normal saline, albumin). |

| | |
|---|---|
| **Common Scenarios** | ■ Severe aortic stenosis |
| | ■ Severe diastolic dysfunction (e.g., HF with preserved EF, amyloid) |
| | ■ Right ventricular failure |
| | ■ Severe pulmonary HTN |
| | ■ Severe tricuspid regurgitation |
| | ■ Submassive/massive pulmonary embolism |
| | ■ Inferior myocardial infarction |
| | ■ Significant vasodilator therapy (e.g., nitroglycerin drip) |
| | ■ Constrictive pericarditis |
| | ■ Extreme tachycardia |
| | ■ Atrial fibrillation/flutter |
| **Note(s)** | ■ The degree of preload dependence varies between patients with the same pathology such as severe aortic stenosis. It is often difficult without invasive hemodynamic monitoring to determine the degree to which a patient is preload dependent. The ideal net negative diuresis goal should be determined via careful uptitration based on hemodynamic stability (e.g., blood pressure response, perfusion of extremities, strength of palpable pulse). Particularly high-risk and difficult patients should have invasive monitoring (e.g., a SGC). |
| | ■ For patient comfort, in the absence of a Foley, diurese earlier in the day when the patient is awake, so they are not constantly awakening during the night. |

## MISTAKE: ORAL LASIX IN ACUTE DECOMPENSATED HEART FAILURE

| | |
|---|---|
| **Case Example** | A patient was recently discharged from the hospital after an HF exacerbation with 40 mg PO furosemide. A week later, she returns to the emergency department with SOB and leg swelling. You decide to continue her oral furosemide at double her home dose. |
| **Reasoning Error(s)** | ■ Not considering bioavailability when prescribing medications |
| | ■ Lack of knowledge regarding the oral bioavailability of furosemide |
| | ■ Lack of knowledge that volume overload leads to gut edema that can impair the absorption of certain drugs |
| **How to Avoid the Mistake** | ■ Understand that the oral bioavailability of furosemide is erratic (widely variable not only between patients but even for the same patient) and decreased in the setting of gut edema. |
| | ■ Always think through the route of administration and associated bioavailability when prescribing any medication. |
| | ■ Always begin inpatient therapy for acute decompensated HF with intravenous (IV) diuretics. |
| | ■ Counsel and educate patients on the limitations of oral furosemide therapy. |
| **Antidote** | ■ IV diuresis |
| | ■ Switch to torsemide or bumetanide, which have nearly 100% oral bioavailability. |
| **Common Scenarios** | ■ Not applicable |

**Note(s)**
- The TRANSFORM-HF Trial is an ongoing (as of July 2022) pragmatic open-label study comparing various outcomes, including mortality and HF hospitalization rates, with oral torsemide versus oral furosemide in the outpatient setting.
- Furosemide is the only common loop diuretic with erratic bioavailability; torsemide, bumetanide, and ethacrynic acid all have bioavailability that approach 100%, even in the presence of significant gut edema.
- Consider converting your practice pattern to prescribing torsemide as the outpatient diuretic of choice given more reliable absorption.

## MISTAKE: WITHHOLDING DIURESIS FOR ANY RISING CREATININE

**Case Example**
A patient presents with acute decompensated HF, and you initiate diuresis only to find that the creatinine climbs from 1.5 to 1.8 the next morning. You pause diuresis despite a volume exam consistent with overload. The patient's oxygen requirements stabilize at 6 L nasal cannula and improves with further diuresis.

**Reasoning Error(s)**
- Solely relying on the creatinine as a marker of volume status
- Perception that a rise in creatinine solely indicates worsening renal function. In fact, during diuresis, transient rises in creatinine are common and reflect intravascular volume shifts secondary to diuresis.
- Considering any increase in creatinine, regardless of magnitude, to reflect worsening renal function or volume depletion
- Lack of experience with a common laboratory phenomenon during diuresis

**How to Avoid the Mistake**
- Use multiple exam and lab findings to determine volume status. For example, check JVP, lower extremity edema, oral mucosa, creatinine, bicarbonate, and urine output.
- Verify that the creatinine increase reflects a real AKI (defined as an increase in creatinine of at least 0.3× or 1.5× baseline).
- Consider the aggressiveness of diuresis (e.g., once a day versus three times a day). Even when volume overloaded, as a patient's overall volume status improves, intravascular volume shifts may take longer, thereby giving rise to very transient prerenal states.

**Antidote**
- Continue diuresing!

**Common Scenarios**
- Not applicable

**Note(s)**
- A term we use when diuresing through slight increases in creatinine is "permissive hypercreatinemia."
- If the creatinine begins rising after significant diuresis, this may truly be due to intravascular volume depletion. Correlate with other markers of volume and do workup of causes of AKI as clinically appropriate.
- In the DOSE trial, worsening renal function during diuresis was not associated with worse long-term renal outcomes.

**Further Reading**
- The DOSE trial is a classic landmark study for your reading list: Felker GM, et al. Diuretic strategies in patients with acute decompensated heart failure. *N Engl J Med.* 2011;364:797-805.

## MISTAKE: WITHHOLDING DIURESIS FOR ALL HYPOTENSION IN ACUTE DECOMPENSATED HEART FAILURE

| | |
|---|---|
| **Case Example** | A 78-year-old male with HFrEF (EF = 15%) is admitted for acute decompensated HF. His home medications include metoprolol succinate 100 mg, Entresto (sacubitril/valsartan) 97–103 mg BID, spironolactone 25 mg, and torsemide 50 mg. His blood pressure is 90/58 mmHg, and you are hesitant to diurese despite seeing that the patient is in significant respiratory distress. On closer review of his outpatient clinic notes, his systolic blood pressures are usually in the high 80s. |
| **Reasoning Error(s)** | ■ Failing to recognize that patients with low EF do not mount robust blood pressures at baseline<br>■ A non–evidence-based but well-intentioned thought that diuresis will significantly lower blood pressures in volume-overloaded patients |
| **How to Avoid the Mistake** | ■ Understand a patient's baseline. It is common for severe HFrEF patients to live with systolic pressures in the 90s, often due to the copious use of guideline-direct medical therapy (GDMT).<br>■ Realize that judicious diuresis does not generally cause hypotension in volume-overloaded patients, since the excess extravascular volume fills the decrease in intravascular volume. |
| **Antidote** | ■ Diurese judiciously (not overly aggressive in frequency, allowing for adequate equilibration of fluid between compartments). |
| **Common Scenarios** | ■ Not applicable |
| **Note(s)** | ■ It is rarely wrong to start with gentle diuresis in the setting of hypotension or borderline blood pressures to observe the patient's response.<br>■ Always consider preload dependence when diuresing, irrespective of blood pressure. |

## MISTAKE: UNDERDOSING DIURETICS IN ACUTE KIDNEY INJURY AND/OR CHRONIC KIDNEY DISEASE

| | |
|---|---|
| **Case Example** | A patient presents with volume overload and a creatinine of 1.9 (estimated glomerular filtration rate [eGFR] 48). You diurese the patient with IV Lasix 20 and a few hours later see minimal urine output. You give another dose of IV Lasix 20, again to little effect. |
| **Reasoning Error(s)** | ■ Not accounting for the renal function (integrity of target mechanism for diuretics)<br>■ Forgetting to use synergistic effects of thiazides with loop diuretics |
| **How to Avoid the Mistake** | ■ Always consider renal impairment (acute and chronic) and whether diuretic doses need to be adjusted (increased) to compensate for poor renal function (GFR).<br>■ Ensure proper conversion between diuretics. Table 8.1 notes the conversion factors between common diuretics.<br>■ An estimation of IV Lasix dosing in significant CKD can be estimated with the formula:<br>   ■ *Lasix dose (mg) = Creatinine * 30*<br>■ Consider using sequential nephron blockade (i.e., of the loop of Henle and distal convoluted tubule) with addition of a thiazide to a loop diuretic. |

TABLE 8.1 ■ **Equivalency Among Common Diuretics**

| Diuretic | PO (mg) | IV (mg) |
|----------|---------|---------|
| Furosemide | 40 | 20 |
| Torsemide | 20 | 20 |
| Bumetanide | 1 | 1 |

| | |
|---|---|
| **Antidote** | ■ Give additional diuretics prior to the next scheduled dose. |
| **Common Scenarios** | ■ Inadequate diuretic dosing for CKD |
| | ■ Diuresing a difficult-to-diurese patient with longstanding CKD with only a loop diuretic |
| **Note(s)** | ■ Diuretics work via an all-or-nothing mechanism where a dose that surpasses the minimum threshold will result in diuresis, and a dose that fails to meet the threshold will have no effect. |
| | ■ Diuretics function by preventing functioning of various electrolyte transporters in the nephrons, thereby affecting the concentration gradients that impact water (urine) reabsorption. This means that a diuretic's effectiveness relies on good kidney function. If a kidney is not able to filter and create urine properly, diuretics will be less effective (thus higher doses are required). |
| | ■ Proper diuretic response is usually demonstrated by a minimum urine sodium of approximately 50–70 mEq. |

## MISTAKE: DISMISSAL OF FeNa AS A VALUABLE TEST FOR GUIDING DIURESIS IN HEART FAILURE

| | |
|---|---|
| **Case Example** | A 78-year-old female with HFpEF (EF = 65%) and severe dementia is admitted for acute decompensated HF. There are no records available in the system, and the patient is unable to provide her home diuretic dosage. Noting that the patient's creatinie is 2.5, you start diuresis aggressively with 80 of IV Lasix. You check her urine output a 3 hours later and notice approximately 400 mL and are unsure whether the patient is responding adequately to your diuretic dosing. You decide to await the final urine output by 6 hours and are dismayed to find a total urine output of 900 mL. |
| **Reasoning Error(s)** | ■ Only associating the value of urine sodium as part of the FeNa for determining the type of acute kidney injury and dismissing its value in HF given the presence of diuretics |
| | ■ Lack of knowledge in how to use the urine sodium for managing HF |
| **How to Avoid the Mistake** | ■ Rather than associating diagnostic tests with reflexive purposes, think critically about the information that each test can provide and whether that may be useful to your specific information needs. |
| | ■ Understand that diuretics should increase the urine sodium; thus checking the urine sodium 1–2 hours after dosing a diuretic can provide early insight into diuretic responsiveness, thereby guiding dosing changes earlier than awaiting urine output. |

**Antidote**   ■  Not applicable

**Common Scenarios**   ■  Not applicable

**Note(s)**   ■  Diuretic responsiveness is generally indicated by a urine sodium of at least 50 mEq/L but can be more formally assessed via the natriuretic response prediction equation (NRPE), a recently developed and validated tool to guide diuretic therapy. Sodium outputs were categorized into poor output (<50 mmol), suboptimal (<100 mmol), and excellent (>150 mmol).

    ■  Sodium Output (mmol) =

$$\text{eGFR} \times \left(\frac{\text{BSA}}{1.73}\right) \times \left(\frac{\text{Serum Cr}}{\text{Urine Cr}}\right) \times 60 \text{ min} \times 3.25 \text{ h} \times \frac{\text{Urine Na}}{1000 \text{ mL}}$$

  ■  Lasix was named as such because it <u>LA</u>sts <u>SIX</u> hours.

**Further Reading**   ■  Validation of the NRPE: Gleason O, et al. Validation of natriuretic response prediction equation in patients with decompensated heart failure. *J Card Fail*. 2020;26(10):S2.

    ■  Study comparing use of the NRPE versus clinical judgment to guide diuretic therapy: Rao VS, et al. Natriuretic equation to predict loop diuretic response in patients with heart failure. *JACC*. 2021;77(6):695-708.

## MISTAKE: INCREASING DIURETIC DOSAGE RATHER THAN FREQUENCY IN NONREFRACTORY DIURESIS

**Case Example**    A patient's overall urine output in response to 60 IV Lasix is 1 L. Your daily net negative goal is 2–3 L, and thus you increase the Lasix to 120 mg IV. You continue to see approximately 1-L urine output following that dose.

**Reasoning Error(s)**   ■  Lack of understanding the diuretic response curve (Fig. 8.2)

    ■  Forgetting that diuresis is a function of both achieving the threshold dose and duration of diuretic effect (i.e., frequency)

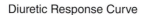

### Diuretic Response Curve

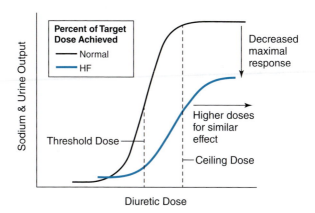

**Fig. 8.2**   Diuretic dose-response curve.

**How to Avoid the Mistake**
- Understand the threshold and ceiling phenomena for diuretics.
- Diurese more frequently rather than increasing diuretic dosages once the threshold dose is discovered.

**Antidote**
- Increase the frequency of diuresis or consider using drip diuresis.

**Common Scenarios**
- Not applicable

**Note(s)**
- Though adverse effects such as hearing loss are rare with diuresis, the effects are indeed real. Do not use higher doses than necessary—it increases patient risk in exchange for little to no benefit.
- Of course, if the diuretic threshold has not been reached and the patient is producing minimal urine, then the diuretic dosage should be increased.
- Confirming diuretic responsiveness can be done via checking the urine sodium (generally >50 mEq/L) and/or using the natriuretic response prediction equation (see page 185).

## MISTAKE: BLIND FAVOR OF BOLUS DIURESIS OVER DRIP DIURESIS

**Case Example**
You are aggressively diuresing a patient with Lasix 80 mg IV three times a day for a goal net negative of 3 L/day. However, in the midst of being called to a rapid and a cardiac arrest, you forget to order the third dose of Lasix before leaving the hospital.

**Reasoning Error(s)**
- Forgetting that bolus and drip diuresis achieve similar outcomes
- Forgetting that bolus and drip diuresis can be combined with occasional success in refractory diuresis
- Lack of comfort or familiarity with drip dosing of diuretics

**How to Avoid the Mistake**
- Consider drip diuresis as an alternate or adjuvant strategy to bolus dosing.
- Understand proper dosing of drip diuresis.
  - Usually begins at 5 mg/h and titrate up to 20 mg/h
  - The goal is to provide a 24-hour dose of diuretic equal to or higher than what the patient has received in boluses thus far. For example, if a patient was refractory to 120 mg IV Lasix BID, then the 24-hour diuretic dose was 240 mg, thus the Lasix drip should begin at a minimum of 10 mg/h (higher if using this method for refractory diuresis).

**Antidote**
- Not applicable

**Common Scenarios**
- Not applicable

**Note(s)**
- Drip diuresis maintains a steadier level of diuretic in the body, as opposed to the significant peaks experienced after bolus dosing. This may lead to decreased side effects such as renal impairment and ototoxicity, as the maximum dose exposure is often significantly lower, though there is no clear evidence to support this.
- As seen in the DOSE trial, the overall diuretic efficacy is similar between the two methods, although higher doses resulted in quicker symptomatic improvement at the expense of *temporary* increased renal impairment.

**Further Reading**

■ The DOSE trial is a classic landmark study for your reading list: Felker GM, et al. Diuretic strategies in patients with acute decompensated heart failure. *N Engl J Med.* 2011;364:797-805.

## MISTAKE: FORGETTING TO BOLUS WHEN INITIATING DRIP DIURESIS

**Case Example**

In the setting of ototoxicity for a patient, you decide to use drip diuresis at 5 mg/h to reduce the exposure to high peak concentrations of diuretic. Hours later, the urine output is minimal.

**Reasoning Error(s)**

■ Forgetting that the drip diuretic is dosed to maintain a steady concentration of diuretic. As such, it would likely not be enough to only start a drip since the minimum effective threshold concentration must be surpassed.

**How to Avoid the Mistake**

■ Consider the mechanism of achieving the desired outcome when using less familiar methods of medication administration.
■ Always bolus before initiating a drip.

**Antidote**

■ Provide a diuretic bolus!

**Common Scenarios**

■ Forgetting to bolus prior to drip diuresis

**Note(s)**

■ The dose of a diuretic bolus should be the minimal necessary to reach the threshold effect.

## MISTAKE: USING THIAZIDES IN MODERATE TO SEVERE HYPONATREMIA

**Case Example**

A 74-year-old female with HFrEF (EF = 20%) and CKD III is admitted to you for profound volume overload. Given the history of CKD and initial difficulty diuresing, you add metolazone 5 mg daily. The patient's sodium levels are as follows: 136 (admission) → 136 → 134 (after metolazone) → 132 → 129.

**Reasoning Error(s)**

■ Forgetting to consider the hyponatremia-inducing effects of thiazides
■ Attributing a new hyponatremia (after thiazide use) to hypervolemia
■ Lack of attention to the sodium level on daily labs

**How to Avoid the Mistake**

■ Understand the potentially strong sodium-wasting effects of thiazides (metolazone in particular).
■ Consider the timeline of hyponatremia (did it start before or after thiazide use?).
■ Pay attention to the sodium level on daily labs.

**Antidote**

■ Withhold thiazides

**Common Scenarios**

■ Not applicable

**Note(s)**

- Older methods of inducing diuresis include the use of urea and hypertonic saline.
  - Urea is an osmole that is 100% secreted, and water follows urea via osmotic diuresis as more commonly seen in hyperglycemia. This may also lead to hypernatremia (or in the case of hyponatremia, correct it).
  - Hypertonic saline may augment diuresis with loop diuretics in refractory cases via a mechanism still under investigation (it is thought that hypochloridemia induces diuretic resistance and hypertonic saline corrects that). The typical dose used is 150 mL of 3% saline in conjunction with a large dose of Lasix.

**Further Reading**

- Early article discussing the use of urea as a diuretic: Crawford H, et al. The use of urea as a diuretic in advanced heart failure. *Arch Intern Med*. 1925;36(4):530-541.
- Study investigating the safety and efficacy of diuresing with hypertonic saline: Griffin M, et al. Real world use of hypertonic saline in refractory acute decompensated heart failure: a US center's experience. *JACC Heart Fail*. 2020;8(3):199-208.

## MISTAKE: NOT SCREENING FOR DIURESIS-ANTAGONISTIC MEDICATIONS

**Case Example**
A frequently seen patient is admitted to you for acute HF exacerbation. You know the drill and begin IV diuresis with twice the patient's home dose of Lasix. You notice that the patient's urine output is not nearly as robust as on prior admissions, yet the kidney function appears at baseline. The medical student notes that during her medication reconciliation, the patient had admitted to newly taking ibuprofen for lower back pain.

**Reasoning Error(s)**

- Forgetting a thorough medication reconciliation focusing on medications that antagonize diuresis
- Lack of knowledge of medications that antagonize diuresis

**How to Avoid the Mistake**

- Understand why certain medications antagonize diuresis. Medications that either decrease GFR or increase water/salt retention offer the opposite effect of diuresis.
- Always perform a thorough medication reconciliation.
- Learn and recognize common medications that antagonize diuresis.

**Antidote**

- Stop the antagonistic medications.

**Common Scenarios**

- Nonsteroidal antiinflammatory drugs (NSAIDs)
- RAAS blockers (ACEIs, ARBs)

**Note(s)**

- Though RAAS blockade does antagonize diuresis to a limited extent, their twofold benefit in HF (short term: afterload reduction, which also benefits diuresis; long term: mortality benefit) outweighs the antagonism and may be continued during diuresis.

## MISTAKE: DELAY IN REDOSING DIURETICS IN RESISTANT OR REFRACTORY DIURESIS

**Case Example**

You diurese a patient with IV Lasix 40 mg and ask the nurse to check the total urine output after 6 hours. You are disappointed to see minimal urine output and increase the next dose of IV Lasix to 80 mg, noticing 2 L of urine output another 6 hours after Lasix administration.

**Reasoning Error(s)**

- In a fixed mindset that diuretics are dosed no earlier than every 6 hours (the duration of action of Lasix)
- Lack of timely information on the patient's diuretic responsiveness

**How to Avoid the Mistake**

- Understand the pharmacodynamics of diuretics (on/off "switch" phenomenon hinging upon adequately meeting the diuretic threshold dose).
- Frequently assess for key signs of diuretic responsiveness and resistance: urine output, urine sodium, oxygenation status.

**Antidote**

- Administer higher-dose diuretics (and/or combination therapy such as thiazides) prior to the next scheduled time.

**Common Scenarios**

- Not applicable

**Note(s)**

- While the degree by which to increase diuretic dosing is largely up to the clinician, the only evidence that we have for an effective strategy comes from the DOSE trial, which increased doses by a factor of 2.5. Once an effective dose is found, you may consider gently decreasing the dose to find the minimum effective diuretic dose, which provides robust urine output at the lowest risk of adverse effects.
- Medications that may offer a synergistic effect on diuresis include acetazolamide, thiazides, and potassium-sparing diuretics such as spironolactone. Though most commonly only thiazides are used to augment diuresis, it is worthwhile to attempt using one or more agents that blockade other parts of the nephron (e.g., proximal tubules).

## MISTAKE: DIURESING TO DOCUMENTED "DRY WEIGHT" RATHER THAN CLINICAL JUDGMENT

**Case Example**

Your patient Mr. Jones has been aggressively diuresed for over a week since he presented in decompensated HF prior to an elective right heart catheterization to measure his pulmonary pressures. His standing weight has decreased from 134 kg to 112 kg. You notice that the last dry weight in his chart from a year ago is 110.8 kg and stop diuresis despite trace edema in the lower extremities. The next day on his right heart cath, his PCWP is found to be 21 mmHg.

**Reasoning Error(s)**

- Trusting documented weights without critical appraisal of the quality of data
- Putting one's clinical volume assessment second to a documented weight
- Forgetting that HF is a cachectic disease

| | |
|---|---|
| **How to Avoid the Mistake** | ■ Trust but verify charted weights. Was the patient truly diuresed to euvolemic prior to discharge (e.g., some clinicians may discharge before fully reaching a dry weight with plans to diurese more in the outpatient setting)? Was the weight a standing weight or a bed weight (which has significant variability and inaccuracy)? |
| | ■ Understand that HF is a cachectic disease. Over time, patients will lose lean body mass. Pay close attention to the date of the last recorded dry weight—the more recent the weight, the more likely to be accurate. |
| | ■ Ultimately, your clinical assessment of a patient's volume status based on exam and laboratory data should guide your decision on when to pause diuresis. |
| **Antidote** | ■ Not applicable |
| **Common Scenarios** | ■ Not applicable |
| **Note(s)** | ■ Lab values that signal reaching or nearing dry weight include contraction alkalosis (increasing bicarbonate), AKI (rising creatinine and urea levels), and hypernatremia. |

## MISTAKE: FREQUENT MANUAL POTASSIUM REPLETION DURING DIURESIS

| | |
|---|---|
| **Case Example** | After 3 consecutive days of significant diuresis resulting in K = 3.2, 3.4, 3.4 with subsequent repletion with both PO and IV potassium, the patient becomes tired of swallowing the large potassium pills and notes some throat irritation. During the next IV potassium administration, he rips out the IV line, noting that "it burns!" |
| **Reasoning Error(s)** | ■ Forgetting to consider patient comfort. IV potassium burns during administration, and oral potassium is caustic and irritating to the throat (particularly in patients with esophagitis and GERD). |
| | ■ Lack of familiarity using a potassium-sparing diuretic to counterbalance potassium-wasting effects of loop diuretics. |
| **How to Avoid the Mistake** | ■ If a patient requires significant or repeated potassium repletions, consider addition of a potassium-sparing diuretic such as spironolactone to help reduce the amount of manual potassium repletion. |
| | ■ Utilize IV potassium repletions when potassium levels are very low or repletion is urgent |
| **Antidote** | ■ Spironolactone (or other potassium-sparing diuretic) |
| **Common Scenarios** | ■ Repeated PO or IV potassium repletion |
| **Note(s)** | ■ Spironolactone is the drug of choice in diuresis accompanied by persistent hypokalemia. |
| | ■ The diuretic effect of potassium-sparing diuretics is weak but synergistic, thus you may even see an increase in diuresis. |

## MISTAKE: ACETAZOLAMIDE TO CORRECT METABOLIC ALKALOSIS WITHOUT CHECKING POTASSIUM

**Case Example**  You notice that a patient who has been diuresed for over a week has a bicarbonate level of 44. Alarmed, you administer 500 mg of Diamox (acetazolamide). Two hours later, however, the patient goes into monomorphic ventricular tachycardia, which degenerates into ventricular fibrillation, and dies.

**Reasoning Error(s)**
- Lack of understanding of how potassium balance affects bicarbonate homeostasis
- Focus on the treatment goal without considering potential adverse effects

**How to Avoid the Mistake**
- Understand the direct relationship between serum potassium and the ability of the kidneys to excrete bicarbonate. Potassium also causes bicarbonate to shift into the cells.
- Carefully monitor potassium levels before and after acetazolamide administration.
- Always consider adverse effects to every diagnostic or therapeutic action, no matter how trivial.

**Antidote**
- Potassium repletion

**Common Scenarios**
- Not applicable

**Note(s)**
- Repletion of potassium corrects metabolic alkalosis. This is a good first step prior to administering acetazolamide.
- Avoid potassium citrate, as the citrate causes worsening alkalosis. Use potassium chloride instead.
- MRAs (e.g., spironolactone) may help correct metabolic alkalosis as well through antagonism of a mechanism that causes bicarbonate retention and increased aldosterone levels.
- Potassium repletion is ineffective in coexisting magnesium deficiency. Thus replete magnesium levels or consider administering both potassium and magnesium if magnesium levels are unknown. Notably, loop diuretics commonly cause magnesium wasting.

## MISTAKE: LACK OF CONSIDERATION FOR NASAL INTERMITTENT POSITIVE-PRESSURE VENTILATION IN ALL PATIENTS WITH ACUTE DECOMPENSATED HEART FAILURE

**Case Example**  A 72-year-old female with HFrEF (EF = 25%) presents with worsening shortness of breath. Her oxygen saturation is 91%, and she recovers soon after you put her on 6 L nasal canula. You diurese her appropriately, and she improves in a few days.

**Reasoning Error(s)**
- Lack of knowledge regarding the mortality and symptomatic benefit of nasal intermittent positive pressure ventilation (NIPPV) in acute decompensated HF
- Belief that NIPPV is only useful for patients requiring high oxygen support
- Inadequate NIPPV equipment availability

| | |
|---|---|
| **How to Avoid the Mistake** | ■ Understand that NIPPV carries a significant in-hospital mortality benefit and time to symptomatic improvement. |
| | ■ Understand that NIPPV is useful regardless of the degree of oxygen support required. |
| | ■ Plan ahead with regard to NIPPV availability. |
| **Antidote** | ■ Trial NIPPV as able |
| **Common Scenarios** | ■ BiPAP |
| | ■ CPAP |
| **Note(s)** | ■ NIPPV (specifically CPAP or BiPAP) is the only intervention to date that has rigorous evidence demonstrating a mortality benefit for acute decompensated HF. In a Cochrane Review meta-analysis, NIPPV decreased in-hospital mortality by 49% (11% versus 18%) with a number needed to treat of 17. |
| | ■ Interestingly, the 2013 AHA/ACC Guidelines on Heart Failure, as well as the 2017 Focused Update, do not address noninvasive ventilation whereas the 2016 European Guidelines recommend its use. |
| **Further Reading** | ■ Meta-analysis demonstrating a mortality benefit to utilization of NIPPV in acute decompensated HF: Berbenetz N, et al. Non-invasive positive pressure ventilation (CPAP or bilevel NPPV) for cardiogenic pulmonary oedema. *Cochrane Database Syst Rev.* 2019. |

## MISTAKE: USE OF NASAL INTERMITTENT POSITIVE-PRESSURE VENTILATION IN ACUTE DECOMPENSATED HEART FAILURE WITH SOFT BLOOD PRESSURES

| | |
|---|---|
| **Case Example** | An 80-year-old male presents with decompensated HF. Initial blood pressure is 91/59 and oxygen saturation is 86% with significant respiratory distress. You place the patient in BIPAP, and he becomes hypotensive to 82/52. |
| **Reasoning Error(s)** | ■ Forgetting that positive pressure may induce hypotension, though anecdotally this is often in patients with other risk factors for hypotension such as right ventricular failure or hypovolemia |
| | ■ Lack of close monitoring when using NIPPV in patients with soft blood pressure |
| **How to Avoid the Mistake** | ■ Understand that positive pressure increases intrathoracic pressure and may lead to decreased venous return and hypotension. |
| | ■ Close blood pressure monitoring is needed. |
| **Antidote** | ■ If hypotensive, switch to alternate respiratory support method. |
| **Common Scenarios** | ■ Not applicable |
| **Note(s)** | ■ The risk of hypotension with NIPPV increases with higher degrees of positive pressure. |

## MISTAKE: USE OF INEFFECTIVE OR EVIDENCE-LACKING STRATEGIES FOR DIURESIS

| | |
|---|---|
| **Case Example** | A patient is admitted to your decompensated HF. Rather than diuresing, you decide to initiative ultrafiltration. Another patient with severe electrolyte derangements that urgently needed dialysis dies due to the lack of available dialysis machines. |
| **Reasoning Error(s)** | ■ Lack of knowledge regarding the efficacy or evidence for an intervention<br>■ Forgetting to consider adverse effects and thinking there is "nothing to lose"<br>■ Not considering the impact of medical practice beyond the individual patient at hand |
| **How to Avoid the Mistake** | ■ Strive to understand the evidence and rationale for every clinical action.<br>■ Consider potential adverse effects and monetary costs for all interventions.<br>■ Recognize that each intervention that is used frivolously causes the potential lack of a beneficial therapy in another patient (e.g., due to limited dialysis machines or cost of a medication). |
| **Antidote** | ■ Not applicable |
| **Common Scenarios** | ■ Ultrafiltration<br>■ Low-dose dopamine<br>■ Nesiritide<br>■ Tolvaptan |
| **Note(s)** | ■ There are several ongoing studies investigating the role of tolvaptan as an adjunct to loop diuretics in decompensated HF. However, there is yet to be robust evidence to support the pricey intervention. |

# Treatment: Guideline-Directed Medical Therapy

## MISTAKE: LIMITED GDMT THERAPY IN THE SETTING OF SOFT BLOOD PRESSURES

| | |
|---|---|
| **Case Example** | A 52-year-old female with HFrEF (EF = 25%) visits your office for HF management. She is currently on metoprolol succinate 25 mg, lisinopril 20 mg, and spironolactone 25 mg. Her blood pressure is 92/61, in line with her usual blood pressures over the last year. Although you wish to increase her GDMT, you are hesitant given her soft blood pressures. The patient voices that she is asymptomatic and that she heard from a friend who is "a doctor" that GDMT doses should be increased as tolerated. You defer uptitration, and she leaves to establish care with another cardiologist. A year later, the patient is admitted to you for decompensated HF at which time she notes that her new cardiologist is "so much better" and that her GDMT is significantly higher now without symptoms. |

**Reasoning Error(s)**
- Hesitancy about inducing hypotension with GDMT (the principle of do no harm)
- Lack of recognition that baseline blood pressures may be soft in HFrEF patients
- Lack of experience safely optimizing GDMT in patients with soft blood pressures
- Comfort with non–evidence-based threshold blood pressure of 90 mmHg

**How to Avoid the Mistake**
- Understand that patients with low EF often live with relatively soft blood pressures due to decreased cardiac output.
- Given the significant benefits of GDMT, overcome the fear of inducing hypotension and challenge patients to see how much GDMT they can tolerate. In other words, if you are not inducing any hypotension at all, you are not optimizing GDMT well enough!
- Rethink the principle of do no harm. Withholding life-changing medicine is more harmful than potentially briefly inducing hypotension.
- Consider inpatient GDMT optimization given the more controlled environment and monitoring in case the patient does become hypotensive.
- Use strategies to minimize the hypotension-inducing effects of GDMT.

**Antidote**
- If hypotensive, decrease or stop offending agents.
- Consider gentle fluids (e.g., 500 mL) if not decompensated.

**Common Scenarios**
- Not applicable

**Note(s)**
- Key strategies for maximizing tolerance of GDMT in patients with soft blood pressures:
  - Perform a thorough medication reconciliation and stop any unnecessary medications that lower blood pressure.
  - Use medications that have the least blood pressure lowering effects possible when first optimizing GDMT since the most common limiting factor for GDMT optimization is blood pressure. For example, use metoprolol succinate rather than carvedilol!
  - Separate timing of GDMT medications (e.g., can divide metoprolol succinate doses into BID)
  - Guide GDMT optimization largely by symptoms in context (e.g., if the patient is sedentary most of the day, brief dizziness when standing twice a day may be acceptable depending on functional status and home support).
- Per Dr. Miriam Bozkurt (former president of Heart Failure Society of America), GDMT optimization is likely possible for blood pressures >80 mmHg.
- Contrary to popular belief among many physicians, metoprolol does decrease blood pressure though to a smaller degree than carvedilol, as evidenced by several small studies comparing their antihypertensive effects.

| Further Reading | ■ Wonderful short article on how to implement GDMT despite soft blood pressures: Bozkurt M. Response to Ryan and Parwani: Heart failure patients with low blood pressure: how should we manage neurohormonal blocking drugs? *Circ Heart Fail.* 2012;5:820-821. |

## MISTAKE: FORGETTING TO ACTIVELY UPTITRATE GDMT TO TARGET DOSES

| Case Example | You see a new patient in clinic who presents for management of HFrEF (EF = 15%). You promptly start the patient on Entresto 24/26 mg BID, COREG (carvedilol) 3.125 mg BID, and eplerenone 25 mg daily over the course of the first month. You attempted to prescribe a sodium-glucose cotransporter-2 (SGLT2) inhibitor but met barriers with the patient's insurance. Over the course of 2 years, the patient's LVEF improves to 20%. A fellow working in your clinic notes one day that the patient's GDMT doses should be increased. You wonder to yourself whether the patient's LVEF may have recovered significantly more had the patient been on target doses of GDMT. |
| Reasoning Error(s) | ■ Lack of understanding that GDMT benefits stem from both a class and dose-dependent effect <br> ■ Difficulty coordinating frequent follow-ups and lab draws to safely uptitrate GDMT in the outpatient setting |
| How to Avoid the Mistake | ■ Understand the target doses for each GDMT. <br> ■ Always think about optimizing GDMT whenever possible, especially in the inpatient setting. |
| Antidote | ■ Not applicable |
| Common Scenarios | ■ Not applicable |
| Note(s) | ■ Target doses for the four cornerstone GDMT are shown in Table 8.2. <br> ■ The MOCHA study from 1996 demonstrates a beautiful graphical representation of the dose-dependent benefits of carvedilol on LVEF recovery. It's such a neat study that we will refrain from showing you the graph here so you can see it for yourself! |
| Further Reading | ■ MOCHA study: Bristow MR, et al. Carvedilol produces dose-related improvements in left ventricular function and survival in subjects with chronic heart failure. *Circulation.* 1996;94(11):2807-2816. |

## MISTAKE: DEFERRING GDMT INITIATION/UPTITRATION TO THE OUTPATIENT SETTING

| Case Example | A 48-year-old male with no past medical history presents with subacute shortness of breath. A TTE reveals a newly reduced LVEF of 35%. You start the patient on lisinopril 10 mg daily but decide to defer the rest of GDMT initiation and uptitration to the outpatient setting. A month later, the patient is readmitted to you for HF exacerbation. You notice that the patient is still only on lisinopril 10 mg daily. |

TABLE 8.2 ■ Target Doses for Common GDMT

| GDMT | Target Dose |
|------|-------------|
| Lisinopril | 40 mg daily |
| Losartan | 150 mg daily |
| Valsartan | 160 mg BID |
| Entresto (sacubitril/valsartan) | 97/103 mg BID |
| Metoprolol succinate | 200 mg BID |
| Carvedilol | 25 mg BID |
| Spironolactone | 25 mg daily |
| Eplerenone | 50 mg daily |
| Dapagliflozin | 10 mg daily |
| Empagliflozin | 25 mg daily |

| | |
|---|---|
| **Reasoning Error(s)** | ■ Putting too much trust in the outpatient system and lack of awareness regarding effectiveness of GDMT management outpatient<br>■ Lack of desire to titrate GDMT because historical practice was to defer to outpatient<br>■ Fear of adverse events while uptitrating GDMT inpatient<br>■ Forgetting that the controlled environment inpatient is ideal for quicker titration. Usually in the outpatient setting, multiple time-consuming visits and lab draws must be coordinated to ensure safe uptitration. |
| **How to Avoid the Mistake** | ■ Understand that the inpatient setting is the safest setting for GDMT manipulation if adverse events were to happen<br>■ Take the initiative and initiate/uptitrate GDMT as able in the inpatient setting<br>■ Recognize the systemwide shortcomings for enrolling patients on appropriate GDMT as born out in studies such as the CHAMP-HF registry demonstrating strikingly low numbers of patients on appropriate GDMT<br>■ Understand that GDMT benefits are derived from not only a class effect but are also dose-dependent, requiring multiple steps to reach target doses. |
| **Antidote** | ■ Not applicable |
| **Common Scenarios** | ■ Not applicable |
| **Note(s)** | ■ The CHAMP-HF (Change the Management of Patients with Heart Failure) Registry provided insight into the gaps underlying the usage and correct dosage of GDMT for patients with HFrEF (Fig. 8.3).<br>■ 73.4%, 67%, and 33.4% of patients without contraindications were on ACEIs/ARBs/ARNIs, β-blockers, and MRA, respectively.<br>　■ Less than one-third of patients on β-blockers and RAAS blockers were receiving target doses, whereas three-fourths of patients on MRAs were at target doses.<br>　■ A shocking 1% of patients were on all eligible GDMT medications at target doses. |

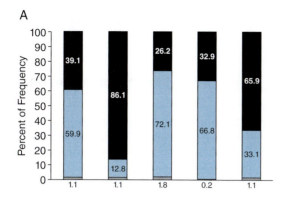

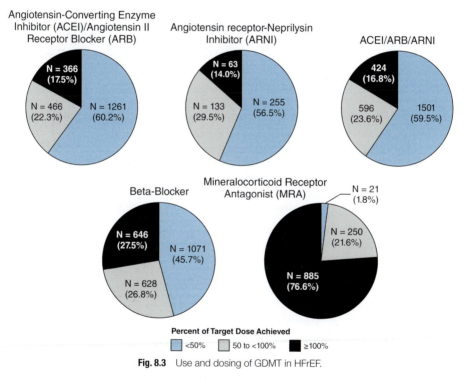

**Fig. 8.3** Use and dosing of GDMT in HFrEF.

**Further Reading**
- The CHAMP-HF Registry: Greene SJ, et al. Medical therapy for heart failure with reduced ejection fraction: the CHAMP-HF Registry. *JACC.* 2018;72(4):351-366.

## MISTAKE: HOLDING ALL GDMT DURING ACUTE DECOMPENSATED HEART FAILURE

**Case Example**
A patient comes in with HF exacerbation, clearly volume overloaded and with warm extremities on exam, maintaining a pulse pressure of 40 mm Hg. You hold their β-blocker. Prior to discharge, you accidentally forget to restart the patient's metoprolol succinate, instead prescribing metoprolol tartrate.

**Reasoning Error(s)**
- Lack of consideration of the mechanism of each GDMT and its effect (supportive, antagonistic, neutral) on your patient with acute decompensated HF (ADHF)
- Equating all HF exacerbations as synonymous with cardiogenic shock
- Exposure to non–evidence-based practice of holding all GDMT during ADHF
- Forgetting to restart GDMT that was held during hospitalization and/or restart the wrong GDMT (e.g., metoprolol tartrate)

**How to Avoid the Mistake**
- Only withhold GDMT for either impending cardiogenic shock or if it interferes with renal function (many patients with ADHF present with AKI, and ACEI/ARBs can antagonize diuresis). Generally, β-blockers, MRAs, and SGLT2 inhibitors can be continued.
- Think about the mechanism of each GDMT and whether it would support (e.g., spironolactone's potassium-sparing effects during aggressive diuresis), antagonize (e.g., negative inotropy of β-blockers when pending cardiogenic shock), or have minimal effect (e.g., β-blockers in a patient with robust blood pressures) in a patient with ADHF.

**Antidote**
- Not applicable

**Common Scenarios**
- Holding GDMT during HF exacerbation
  - β-Blockers
  - MRAs (e.g., spironolactone)
  - SGLT2 inhibitors
  - Isosorbide dinitrate/hydralazine
  - Ivabradine
- Holding ACEIs/ARBs in the setting of COVID infection

**Note(s)**
- ACEIs/ARBs are nearly always held upon admission for ADHF given the prevalence of AKI and potentially antagonistic effects on diuresis.
- There are several studies such as the B-CONVINCED study that demonstrate increased mortality and morbidity when GDMT, in particular β-blockers, is held unnecessarily during hospitalization.

## MISTAKE: DISCONTINUING GDMT IN RECOVERED HFrEF

**Case Example**
A patient's EF rises from 30% tto 55% with the use of Entresto, spironolactone, and metoprolol succinate. Given concerns of polypharmacy, you discontinue the Entresto and metoprolol succinate at a follow-up visit. Three months later, the patient's EF is now 40%.

| | |
|---|---|
| **Reasoning Error(s)** | ■ Relying on well-intentioned common sense or intuition (one might reasonably expect that withdrawing the medications after recovery would do no harm given the EF has recovered) rather than evidence-based medicine |
| **How to Avoid the Mistake** | ■ Consider all GDMT medications as lifetime medications unless intolerance (e.g., allergic reactions, hypotension) develop. |
| | ■ Confirm intuitive clinical reasoning with evidence prior to implementing clinical practice. |
| **Antidote** | ■ Restart GDMT. |
| **Common Scenarios** | ■ β-Blockers |
| | ■ ACEIs/ARBs |
| | ■ MRAs (e.g., spironolactone) |
| | ■ SGLT2 inhibitors |
| | ■ Isosorbide dinitrate/hydralazine |
| | ■ Ivabradine |
| **Note(s)** | ■ There are currently no outcomes data after discontinuation of newer (e.g., SGLT2) or niche (e.g., ivabradine) GDMT. However, based on robust data on other GDMT, these should also be considered lifetime medications until evidence is available suggesting potential discontinuation without adverse effects. |

## MISTAKE: HOLDING OR WITHDRAWING ACEIs/ARBs FOR INCREASING CREATININE AFTER INITIATION

| | |
|---|---|
| **Case Example** | A 72-year-old male admitted for shortness of breath is found to have a newly reduced LVEF to 25%. As part of his HF regimen, you start him on valsartan 40 mg BID. The next morning, you notice that his creatinine has risen from 0.9 to 1.3. Fearing damage to the kidneys, you hold the patient's valsartan. He is discharged on metoprolol succinate and spironolactone. A month later, you see him in outpatient clinic and notice that his valsartan had been restarted in the hospital discharge follow-up clinic. You check labs and notice that the patient's creatinine is at baseline. |
| **Reasoning Error(s)** | ■ Misunderstanding that a rise in creatinine in the setting of RAAS blocker initiation reflects kidney damage |
| | ■ Misattribution of a rise in creatinine to changes in volume status (e.g., prerenal) |
| **How to Avoid the Mistake** | ■ Understand that ACEIs and ARBs cause efferent arteriolar dilation, which reduces glomerular filtration pressure and increases the creatinine transiently until the arterioles normalize. In other words, the creatinine reflects an alteration in hemodynamics rather than nephrotoxicity. |
| | ■ Remember that the rise in creatinine in the setting of an RAAS blocker is usually transient. |
| **Antidote** | ■ Not applicable |
| **Common Scenarios** | ■ Not applicable |

**Note(s)**
- The rise in creatinine with ACEI or ARB initiation is usually modest and transient. Importantly, a sharp rise (i.e., >30%) in creatinine within 1 week, especially in the setting of uncontrolled HTN, may signal the presence of renal artery stenosis (typically bilateral to cause such an effect).
- ARBs are better tolerated overall, carrying a lower risk of angioedema and cough. Best of all, they are now very inexpensive, and many physicians prefer to use them as first-line treatment.

## MISTAKE: NOT TRIALING AN ARB AFTER ACEI ANGIOEDEMA

**Case Example**
A female with HFrEF who had been prescribed lisinopril 1 week ago is admitted to the ICU with angioedema. At bedside, you observe that the patient is nasally intubated with a large swollen tongue protruding out of her mouth. Over the course of the next week, the patient slowly improves on high-dose steroids. Prior to discharge, you wonder whether you should challenge the patient with an ARB given the mortality benefit in HFrEF.

**Reasoning Error(s)**
- Fear of recurrent angioedema with ARB use
- Forgetting about the potential long-term benefits of ARB therapy and weighing the risk-benefit of an ARB challenge

**How to Avoid the Mistake**
- Understand that the risk of angioedema with ARBs in patients who had angioedema due to ACEIs is relatively low (5–10%).
- Discuss the risks and benefits of trialing an ARB with the patient, focusing on the huge long-term benefits that ARB therapy may have on the patient's HF.
- Challenge with an ARB in a controlled setting (e.g., inpatient).

**Antidote**
- Not applicable

**Common Scenarios**
- Not applicable

**Note(s)**
- Given the robust evidence for ARBs in HFrEF therapy and the inexpensive cost, it is reasonable to prescribe ARBs from the offset. It is also easier to transition from an ARB to Entresto due to the lack of a washout period.

**Further Reading**
- Great short article addressing the data around whether patients who have had angioedema can be prescribed ARBs: Sharma P, et al. Can an ARB be given to patients who have had angioedema on an ACE inhibitor? *Cleveland Clin J Med.* 2013;80(12):755-757.

## MISTAKE: NOT USING OR DISCONTINUING LOW-DOSE ACEI/ARB THERAPY IN CKD/ESRD

**Case Example**
A patient with HFrEF and end-stage renal disease (ESRD) presents to your HF clinic to establish care. You notice that the patient is on 10 mg losartan and decide to stop it for fear of hyperkalemia given the patient's ESRD. The patient's primary care physician reaches out and notes that the patient has been tolerating the medication well, making you question your decision.

| | |
|---|---|
| **Reasoning Error(s)** | ■ Well-intentioned fear of adverse events |
| | ■ Lack of knowledge about empiric data on tolerability of ACEIs/ARBs in renal dysfunction |
| | ■ Lack of patient-centered risk-benefit discussion |
| **How to Avoid the Mistake** | ■ In the setting of such huge benefit for HFrEF, be willing to find a way to incorporate the medications safely rather than stopping in fear. |
| | ■ Understand that patients generally tolerate low doses of ACEIs/ARBs well even in ESRD. |
| | ■ Consider potassium binders such as Lokelma (sodium zirconium cyclosilicate) to help with hyperkalemia though a small dose usually does not significantly affect the potassium. |
| | ■ Realize the necessity of thorough risk-benefit discussion with patients, emphasizing potential long-term benefits in HFrEF versus temporary adverse event(s). |
| **Antidote** | ■ Not applicable |
| **Common Scenarios** | ■ Not applicable |
| **Note(s)** | ■ Though the large-scale trial data for HFrEF mortality benefit with ACEIs and ARBs excluded hemodialysis patients, small studies have reproduced the beneficial effects seen and it is generally assumed that the benefit is no different in ESRD. |
| | ■ Work from Clyde Yancy's group has recently focused on disparities in HFrEF therapy use, such as in the setting of renal dysfunction. The patients who need the therapies the most are often not optimally treated with life-saving medications such as ACEI/sARBs. |
| **Further Reading** | ■ Patel R, et al. Kidney function and outcomes in patients hospitalized with heart failure. *JACC*. 2021;78(4):330-343. |

## MISTAKE: MAINTAINING ACEIs/ARBs INSTEAD OF ARNIs

| | |
|---|---|
| **Case Example** | You have been following a patient with HFrEF for years. The patient's GDMT is at optimal doses on all the right classes of medications. She has done well enough to where an ICD was not indicated for primary prevention given EF recovery to 37%. The patient asks you about an ad she saw on television about Entresto, and you realize that you had forgotten to transition the patient to Entresto. |
| **Reasoning Error(s)** | ■ Forgetting that Entresto carries a superior mortality compared to ACEIs in HFrEF |
| | ■ Fear of inducing hypotension given Entresto has much stronger blood pressure–lowering effect |
| | ■ Logistical barriers such as scheduling to set up multiple appointments for transitioning safely (due to washout of ACEIs, lab draws, and so forth) |

| How to Avoid the Mistake | ■ Understand the superiority of Entresto in HFrEF, best evidenced by the PARADIGM-HF trial. |
| | ■ Transition starting with the low dose of Entresto (24/26 mg) to watch for hypotension. Though goals are tailored to the patient, generally transition to Entresto is not recommended if blood pressures are <100 mmHg. |
| | ■ Inpatient hospitalizations are great opportunities to transition patients safely to Entresto. |
| Antidote | ■ Not applicable |
| Common Scenarios | ■ Not applicable |
| Note(s) | ■ The bioavailability of valsartan is increased when combined with sacubitril. In terms of predicting antihypertensive effects, the 26 mg and 103 mg of valsartan within Entresto equate to 40 mg and 160 mg of stand-alone valsartan. |
| | ■ Remember that transitioning from an ACEI to Entresto requires a minimum 36-hour washout period. Multiple studies have shown increased adverse events in the setting of dual ACEI/ARB therapy. |
| Further Reading | ■ We recommend reading the PARADIGM-HF and PIONEER-HF trials. PARADIGM-HF was the landmark trial showing the superiority of Entresto compared to ACEIs, and PIONEER-HF demonstrated that inpatient initiation of Entresto was associated with improved reduction in NT-proBNP, suggesting at least a subclinical benefit to early initiation. |

## MISTAKE: TRANSITIONING TO ARNIs FROM ACEIs WITHOUT A WASHOUT PERIOD

| Case Example | A patient presents to your HFrEF clinic for GDMT optimization. You notice that the patient has been on Ramipril for years and eagerly transition the patient to Entresto. The next day, you receive an alert that the patient was admitted for hypotension. |
| Reasoning Error(s) | ■ Lack of knowledge about the increased adverse events with combination ACEI/ARB therapy |
| | ■ Forgetting that Entresto contains an ARB |
| | ■ Lack of knowledge regarding the duration required to reach negligible levels of ACEIs |
| How to Avoid the Mistake | ■ Always understand what components compose combination medications. |
| | ■ Remember that ACEIs require 36 hours for a complete washout. Studies such as the ONTARGET Trial noted an increase in renal dysfunction, hyperkalemia, and hypotension in patients who received combination ACEI/ARB therapy. |
| Antidote | ■ Not applicable |
| Common Scenarios | ■ Not applicable |

| | |
|---|---|
| **Note(s)** | ■ Entresto is contraindicated in pregnancy, as are ACEIs/ARBs. |
| | ■ Avoid Entresto in severe liver dysfunction (Child-Pugh Class C) due to potential adverse effects (not studied in this population). |

## MISTAKE: LIBERAL VASODILATOR USE IN SEVERE AORTIC STENOSIS

| | |
|---|---|
| **Case Example** | A 70-year-old female with HFrEF (EF = 20%) and severe aortic stenosis presents to your office for GDMT optimization. A big proponent of reaching target doses, you eagerly increase the dose of losartan from 10 mg to 40 mg. The same evening, the patient calls your emergency line from home noting extreme dizziness and chest pain and is soon taken to the emergency department. The patient is found hypotensive to 83/60. |
| **Reasoning Error(s)** | ■ Not realizing or forgetting that a medication is a vasodilator, especially if the main use of the medication is for another purpose (e.g., HFrEF mortality benefit) |
| | ■ Lack of recognition or knowledge of a patient's preload-dependent states |
| | ■ Using typical dosages of vasodilators in preload-dependent states |
| **How to Avoid the Mistake** | ■ Understand the mechanism of hypotension from vasodilators: decreases in preload due to expansion of the venous blood bed. |
| | ■ Recognize common vasodilators: calcium channel blockers, nitrates, hydralazine, ACEIs/ARBs. |
| | ■ Recognize and exercise increased caution with vasodilators in preload-dependent states such as aortic stenosis and severe pulmonary HTN. |
| **Antidote** | ■ Administer fluid bolus and hold vasodilators. |
| **Common Scenarios** | ■ Severe pulmonary HTN |
| | ■ Severe tricuspid regurgitation |
| | ■ Right ventricular failure |
| **Note(s)** | ■ Not only can vasodilators in preload-dependent states cause systemic hypotension, but they can also cause decreased coronary artery perfusion pressure (e.g., in states such as aortic stenosis where the LVEDP is high and oxygen demand is greater). |
| | ■ While liberal use is dangerous, it is equally inappropriate to withhold vasodilators completely. Judicious use of small doses can certainly help optimize hemodynamics! |

## MISTAKE: PRESCRIBING METOPROLOL IN THE SETTING OF HYPOTENSION

| | |
|---|---|
| **Case Example** | A 75-year-old female with HFrEF (EF = 15%) is admitted for decompensated HF. While diuresing, you attempt to optimize her GDMT as able. This morning, the patient's blood pressure is 81/60. Your senior tells you to increase the patient's metoprolol tartrate from 12.5 mg q6h to 25 mg q6h. An hour after administering the first dose, the patient's blood pressure drops to 75/55 and she complains of lightheadedness. |

| | |
|---|---|
| **Reasoning Error(s)** | ■ Misconception that metoprolol has "no" or "minimal" blood pressure effect |
| **How to Avoid the Mistake** | ■ Understand that metoprolol's average blood pressure effect is difficult to study given the varied dosing but that large meta-analyses have shown an average blood pressure–lowering effect between 5 and 10 mmHg with metoprolol of ≥50 mg. |
| **Antidote** | ■ Administer fluids to temporize if able. |
| **Common Scenarios** | ■ Not applicable |
| **Note(s)** | ■ Fractioned metoprolol (tartrate formulation) has a duration of action between 6 and 12 hours, whereas metoprolol succinate lasts for 24 hours. IV metoprolol tartrate pushes have a faster onset of action (5 minutes) but is shorter overall (approximately 5–8 hours). |

## MISTAKE: RAPID UPTITRATION OF β-BLOCKER DOSING (PARTICULARLY IN NEW HEART FAILURE)

| | |
|---|---|
| **Case Example** | A 45-year-old male with no significant past medical history presents with gradually worsening shortness of breath. A TTE reveals (LVEDD 5.1, IVS 1.0, LVPW 1.1, LVEF 25%), and you eagerly start the patient on metoprolol succinate 50 mg. You remember that achieving target doses is important for GDMT management and, over the course of the next 2 days, uptitrate to metoprolol succinate 200 mg. Unfortunately, a rapid response is called during the night on the patient who went into flash pulmonary edema due to cardiogenic shock. |
| **Reasoning Error(s)** | ■ Lack of consideration or knowledge about whether a patient is β-blocker naïve<br>■ Lack of experience or knowledge uptitrating β-blockers<br>■ Lack of complete knowledge regarding a patient's heart function (e.g., TTE has not yet resulted) and/or the acuity of the changes to function |
| **How to Avoid the Mistake** | ■ Elicit a careful history and medication reconciliation to determine whether a patient is β-blocker naïve.<br>■ Consider performing a quick bedside cardiac ultrasound to ensure that the patient's LV function is not newly severely depressed, which would be a relatively strong contraindication for initiating β-blockers early in the hospitalization.<br>■ Contextualize the risk and benefit of uptitrating β-blockers for patients. A patient with long-standing HFrEF is more adjusted to their low output state and will tolerate β-blockers (let alone higher doses) better. On the other hand, a patient with newly reduced EF (perhaps in the setting of ACS) is unaccustomed to the decrease in cardiac output, and β-blocker titration should be more gradual.<br>■ Determine whether the reduction in EF is likely recent by noting the LV end diastolic diameter (LVEDD). A weak ventricle will dilate over time to attempt to reposition itself on the Frank-Starling curve, thus a normal LVEDD suggests that the EF reduction is relatively recent. |

| | |
|---|---|
| **Antidote** | ■ Withhold further β-blockers. |
| | ■ AVOID fluids as their cardiac output is very poor in the setting of iatrogenic cardiogenic shock. |
| | ■ Consider use of pressors, particularly those that have mechanisms beyond catecholaminergic drive (since β-blockers block the receptors those inotropes work on). |
| **Common Scenarios** | ■ Not applicable |
| **Note(s)** | ■ The COMMIT-CCS 2 trial is often cited incorrectly as evidence to support overly cautious or limited β-blocker therapy in the setting of ACS. It must be noted that the protocol for uptitration of metoprolol in the trial is heavily criticized given that it uptitrated β-blocker naïve patients in the setting of new ACS up to the maximal dose of 200 mg metoprolol succinate very aggressively. This actually provides evidence for slower uptitration! |

## MISTAKE: WITHHOLDING β-BLOCKERS IN BRONCHOSPASTIC DISEASE

| | |
|---|---|
| **Case Example** | A 65-year-old male with long-standing COPD ($FEV_1$/FVC 62%) and newly discovered HFrEF (EF = 20%) presents to your outpatient clinic for follow-up. The patient is already on Entresto, and you consider which additional GDMT to add, settling on spironolactone and empagliflozin and deferring on β-blockers given the patient's COPD. Your attending raises his eyebrows as you present your plan. |
| **Reasoning Error(s)** | ■ Fear of adverse effects (e.g., bronchospasm) |
| | ■ Lack of knowledge regarding the occurrence rate of bronchospasm due to β-blockers |
| | ■ Treatment of bronchospastic disease as one entity rather than a spectrum of severity |
| | ■ Thinking about all β-blockers as equal in bronchospastic potential |
| **How to Avoid the Mistake** | ■ Understand not only the possible side effects but also the probability of the major side effects. Bronchospasm from β-blockers is exceedingly rare in the absence of preexisting bronchospastic lung disease and rare even in mild and moderate disease. |
| | ■ Think about diseases as on a spectrum of severity. It is rare for any disease to present with the same severity across patients. COPD and asthma are common comorbidities in many patients with HFrEF, and these patients should have judicious β-blocker therapy whenever possible. |
| | ■ Understand that not all β-blockers hold the same bronchospastic ability. Among the three β-blockers with mortality benefit in HFrEF, the ideal choice is bisoprolol followed by metoprolol then carvedilol, in the order of bronchospastic potential. This is because the selective $\beta_1$-antagonists are less likely to affect $\beta_2$-receptors on the smooth muscle surrounding the airways and only do so in off-target effects in a dose-dependent manner. Carvedilol, on the other hand, is nonselective and includes effect on $\beta_2$-receptors. |
| **Antidote** | ■ Not applicable |

**Common Scenarios** ■ Not applicable

**Note(s)**
- Relative contraindications to β-blockers include *severe* bronchospastic disease, significant first-degree heart block (defined as PR ≥ 0.24 ms by the FDA), and bradycardia.
- Absolute contraindications to β-blockers include second- and third-degree heart block (in the absence of a pacemaker) and severe bradycardia (HR <45 per the FDA).
- The FDA label for metoprolol succinate notes that bronchospastic disease is generally a contraindication. However, this is outdated and based on very old studies. Newer studies such as the BICS (Bisoprolol in COPD) study call into question the extent of danger of β-blockers in COPD (particularly when not severe).
- It is worthwhile to note that the large studies of various GDMT in HF were done in a sequential manner, meaning that newer therapies such as SGLT2 inhibitors were done in populations who were mostly on older therapies such as β-blockers. Thus, in one sense, the benefit of newer GDMT is in patients who are already on older therapies. However, small studies demonstrate that this is not necessarily the case.

**Further Reading**
- Quick summary regarding the latest evidence regarding β-blocker use in HFrEF patients with COPD: Lipworth B, et al. Beta blockers in COPD: time for reappraisal. *Eur Resp J* 2016;48:880–888.

## MISTAKE: TREATING COCAINE AS AN ABSOLUTE CONTRAINDICATION TO β-BLOCKER THERAPY

**Case Example**     A chronic IV drug user (cocaine, heroin) presents to you after using cocaine with SOB. A TTE demonstrates a reduced EF of 20%, which you believe is chronic given the LVEDD is 6.3. The patient takes no medications, and you decide that it would be ineffective to prescribe any medications for him, particularly β-blockers, in the setting of his cocaine use. Two months after discharge, you hear that the patient died from sudden cardiac death.

**Reasoning Error(s)**
- Well-intentioned and logical thinking based on known pathophysiologic mechanisms but with lack of corroborating empiric data
- Judgmental bias (e.g., assuming the patient would not take their β-blockers because of their association with illicit drug use)

**How to Avoid the Mistake**
- Understand the data around the use of β-blockers in cocaine users. Based on several meta-analyses, there does not appear to be any significant worsening in clinical outcomes (e.g., unopposed coronary vasospasm) with the use of β-blockers in cocaine users.
- Use historical precedent (actions) rather than stereotypes to determine likely medication adherence. However, in the absence of a significant contraindication (e.g., breeding resistance with inconsistent use of antiretroviral agents in HIV), there is little downside to prescribing medications to even nonadherent patients as they may change their habits and deserve the chance.

**Antidote**     ■ Not applicable

| Common Scenarios | ■ Not applicable |
|---|---|
| Note(s) | ■ Nonselective β-blockers with activity on α- and β-receptors, such as carvedilol, are theoretically even lower risk for adverse events in cocaine use (which targets the α-, β-, and dopaminergic receptors). |
| | ■ In patients presenting with chest pain after cocaine use, benzodiazepines are an effective treatment. |
| Further Reading | ■ Cochrane meta-analysis on use of β-blockers in cocaine users: Lo KB, et al. Clinical outcomes after treatment of cocaine-induced chest pain with beta-blockers: a systematic review and meta-analysis. *Am J Med.* 2019;132(4):505-509. |

## MISTAKE: WITHHOLDING ACEIs/ARBs/ARNIS AND/OR SPIRONOLACTONE FOR MILD HYPERKALEMIA

| Case Example | A 74-year-old male with HFrEF (EF = 20%), COPD, and CKD III presents to you for follow-up. His current GDMT regimen includes bisoprolol, losartan, and sotagliflozin. You want to start spironolactone but worry given the CKD and potassium level of 4.9. |
|---|---|
| Reasoning Error(s) | ■ Lack of pursuit for ways to find solutions to hurdles in patient care |
| | ■ Rigidity regarding K >5.0 as a cutoff beyond which increased adverse events occur, leading to fear that potassium level will surpass 5.0 with the addition of certain GDMT |
| | ■ Forgetting methods of decreasing total body potassium |
| | ■ Patient disinterest in additional medications |
| How to Avoid the Mistake | ■ Always think about creative methods to achieve the results that you want. Where there is a will, there is a way! |
| | ■ Understand that asymptomatic and well-tolerated potassium levels vary somewhat between patients and that a K >5.0 cutoff is not one nature has created as a rigid threshold beyond which adverse events occur. In other words, K >5.0 reflects a bias of beauty in that the number is visually appealing and easy. In patients with severe CKD or ESRD, their bodies are more tolerant of hyperkalemia given chronically high levels. |
| | ■ Consider the use of potassium binders such as Lokelma (sodium zirconium cyclosilicate) or patiromer, as well as low-potassium diets. Other methods include using medications that may have stronger potassium-wasting effects, such as chlorthalidone, over common medications such as hydrochlorothiazide. |
| | ■ Counsel the patient on the importance of GDMT and long-term outcomes and how that likely outweighs the addition of one more medication to their regimen. |
| Antidote | ■ Not applicable |
| Common Scenarios | ■ Not applicable |

| | |
|---|---|
| **Note(s)** | ■ In the EMPHASIS-HF trial, which demonstrated the mortality benefit of eplerenone in HFrEF, patients were started on eplerenone with a baseline K of as high as 4.9. Hyperkalemia was defined as K >5.5. Thus, the commonly used threshold of K >5.0 is an arbitrary, non–evidence-based threshold that should generally not deter addition of lifesaving medications. |
| | ■ In fact, numerous landmark GDMT trials such as SOLVD, CHARM, RALES, and PARADIGM-HF were designed with hyperkalemia defined as K >5.5 for safety data. Unsurprisingly, in trials that involved the combination of multiple potassium-increasing agents (e.g., RALES, which studied spironolactone added to ACEI or ARB therapy), the rate of hyperkalemia as defined above was significantly higher (approximately 15–20%); However, this means that 80–85% of patients who are challenged with these lifesaving medications will likely tolerate it! |
| | ■ For comparison of the incidence of hyperkalemia based on potassium cutoffs, we can look at the RALES trial; 19% of patients on ACEI/ARB plus spironolactone surpassed a threshold of K >5.5, whereas 51% of patients did so for K >5.0. Thus, abiding by the commonly used definition of K >5.0 is likely shortchanging many patients of lifesaving medications. |

## MISTAKE: PRESCRIBING SGLT2 INHIBITORS TO PATIENTS WITH FREQUENT UTIs

| | |
|---|---|
| **Case Example** | A 78-year-old female with recurrent hospitalizations (three or four per year) for urinary tract infections presents to your HF clinic. You notice that the patient is optimized on older GDMT but is yet to be on an SGLT2 inhibitor. A week after prescribing canagliflozin, the patient is admitted to the hospital with urosepsis and dies. |
| **Reasoning Error(s)** | ■ Lack of knowledge regarding common contraindications and adverse effects of SGLT2 inhibitors (or any other medications, particularly newer drugs) |
| | ■ Lack of complete information regarding a patient's comorbidities |
| **How to Avoid the Mistake** | ■ Learn the common side effects of medications that you commonly prescribe. |
| | ■ Assess patients for comorbidities that may contribute to increased adverse events with the drug in question. |
| **Antidote** | ■ Not applicable |
| **Common Scenarios** | ■ Urinary tract infections |
| | ■ Genital infections (e.g., yeast) |
| | ■ History of euglycemic diabetic ketoacidosis (DKA) |
| | ■ Severe peripheral arterial disease |
| | ■ GFR <30 mL/min/1.73 m$^2$ |

| | |
|---|---|
| **Note(s)** | ■ New evidence suggests that perhaps the risk of genital and urinary tract infections is not as significantly increased with SGLT2 inhibitors as previously thought. With new therapies, information will be limited and much of the clinical decision-making relies on individualizing the risk-benefit and involving the patient in decision-making. Notably, the above scenarios are all relative contraindications, with the exception of severe CKD. |
| | ■ The risk of amputation with SGLT2 inhibitors, particularly cana-gliflozin (from the CANVAS trial) is also under ongoing exploration. |

## MISTAKE: FORGETTING TO CONSIDER HYDRALAZINE/NITRATES, IVABRADINE, OR ICD THERAPY FOR GDMT

| | |
|---|---|
| **Case Example** | A patient with long-standing HFrEF (EF = 25%) presents to your clinic for follow-up. The patient is optimized on all GDMT, meaning 97–103 mg sacubitril-valsartan, 200 mg metoprolol succinate, 25 mg eplerenone, and 10 mg dapagliflozin. You note that the patient is doing great and send him home. |
| **Reasoning Error(s)** | ■ Lack of knowledge or familiarity with less common GDMT |
| | ■ Not assessing for how to optimize GDMT at each patient interaction |
| **How to Avoid the Mistake** | ■ Always assess for GDMT optimization in HF (both systolic and diastolic!) patients. The more you think through the possible options, the easier it will be to remember the less common GDMT agents. |
| **Antidote** | ■ Not applicable |
| **Common Scenarios** | ■ Hydralazine plus long-acting nitrates (self-reported Black patients, patients with severe CKD/ESRD intolerant of other GDMT) |
| | ■ Ivabradine (HR ≥70 after all other GDMT optimized) |
| | ■ ICD (EF <35%, ideally after 3 months of GDMT optimization) |
| **Note(s)** | ■ The A-HeFT Trial demonstrated a percent reduction in HF mortality with the addition of hydralazine and a long-acting nitrate in patients who self-reported as Black and were on optimal GDMT. Though off-label, some HF specialists trial patients on hydralazine and a long-acting nitrate even if they are not Black given (1) a lot of ancestry is mixed (especially prevalent in certain populations such as Dominican patients) and (2) the lack of options in patients with severe CKD/ESRD. |
| | ■ The SHIFT Trial demonstrated a 2% absolute reduction in HF-driven mortality and 5% absolute reduction in HF hospitalizations with the addition of ivabradine to patients who had a resting heart rate of ≥70 and on optimized GDMT. |
| **Further Reading** | ■ An excellent read on rethinking (extending) the timeline for ICD implantation: DeFilippis EM, et al. Waiting period before implant-able cardiac-defibrillator implantation in newly diagnosed heart failure with reduced ejection fraction. *Circ Heart Fail.* 2017;10:e004478. |
| | ■ Though yet to be incorporated into guidelines, the recent DAN-ISH Trial in 2016 cast increasing uncertainty on the benefit of ICD therapy in patients with non-ischemic cardiomyopathy: Kober L, et al. Defibrillator implantation in patients with nonischemic systolic heart failure. *N Engl J Med.* 2016;375(13):1221-1230. |

## MISTAKE: LACK OF PATIENT-CENTERED CONSIDERATION FOR A LIFEVEST FOR SEVERE ISCHEMIC HFrEF DURING GDMT OPTIMIZATION

**Case Example**

A 52-year-old female is admitted with a large anterior myocardial infarction and sent straight to the catheterization laboratory. She receives two stents to the mid-LAD and receives a TTE afterward, which demonstrates a newly reduced EF of 25%. Prior to discharge, you initiate her on losartan, metoprolol, and spironolactone and ensure she has good follow-up. When she misses her appointment with you, you discover that she died from sudden cardiac death 2 weeks after leaving the hospital.

**Reasoning Error(s)**

- Forgetting to think about how to treat a patient beyond the immediate hospitalization
- Lack of knowledge about the data surrounding sudden cardiac death post-MI
- Lack of belief in use of a wearable cardiac defibrillator (WCD) due to mixed data regarding its real-world effectiveness
- Not considering whether the patient is compliant to wearable vest therapy

**How to Avoid the Mistake**

- Remember to think of treatment for the acute scenario at hand but also long term (how to prevent complications and recurrent episodes).
- Understand that sudden cardiac death risk is highest in the first week and month after a large MI. A short-term WCD may be reasonable in high-risk patients (lower LVEF).
- Consider a patient-centered discussion about some of the mixed data surrounding a WCD. Given some relatively strong recent data on the lifesaving benefits of WCD after new ischemic cardiomyopathy, it is likely inappropriate to withhold a discussion with the patient.
- Inquire regarding patient's willingness, ability, and social support for wearing the portable cardiac defibrillator.

**Antidote**

- Not applicable

**Common Scenarios**

- Not applicable

**Note(s)**

- The VALIANT trial provided a great look into the frequency and associated factors of sudden cardiac death in patients with systolic dysfunction after myocardial infarction. The risk of SCD was highest in the first week after MI, and greatest among patients with the lowest EF. After the first week, the risk falls sharply within the first month but the absolute risk of SCD within the first month is still high (2.3% in the highest risk group with LVEF ≤30%).

## MISTAKE: FORGETTING AEROBIC EXERCISE PRESCRIPTIONS IN HFrEF AND HFpEF

**Case Example**

A 71-year-old female with NICM (EF = 15%) presents to your clinic for follow-up. Since the patient has no specific concerns, you continue optimizing her GDMT. Each visit, you forget to prescribe or counsel on exercise therapy.

| | |
|---|---|
| **Reasoning Error(s)** | ■ Lack of knowledge regarding the effectiveness of aerobic exercise in HF |
| | ■ Exclusive focus on medical therapy that leads to forgetting nonmedical interventions |
| | ■ Fear that exercise therapy may be dangerous for the patient with a frail heart |
| | ■ Thinking that the patient will be able to complete aerobic exercise therapy |
| **How to Avoid the Mistake** | ■ Understand the effectiveness of aerobic exercise. Studies have shown a reduction in hospitalizations and likely mortality with supervised exercise programs. Notably, its safety has been proven extensively and there is no evidence of adverse LV remodeling with exercise. |
| | ■ Always think about both medical and nonmedical treatment options. |
| | ■ Exercise training prescriptions should be individualized to the ability of the patient. Every step counts! |
| **Antidote** | ■ Not applicable |
| **Common Scenarios** | ■ Not applicable |
| **Note(s)** | ■ The HF-ACTION Trial is one of the largest trials assessing the role of exercise in chronic systolic HF. Importantly, it demonstrated that a relatively intense exercise regimen was safe for patients with severe HR (mean EF = 25%). Furthermore, it demonstrated a decrease in hospitalizations and probably mortality (a trend). |
| **Further Reading** | ■ Taylor RS. Exercise-based rehabilitation for heart failure. *Cochrane Database Syst Rev.* 2014;4:CD003331. |

## MISTAKE: NOT CONSIDERING GDMT FOR HFpEF

| | |
|---|---|
| **Case Example** | An 80-year-old female with HFpEF (EF = 65%) presents to your clinic after being hospitalized for decompensated HF. You undertake a lengthy discussion with the patient regarding the lack of medical therapies for HFpEF and the patient breaks out in tears, noting that their granddaughter will go to college soon. |
| **Reasoning Error(s)** | ■ Lack of knowledge regarding the latest advancements in HFpEF treatment |
| | ■ One-sided interpretation of HFpEF medical therapy based on limited positive data |
| **How to Avoid the Mistake** | ■ Learn the most recent developments in HFpEF medical therapy. These include the PARAGON-HF trial, which had a subanalysis demonstrating a reduction in HF mortality and hospitalization, leading the US FDA to announce Entresto as the first FDA-approved medical therapy for HFpEF in early 2021. A post hoc reanalysis of the TOP-CAT trial also demonstrated a mortality and hospitalization reduction with spironolactone. Most recently, the EMPEROR-PRESERVED trial in late 2021 demonstrated significant benefit for empagliflozin, regardless of diabetes status. |
| | ■ Though the evidence for HFpEF medical therapies is far from perfect, it opens the doors, and without a clear signal of increased significant adverse events, there is little reason to not trial patients on these therapies since there is a dearth of therapies available. Patient-centered discussions are key. |

| | |
|---|---|
| **Antidote** | ■ Not applicable |
| **Common Scenarios** | ■ Not applicable |
| **Note(s)** | ■ The TOPCAT trial was likely an unfortunate example of faulty ethics. Two of the four trial arms (Russia and Georgia) did not have evidence of a urinary metabolite of spironolactone, suggesting that the patients may not have received (consistently, at least) spironolactone. The aforementioned post hoc reanalysis took into consideration only the two arms (North and South America) that demonstrated clear evidence of patients taking spironolactone as intended. |
| | ■ Men who cannot tolerate spironolactone due to gynecomastia or breast tenderness may be switched to eplerenone, which has been shown in the EMPHASIS-HF trial to have approximately the same mortality benefit as spironolactone in HFrEF. |
| **Further Reading** | ■ A wonderful comprehensive review on HFpEF from its history to definitions to treatments and future directions by one of the legends of HFpEF, Dr. Marc Pfeffer: Pfeffer MA, et al. Heart failure with preserved ejection fraction in perspective. *Circ Res.* 2019;124(11):1598-1617. |

# Treatment: Vasopressors and Inotropes

## MISTAKE: USE OF β-BLOCKERS WHILE ON CATECHOLAMINERGIC PRESSORS OR INOTROPES

| | |
|---|---|
| **Case Example** | A patient with ischemic cardiomyopathy and chronic atrial fibrillation is admitted to you in cardiogenic shock. You continue her home metoprolol in fractionated form at 12.5 mg q6h to decrease the likelihood of her undergoing rapid ventricular response (RVR). You concurrently start Levophed (norepinephrine bitartrate) at 5 µg/min but notice that the patient is continuing to deteriorate. |
| **Reasoning Error(s)** | ■ Forgetting that there is overlap in the target receptors and receptors blocked |
| | ■ Lack of understanding regarding the physiology of the medications being used |
| **How to Avoid the Mistake** | ■ Understand that β-blockers, depending on selectivity, may inhibit $\beta_1$-, $\beta_2$-, and $\alpha_1$-receptors. Catecholamines such as norepinephrine, epinephrine, and dobutamine have effects on β- and α-receptors, and their actions are antagonized by β-blockers. However, the net effect depends on the relative dosages used; higher doses of inotropes are likely to overwhelm low doses of β-blockers. |
| | ■ Always strive to understand the basic physiology of medications utilized and pick the ideal pressors or inotropes for each clinical scenario (Table 8.3). |
| **Antidote** | ■ Switch to noncatecholaminergic inotropes: milrinone (phosphodiesterase inhibitor) or levosimendan (calcium sensitizer). |
| **Common Scenarios** | ■ Not applicable |

TABLE 8.3 ■ **Common Tricky Scenarios**

| Scenario | Ideal Pressor/ Inotropes | Alternate Pressors/ Inotropes | Less Than Ideal Pressors/Inotropes |
|---|---|---|---|
| LV outflow track obstruction (e.g., aortic stenosis and hypertrophic cardiomyopathy) | Phenylephrine | Norepinephrine | Dobutamine |
| Obstructive shock (pulmonary hypertension and pulmonary embolism) | Vasopressin (theoretical rather than practical) | Norepinephrine, dobutamine | Phenylephrine, dopamine |
| Cardiogenic shock | Dobutamine, milrinone | Dopamine, epinephrine (low) | Phenylephrine, epinephrine (high) |
| Septic shock | Norepinephrine | Phenylephrine, vasopressin | Epinephrine |
| Arrhythmias and ectopy | Phenylephrine | Norepinephrine, dobutamine | Dopamine, epinephrine |
| Concomitant β-blockade | Phenylephrine, vasopressin | Dopamine, milrinone | Norepinephrine, epinephrine, dobutamine |
| Active ischemia | Dobutamine | Dopamine, norepinephrine | Phenylephrine, epinephrine |

**Note(s)**

- Some physicians do use β-blockers in the presence of significant inotropes to suppress ectopy, though often higher doses of inotropes are required to adequately increase cardiac output. There is no clear evidence that this approach is clinically effective.
- Milrinone is renally cleared and thus should be avoided in patients with significant renal dysfunction. Signs of toxicity include dizziness, wheezing, chest pain or tightness, and severe arrhythmias.

## MISTAKE: LIBERAL USE OR INCORRECT CHOICE OF INOTROPES IN PATIENTS WITH ARRHYTHMIC SUBSTRATE AND/OR ISCHEMIA

**Case Example**

A 70-year-old male with HFrEF (EF = 20%) and long-standing atrial fibrillation is admitted for decompensated HF. Initial attempts at diuresis are ineffective despite hefty dosage increases, and then you discover rising AST/ALT indicating hypoperfusion. You start the patient on 4 µg/kg/min dobutamine. Half an hour later, the patient is noted to be in atrial fibrillation with RVR to the 180s.

**Reasoning Error(s)**

- Lack of information on patient comorbidities
- Forgetting the arrhythmogenic nature of all inotropes, regardless of mechanism (catecholaminergic or otherwise)
- Not tailoring inotrope choice to each patient and clinical scenario
- Not considering that inotropes increase myocardial oxygen demand, which not only exacerbates supply-demand mismatch (thus increasing infarct size) but also increases arrhythmias.

| | |
|---|---|
| **How to Avoid the Mistake** | ■ Assess patient for comorbidities that would predispose to arrhythmias. These include preexisting arrhythmia history, active or recent ischemia, and preexisting structural heart disease (e.g., scars/fibrosis, enlarged atria). |
| | ■ Understand the arrhythmogenicity of inotropes. From most to least: dopamine = epinephrine > milrinone > norepinephrine = dobutamine. |
| | ■ Judicious utilization (starting with low doses and slowly uptitrating) in patients with arrhythmogenic substrate. Choose inotropes based on individual comorbidities and the clinical disease state at hand. |
| | ■ In ischemia, a careful balance should be undertaken with maintaining perfusion and limiting worsening ischemia from increased myocardial oxygen demand and arrhythmias. Generally, this is until the patient requires inotrope support at least to bridge to mechanical support such as a balloon pump. During this critical period, the lowest possible dose of inotrope should be used. |
| **Antidote** | ■ Not applicable |
| **Common Scenarios** | ■ Preexisting arrhythmias (e.g., atrial fibrillation, ventricular tachycardia, frequent premature beats) |
| | ■ Structural heart disease (e.g., enlarged atria, scars/fibrosis, poor LV function) |
| | ■ Ischemia (active or recent revascularization) |
| **Note(s)** | ■ AVOID epinephrine in active ischemia. First-line inotropes in the setting of ischemia are either dobutamine or dopamine given they do not stimulate $\alpha_1$-receptors, which can significantly worsen ischemia. |
| | ■ Phenylephrine is not an inotrope; as a pure $\alpha$-agonist it should not increase arrhythmogenicity. |

## MISTAKE: AGGRESSIVE WEANING OR SUDDEN DISCONTINUATION OF INOTROPES

| | |
|---|---|
| **Case Example** | A 74-year-old female is hospitalized with cardiogenic shock requiring 10 μg/kg/min of dobutamine. Her hemodynamics soon improve with diuresis and her markers of end organ perfusion improve as well. You drop the dobutamine to 5 μg/kg/min and then an hour later stop it all together. Ten minutes later, the patient becomes unresponsive and is icy cold to the touch. |
| **Reasoning Error(s)** | ■ Lack of experience or knowledge on weaning inotropes safely |
| | ■ In a rush for whatever reason (e.g., to decrease length of hospitalization) |
| **How to Avoid the Mistake** | ■ Understand that inotropes require gradual weaning. Many inotropes have short half-lives and thus abrupt discontinuation or large falls in level will leave the heart in a "daze" (inability to contract adequately given the sudden loss of driving factor) and may precipitate cardiogenic shock. |
| | ■ Ask for help from more experienced physicians if uncomfortable weaning inotropes, especially for those that you have yet to become familiar. |

| | |
|---|---|
| **Antidote** | ■ If hemodynamically unstable, increase the inotrope back up and wean slower |
| **Common Scenarios** | ■ Not applicable |
| **Note(s)** | ■ Long-term inotropes (especially milrinone) are associated with increased mortality. |
| | ■ Some patients cannot be weaned off inotropes, termed inotrope dependence. |

## MISTAKE: HIGH-DOSE PHENYLEPHRINE IN AFTERLOAD-SENSITIVE DISEASES

| | |
|---|---|
| **Case Example** | A patient with severe pulmonary hypertension abruptly becomes hypotensive to 82/60. You react quickly by starting phenylephrine 100 µg/min. Seeing no response, you increase the phenylephrine to 200 µg/min. The blood pressure drops further to 74/55. You realize that the phenylephrine may be antagonizing forward blood flow by contributing to increased afterload and thus worsening the pulmonary hypertension. You stop the phenylephrine and the patient's blood pressure recovers to 84/58. |
| **Reasoning Error(s)** | ■ Failing to recognize an afterload-sensitive disease state |
| | ■ Focusing on the blood pressure–augmenting effects of phenylephrine without considering the mechanism ($\alpha_1$-agonism → constriction → increased afterload) |
| **How to Avoid the Mistake** | ■ Assess each cardiac disease state in terms of preload and afterload. |
| | ■ Associate phenylephrine with arterial vasoconstriction and increased afterload. |
| **Antidote** | ■ Decrease or discontinue phenylephrine. |
| **Common Scenarios** | ■ HF (any type: left, right, systolic, diastolic, valvular) |
| | ■ Severe pulmonary HTN |
| | ■ Massive pulmonary embolism |
| | ■ Severe mitral or aortic regurgitation |
| **Note(s)** | ■ As a pure $\alpha_1$-agonist, phenylephrine increases afterload but does not affect preload, since it has no impact on the venous circulation. |

## MISTAKE: USING DOBUTAMINE OR NOREPINEPHRINE IN HYPOTENSION IN THE SETTING OF LEFT VENTRICULAR OUTFLOW TRACT OBSTRUCTION

| | |
|---|---|
| **Case Example** | An 82-year-old male with critical aortic stenosis is admitted for failure to thrive in the setting of dysphagia and lack of home support. He is also experiencing profuse diarrhea and appears quite dehydrated. For the patient's hypotension to 81/55, you initiate dobutamine. The patient's blood pressure drops even further! |
| **Reasoning Error(s)** | ■ Lack of knowledge regarding best choice of inotrope in left ventricular outflow tract obstruction (LVOTO) |
| | ■ Not reasoning through the full pathophysiology of hypotension in LVOTO, such as thinking about afterload and deciding that phenylephrine should be avoided in hypotensive patients with LVOTO |
| | ■ Misunderstanding the afterload in aortic stenosis as dynamic (it is relatively fixed) |

| | |
|---|---|
| **How to Avoid the Mistake** | ■ Associate phenylephrine as the pressor of choice for hypotension in LVOTO.<br>■ Understand that aortic stenosis is a form of fixed afterload. That is, changes in afterload, such as with phenylephrine, minimally affect the cardiac output.<br>■ Understand that phenylephrine increases diastolic blood pressure and thus coronary perfusion (during diastole). Furthermore, phenylephrine may induce a reflex bradycardia which actually increases LV filling and decreases myocardial oxygen demand in the setting of LVOTO. |
| **Antidote** | ■ Quickly transition to phenylephrine.<br>■ Vasopressin is a reasonable second choice when phenylephrine is not available. |
| **Common Scenarios** | ■ Aortic stenosis<br>■ Hypertrophic obstructive cardiomyopathy<br>■ Any other anatomic variant that causes obstruction at the supravalvular, valvular, or subvalvular level |
| **Note(s)** | ■ Not all hypertrophic cardiomyopathies carry an obstructive phenotype (e.g., some hypertrophic cardiomyopathy may be apical); thus, it is important to characterize the LVOT gradient.<br>■ High doses (generally >15 µg/min) of norepinephrine cannot be used with peripheral intravenous access given its caustic nature. |

## CHAPTER 9

# Arrhythmias

Bliss J. Chang

Mistake: Adenosine in the Setting of Recent Caffeine Ingestion

Mistake: Adenosine in the Setting of Severe Reactive Airway Disease or Heart Block

Mistake: Pushing Adenosine Without a Saline Flush and/or Three-Way Stopcock

Mistake: Using the Same Voltages for Electrical Cardioversion/Defibrillation in All Patients

**Ventricular Tachycardia**

Mistake: Treating an Undifferentiated Wide-Complex Tachycardia as Supraventricular

Mistake: Diagnosing Supraventricular Tachycardia With Aberrancy Based on Termination of a Wide-Complex Tachycardia With Adenosine

Mistake: Forgetting to Assess for Reversible Causes of Ventricular Tachycardia

Mistake: Electrically Cardioverting All Stable Ventricular Tachycardia

Mistake: Withholding Magnesium in Torsade Due to Normal Magnesium Levels

Mistake: Overly Rapid Magnesium Administration in Torsade

Mistake: Forgetting to Treat Sympathetic Discharge in Ventricular Tachycardia

**Miscellaneous**

Mistake: Not STAT Consulting Cardiology for Inappropriate Implantable Cardioverter-Defibrillator Shocks

# Atrial Fibrillation/Flutter: General

## MISTAKE: NOT TREATING THE ETIOLOGY OF ATRIAL FIBRILLATION

| | |
|---|---|
| **Case Example** | You are called to the bedside of an older patient undergoing aggressive diuresis for acute decompensated heart failure (ADHF) who just went into atrial fibrillation with rapid ventricular response (RVR) to the 140s. The patient's heart rate settles with a 5 mg IV push of metoprolol but soon goes back into RVR. This pattern repeats throughout the night. |
| **Reasoning Error(s)** | ■ Only focusing on acutely controlling the rate or rhythm without thinking in the long term<br>■ Lack of understanding the various triggers of atrial fibrillation/flutter |
| **How to Avoid the Mistake** | ■ Always consider the etiology of atrial fibrillation/flutter. In many cases without a long-established history of arrhythmia, there is often a trigger that may be more effective at controlling the arrhythmia than commonly used medical management.<br>■ Think prevention in addition to current management. |
| **Antidote** | ■ Not applicable |
| **Common Scenarios** | ■ Intravascular volume imbalance<br>■ Electrolyte imbalance<br>■ Substance use (e.g., alcohol, cocaine)<br>■ Ischemia<br>■ Recent surgery (particularly cardiac/thoracic)<br>■ Structural heart disease (e.g., mitral regurgitation) |
| **Note(s)** | ■ Evidence of structural heart disease, in particular left atrial enlargement, can be helpful in the management of patients with atrial fibrillation. It may provide clues as to whether the atrial fibrillation is likely new or old, whether the patient has substrate for arrhythmia (is likely to difficult to rhythm control), or the presence of any driving factor that can be corrected. |

**Further Reading**
- Article based on the Framingham Heart Study examining common risk factors and substrates for atrial fibrillation: Kannel WB, et al. Prevalence, incidence, prognosis, and predisposing conditions for atrial fibrillation: population-based estimates. *Am J Cardiol.* 1998:82(8A):2N-9N.

# Atrial Fibrillation/Flutter: Anticoagulation

## MISTAKE: INCORRECT CALCULATION OF THE CHA$_2$DS$_2$-VASc SCORE (WOMEN, HFpEF, VASCULAR DISEASE)

**Case Example**
A 58-year-old female with heart failure with preserved ejection fraction (HFpEF) and new-onset atrial fibrillation presents to your office for a second opinion regarding anticoagulation. She believes that she should not be anticoagulated but notes that she was told she requires it. You calculate her CHA$_2$DS$_2$-VASc score to be 2 and agree that she should not be anticoagulated. The patient astutely asks about whether you are counting her sex as 1 point.

**Reasoning Error(s)**
- Lack of complete understanding of what factors contribute to the CHA$_2$DS$_2$-VASc score, particularly for C (heart failure with reduced ejection fraction [HFrEF] versus HFpEF) and V for "vascular disease"
- Applying the outdated interpretation of the CHA$_2$DS$_2$-VASc score with regard to the significance of female sex
- Lack of complete clinical information for calculating the CHA$_2$DS$_2$-VASc score

**How to Avoid the Mistake**
- Understand the nuances behind what each letter in the CHA$_2$DS$_2$-VASc score represents (see the Notes section).
- Perform a thorough investigation to ensure that you have a full understanding of the major stroke risk factors for each patient. For example, patients should be screened for peripheral arterial disease (PAD) (a significantly underdiagnosed disease) and receive chest imaging that may demonstrate the presence of aortic calcifications when determining whether to add a point for the "V."

**Antidote**
- Not applicable

**Common Scenarios**
- Female biologic sex
- HFpEF
- Vascular disease

**Note(s)**

- Remember, the $CHA_2DS_2$-VASc score only applies to nonvalvular atrial fibrillation. All patients with mitral stenosis and hypertrophic cardiomyopathy with atrial fibrillation should be anticoagulated.
- While the $CHA_2DS_2$-VASc score was developed during an era where HFrEF was more common and on a population that excluded HFpEF patients, a point should be given for "C" in HFpEF as well. HFrEF likely increases the incidence of stroke due to its association with arrhythmia as well as its long-term structural implications (e.g., increased left ventricular filling pressures leading to left atrial dilation). HFpEF is associated with a similar risk of stroke, has a higher rate of associated atrial fibrillation, and leads to left atrial dilation.
- The "V" in the $CHA_2DS_2$-VASc score was defined to include three types of vascular disease: myocardial infarction, PAD, and aortic plaque.
- The latest data from the Danish National Patient Registry demonstrate that female sex is a risk modifier rather than a risk factor. In other words, women with a $CHA_2DS_2$-VASc score ≥2 possess higher stroke risk than their male counterparts whereas women with a $CHA_2DS_2$-VASc score <2 do not achieve stroke risk comparable to their male counterparts. Thus, the new recommendation is for females with nonvalvular atrial fibrillation to be anticoagulated for $CHA_2DS_2$-VASc score ≥3 (with a score of 2 indicating patient-shared decision making similar to a score of 1 in men).

**Further Reading**

- A thoughtful viewpoint on whether HFpEF should count as a point for the $CHA_2DS_2$-VASc score: Mulder BA, et al. What should the C ('congestive heart failure') represent in the $CHA_2DS_2$-VASc score? *Eur J Heart Fail*. 2020;22(8):1294-1297.

## MISTAKE: CHEMICAL AND/OR ELECTRICAL CARDIOVERSION IN CHRONIC ATRIAL FIBRILLATION WITHOUT ANTICOAGULATION

**Case Example**

You are called to the bedside of a patient who went into atrial fibrillation approximately half a day ago. The patient states that she has never experienced palpitations before. You decide to use amiodarone to chemically cardiovert the patient given soft blood pressures. Your treatment works well, and the patient is in sinus rhythm within 1 hour of the amiodarone bolus. However, you notice a new dysarthria and droopy smile.

**Reasoning Error(s)**

- Assuming that the first discovery of atrial fibrillation/flutter is the first time ever the patient has had the arrhythmia
- Trusting the patient's well-intentioned subjective to determine acute versus chronic
- Lack of knowledge regarding the definitions of acute and chronic atrial fibrillation/flutter
- Incorrect belief that chemical cardioversion carries a different risk of thromboembolism than electrical cardioversion
- Believing that the chance of thromboembolism is low enough

| | |
|---|---|
| **How to Avoid the Mistake** | ■ Without clear, strong evidence that the arrhythmia is truly new, assume that the arrhythmia is chronic. Trust but verify history provided by the patient. |
| | ■ Understand that acute atrial fibrillation/flutter is defined as onset <48 hours. |
| | ■ Remember that the risk of thromboembolism postcardioversion remains the same regardless of cardioversion method (electrical, chemical, and even spontaneous cardioversion). Atrial stunning is not due to the electrical current delivered during cardioversion and is intrinsic to the restoration of sinus rhythm. This is evidenced by the lack of atrial stunning with failed cardioversion attempts. |
| | ■ Weigh the risk-benefit carefully. The absolute risk of stroke (not including other thromboembolism) after cardioversion in chronic atrial fibrillation is approximately 5–7%. This is a very high risk of permanent devastating damage. |
| | ■ If cardioversion is required, consider obtaining a transesophageal echocardiography to rule out any obvious clots in the left atrium and left atrial appendage, regardless of how recent the onset of atrial fibrillation appears to be. |
| **Antidote** | ■ If a clear neurologic deficit occurs after cardioversion, consider TPA as the likely etiology is cardioembolic |
| **Common Scenarios** | ■ Spontaneous cardioversion |
| | ■ Electrical cardioversion |
| | ■ Chemical cardioversion |
| | ■ Conversion via overdrive pacing and/or ablation |
| **Note(s)** | ■ Atrial stunning improves rapidly beginning immediately after cardioversion and continues to improve for several weeks thereafter. Factors that affect how quickly atrial stunning resolves include atrial size and duration of atrial fibrillation/flutter. |

## MISTAKE: LACK OF ANTICOAGULATION IMMEDIATELY POSTCARDIOVERSION FOR CHA$_2$DS$_2$-VASc 0

| | |
|---|---|
| **Case Example** | A patient presents in atrial fibrillation. You astutely provide the patient with 3 weeks of apixaban prior to cardioversion. After successful cardioversion, the patient goes home but is readmitted with a stroke 1 week later. |
| **Reasoning Error(s)** | ■ Thinking that anticoagulation is required only in the presence of active atrial fibrillation/flutter |
| | ■ Lack of understanding regarding why anticoagulation is needed immediately postcardioversion |
| | ■ Incorrect belief that anticoagulation in the immediate period after cardioversion is based on the CHA$_2$DS$_2$-VASc score |
| | ■ Only thinking about the acute scenario at hand |

| | |
|---|---|
| **How to Avoid the Mistake** | ▪ Understand that, regardless of cardioversion method, atrial stunning occurs after cardioversion that increases the risk of stroke.<br>▪ Understand that the chance of recurrence of atrial fibrillation/flutter after cardioversion (except ablation of the cavotricuspid isthmus in typical flutter) is high and may not be clinically apparent, thus requiring chronic anticoagulation except in select circumstances.<br>▪ Anticoagulate all patients after cardioversion for a minimum of 4 weeks and then decide long-term anticoagulation based on the patient characteristics (such as $CHA_2DS_2$-VASc).<br>▪ Always think about the potential short- and long-term complications to a procedure and how to minimize them. |
| **Antidote** | ▪ Anticoagulate! |
| **Common Scenarios** | ▪ $CHA_2DS_2$-VASc 0 or 1 |
| **Note(s)** | ▪ The most common site of clot formation in atrial fibrillation is the left atrial appendage. |

## MISTAKE: LACK OF LONG-TERM ANTICOAGULATION POSTCARDIOVERSION

| | |
|---|---|
| **Case Example** | A 70-year-old male with hypertension, type 2 diabetes, and HFpEF (EF = 65%) presents in atrial fibrillation. You astutely provide the patient with 3 weeks of apixaban prior to cardioversion. After successful cardioversion, the patient goes home on 4 weeks of apixaban again to minimize the stroke risk in the setting of atrial stunning. Given the patient has not had a recurrence of atrial fibrillation, the anticoagulation is not continued. Three months later, the patient is admitted with a right middle cerebral artery cardioembolic stroke. |
| **Reasoning Error(s)** | ▪ Thinking that anticoagulation is only required in the presence of active atrial fibrillation/flutter<br>▪ Lack of understanding regarding why or for who anticoagulation is needed long-term post-cardioversion |
| **How to Avoid the Mistake** | ▪ Understand that the chance of recurrence of atrial fibrillation/flutter after cardioversion (except ablation of the cavotricuspid isthmus in typical flutter) is high and may not be clinically apparent, thus requiring chronic anticoagulation except in select circumstances. This is often a difficult concept that requires careful explanation to patients.<br>▪ Decide upon long-term anticoagulation based on the $CHA_2DS_2$-VASc score. |
| **Antidote** | ▪ Anticoagulate! |
| **Common Scenarios** | ▪ Not applicable |
| **Note(s)** | ▪ The only exception to long-term anticoagulation in patients with atrial fibrillation and a high $CHA_2DS_2$-VASc score is left atrial occlusion (e.g., using the Watchman device). Thus, this is an option to reduce stroke risk in patients who cannot tolerate long-term anticoagulation. However, even after left atrial appendage closure, anticoagulation is generally required for a short period, though it may be avoided in patients with absolute contraindications by using 6 months of dual antiplatelet therapy (DAPT). |

## MISTAKE: LACK OF ANTICOAGULATION IN PAROXYSMAL ATRIAL FIBRILLATION

| | |
|---|---|
| **Case Example** | A 55-year-old male with HFrEF (EF = 20%) is discovered to be in paroxysmal atrial fibrillation. Interrogation of his ICD reveals that he has only been in atrial fibrillation on average for 40 seconds every month. The patient asks why he should be on anticoagulation. You realize that he has a great point and discontinue his anticoagulation. The patient is admitted for dysarthria the following month. |
| **Reasoning Error(s)** | ■ Well-intentioned and reasonable but incorrect logic that patients with shorter time in atrial fibrillation do not require anticoagulation<br>■ Lack of knowledge of regarding data on prevalence of stroke in paroxysmal atrial fibrillation |
| **How to Avoid the Mistake** | ■ Understand that while the risk of stroke is likely not truly equivalent in all types of atrial fibrillation/flutter (e.g., paroxysmal versus chronic) based on small studies in patients with long-term arrhythmia monitors, current guidelines recommend anticoagulation without discrimination given the significant stroke risk regardless of type or duration.<br>■ Anticoagulate all patients with any type (duration) of atrial fibrillation equally. The amount of atrial fibrillation that is considered significant is not consistently agreed upon yet. Most agree that hours of atrial fibrillation are significant, but not everyone agrees minutes seen on a pacemaker interrogation or telemetry merit anticoagulation. For now, the decision to anticoagulate is primarily based on the $CHA_2DS_2$-VASc score. |
| **Antidote** | ■ Anticoagulate! |
| **Common Scenarios** | ■ Paroxysmal atrial fibrillation<br>■ Asymptomatic atrial fibrillation |
| **Note(s)** | ■ In the SPORTIF and AMADEUS trials, the rate of stroke on anticoagulation for paroxysmal versus persistent atrial fibrillation was 0.93% versus 1.73%. However, some data suggest that this only applies to patients with lower risk of stroke. |
| **Further Reading** | ■ A statement from the American Heart Association on considering the burden of atrial fibrillation rather than treating it as a binary decision-tree: Chen LY, et al. Atrial fibrillation burden: moving beyond atrial fibrillation as a binary entity: a scientific statement from the American Heart Association. *Circulation*. 2018;137:e623-e644. |

## MISTAKE: USING THE $CHA_2DS_2$-VASc SCORE TO DETERMINE ANTICOAGULATION IN MITRAL STENOSIS, MECHANICAL VALVES, OR HYPERTROPHIC CARDIOMYOPATHY

| | |
|---|---|
| **Case Example:** | A 40-year-old female with severe rheumatic mitral stenosis presents for palpitations and is discovered to be in atrial fibrillation. You calculate her $CHA_2DS_2$-VASc score to be 0 and forego anticoagulation. The patient is admitted a month later with a cardioembolic stroke. |

**Reasoning Error(s)**
- Incorrect belief that CHA$_2$DS$_2$-VASc score applies to all types of atrial fibrillation
- Lack of knowledge of comorbid conditions that always require anticoagulation if tolerated

**How to Avoid the Mistake**
- Understand that the CHA$_2$DS$_2$-VASc score only applies to nonvalvular atrial fibrillation (which is just that induced by mitral stenosis or in the presence of a mechanical valve).
- In patients with atrial fibrillation and mitral stenosis, mechanical valves, or hypertrophic cardiomyopathy, always anticoagulate if tolerated.

**Antidote**
- Not applicable

**Common Scenarios**
- Mitral stenosis
- Mechanical valves
- Hypertrophic cardiomyopathy (does not need to be obstructive)

**Note(s)**
- Notably, anticoagulation for patients with mitral stenosis or mechanical valve(s) should be with warfarin. Newer data have provided convincing safety data on the use of direct-acting oral anticoagulants for atrial fibrillation in hypertrophic cardiomyopathy.
- Many amyloid experts support a very low threshold for anticoagulation in patients with atrial fibrillation and amyloid cardiomyopathy. This is based on an increased risk of stroke seen in this population.

## MISTAKE: ANTICOAGULATION WITH DIRECT ORAL ANTICOAGULANTS FOR VALVULAR ATRIAL FIBRILLATION

**Case Example**
A 40-year-old female with severe rheumatic mitral stenosis presents for palpitations and is discovered to be in atrial fibrillation. You astutely recognize that the CHA$_2$DS$_2$-VASc score does not apply in this case and start the patient on apixaban to save the patient from weekly blood draws. The patient is admitted a month later with a cardioembolic stroke.

**Reasoning Error(s)**
- Misconception that the choice of anticoagulant does not matter for atrial fibrillation
- Inability to discern mechanical from bioprosthetic valves

**How to Avoid the Mistake**
- Understand that limited data have shown direct oral anticoagulants (DOACs) to possess increased stroke risk in the presence of valvular atrial fibrillation. This, in combination with limited safety data (e.g., very small number of patients with valvular atrial fibrillation included in the big DOAC trials), has led to the recommendation against DOAC use in valvular atrial fibrillation.
- Recognize mechanical versus bioprosthetic valves. Always verify the material used in the valve replacement (e.g., with a chest radiograph, through record verification). The most common valve replacement (TAVR) uses a bioprosthetic valve, which would not require anticoagulation. In patients with a bioprosthetic valve and concomitant atrial fibrillation, there is emerging evidence to suggest that DOACs are appropriate choices.

**Antidote**
- Switch to a vitamin K antagonist (e.g., warfarin)

| | |
|---|---|
| **Common Scenarios** | ■ Mitral stenosis |
| | ■ Mechanical valves |
| **Note(s)** | ■ Note that patients with mechanical valves require anticoagulation regardless of the presence of atrial fibrillation. Hopefully they are already on anticoagulation! |
| **Further Reading** | ■ Interesting article on a hypothesis on why DOACs may still merit further study in patients with valvular atrial fibrillation (essentially why the first DOAC, studied in the context of valvular atrial fibrillation dabigatran, may have specific reasons to cause increased thromboembolism): Chan NC, et al. Anticoagulation for mechanical heart valves: will oral factor Xa inhibitors be effective? *Arterioscler Thromb Vasc Biol.* 2017;37(5):743-745. |

## MISTAKE: USING THE SAME INR GOAL FOR MECHANICAL VALVES REGARDLESS OF POSITION

| | |
|---|---|
| **Case Example** | A 40-year-old female with severe rheumatic mitral stenosis presents for palpitations and is discovered to be in atrial fibrillation. After a mechanical mitral valve replacement, you bridge the patient with Lovenox (enoxaparin sodium) to warfarin with an INR goal of 2.0–3.0. The patient presents 1 month later with hemiparesis. |
| **Reasoning Error(s)** | ■ Thinking that anticoagulation is the same in all patients (without nuance) |
| | ■ Lack of understanding the reasoning for varying INR goals |
| **How to Avoid the Mistake** | ■ Understand that the mitral mechanical valves carry increased thrombogenicity compared to aortic mechanical valves. This led to the recommendation for a higher INR goal in the mitral position (i.e., minimum 2.5 as opposed to 2.0). |
| | ■ Individualize INR goals based on the type of valve, position of the valve, and any breakthrough events on anticoagulation. Always reason through what the goal INR should be for each individual patient. |
| | ■ A notable problem with warfarin is the wide drift in INR levels even on stable doses. Therefore, the INR goal should never be on the lower end of the range, as downward drifts are effectively no better than control. Aim for at least the middle of the INR range (e.g., aim for 2.5 for a goal of 2.0–3.0 for atrial fibrillation). |
| **Antidote** | ■ Not applicable. |
| **Common Scenarios** | ■ Mitral mechanical valve (INR goal 2.5–3.5) |
| **Note(s)** | ■ Even on anticoagulation, the risk of thromboembolism in patients with a mechanical valve is greater than that of a bioprosthetic valve (approximately 2% versus 0.7%). |

## MISTAKE: FORGETTING TO CONSIDER LEFT ATRIAL APPENDAGE CLOSURE FOR PATIENTS WITH HIGH BLEEDING RISK

**Case Example**

A 94-year-old female with nonvalvular atrial fibrillation and multiple prior GI bleeds has been continued on apixaban for 2 months since a Holter monitor first demonstrated atrial fibrillation. One day, she is found alone in her house with a massive GI bleed, laying unresponsive in a large pool of hematochezia.

**Reasoning Error(s)**

- Forgetting that it may be possible to avoid anticoagulation in patients with atrial fibrillation and prohibitively high bleeding risk
- Lack of thorough risk-benefit discussion with patient

**How to Avoid the Mistake**

- Understand that the long-term goal of left atrial appendage closure is to free patients from anticoagulation, hence a great choice for patients with prohibitive bleeding risk. The risk of stroke after a Watchman was noninferior to anticoagulation with warfarin in the PROTECT-AF trial.
- Thoroughly inform the patient of all alternatives, risks, and benefits for each clinical action.

**Antidote**

- Not applicable

**Common Scenarios**

- Not applicable

**Note(s)**

- Although left atrial appendage closure/occlusion may obviate the need for long-term anticoagulation, it is generally preferred that the patient is anticoagulated in the short term (generally 45 days as per the PROTECT-AF trial protocol) after device placement due to slightly increased risk of thrombogenic events. In cases where anticoagulation is absolutely prohibited, DAPT may be used instead.
- There are various types of left atrial appendage closure devices: the Watchman, Amplatzer, and WaveCrest. While we have the most data for the Watchman, they are treated as approximately equivalent methods.

## MISTAKE: FAILING TO CONSIDER ANTIPLATELET MONOTHERAPY IN PATIENTS WITH HIGH BLEEDING RISK

**Case Example**

A 94-year-old female with nonvalvular atrial fibrillation and multiple prior GI bleeds has been continued on apixaban for 2 months since a Holter monitor first demonstrated atrial fibrillation. One day, she is found alone in her house with a massive GI bleed, laying unresponsive in a large pool of hematochezia.

**Reasoning Error(s)**

- Lack of awareness of the data and potential usage of antiplatelet therapy alone for stroke reduction in atrial fibrillation
- Lack of knowledge regarding the efficacy of antiplatelet agents in stroke reduction in atrial fibrillation
- Searching for an ideal solution rather than settling for the best solution under a given set of circumstances

| How to Avoid the Mistake | ■ Remember that an alternative off-guideline consideration to left atrial occlusion is the use of only antiplatelet agents (monotherapy) for patients who have an absolute contraindication to anticoagulation and are not operative candidates (or do not wish a left atrial appendage closure). |
|---|---|
| | ■ Understand the efficacy of common agents used to prevent thromboembolism in atrial fibrillation. In the SPAF-I study, warfarin and aspirin (325 mg) reduced the rate of stroke by 67% and 42%, respectively. Later, the SPAF-II study demonstrated the superiority of warfarin over aspirin (1.3% versus 1.9%) for preventing systemic thromboembolism. In the ACTIVE-W study, warfarin was superior to DAPT (aspirin + clopidogrel) in reducing the rate of stroke and had lower bleeding risk. |
| Antidote | ■ Not applicable |
| Common Scenarios | ■ Not applicable |
| Note(s) | ■ Aspirin monotherapy may also be considered for patients with an intermediate $CHA_2DS_2$-VASC score (1 in men, 2 in women). |
| | ■ Notably, warfarin therapy is challenging due to fluctuations in INR. In many large trials, patients were able to obtain therapeutic INR's approximately two-thirds of the time. |
| | ■ The benefit of aspirin or clopidogrel for stroke prevention in atrial fibrillation is marginal, and many electrophysiologists no longer prescribe them for low CHADs patients. The modest effect of aspirin may be for non–atrial fibrillation sources of embolic stroke. |
| Further Reading | ■ The landmark SPAF trial that first investigated the efficacies of aspirin and warfarin in stroke prevention for patients with atrial fibrillation: SPAF Investigators. Stroke Prevention in Atrial Fibrillation Study. *Circulation*. 1991;84:527-539. |

# Atrial Fibrillation/Flutter: Rate Control

## MISTAKE: UNREALISTIC EXPECTATIONS AND TITRATION OF RATE (AND RHYTHM) CONTROL

| Case Example | A 78-year-old female with atrial fibrillation comes to your office for management of persistent palpitations. She is already on metoprolol 100 mg daily and amiodarone 400 mg daily. Despite this regimen, she experiences palpitations twice a week. Given that the patient continues to experience symptoms, you presume that her current therapy is not working and add propafenone. |
|---|---|
| Reasoning Error(s) | ■ Misconception that rate control will perfectly control a patient's heart rate under a specific goal 100% of the time |
| | ■ Misconception that rhythm control agents are binary in efficacy (converts and keeps patient in sinus rhythm versus do not work at all) |

| | |
|---|---|
| **How to Avoid the Mistake** | ■ Understand that the goal of rate and rhythm control is to decrease the severity, frequency, and duration of atrial fibrillation and/or rapid ventricular response. Therapy may not be effective 100% of the time. For example, a patient's rates may be controlled to under 110 on average but they may experience brief periods of faster rates, or a patient may intermittently flip in and out of atrial fibrillation. The goal is to reduce atrial fibrillation burden to the point that symptoms are tolerable.<br>■ Set realistic expectations and optimize therapy based on stepwise improvements rather than in a binary fashion of effective or not.<br>■ Elicit careful patient histories to guide the titration of rate and rhythm control medications. |
| **Antidote** | ■ Not applicable |
| **Common Scenarios** | ■ Intermittent rapid ventricular rates<br>■ Intermittent atrial fibrillation/flutter |
| **Note(s)** | ■ In addition to managing the clinician's expectations, the patient's expectations should also be managed by informing them of realistic outcomes based on the treatments. This may also contribute to psychologic acceptance and improvement of symptomology. |

## MISTAKE: EXCESSIVELY STRICT RATE CONTROL

| | |
|---|---|
| **Case Example** | A 79-year-old female with permanent atrial fibrillation ($CHA_2DS_2$-VASC 6) presents to your office for a routine follow-up. Her heart rate is 106 bpm. She also brought her Apple watch with her, and you are able to see that her average heart rate is between 100 and 105 bpm. She reports no symptoms. You increase her metoprolol succinate dosage from 100 mg to 200 mg daily. She returns 1 week later reporting intermittent lightheadedness. |
| **Reasoning Error(s)** | ■ Lack of knowledge regarding the heart rates ideal for decreasing cardiovascular events<br>■ Discomfort associated with relatively high heart rates (e.g., 100 bpm appears abnormal and may cause discomfort) |
| **How to Avoid the Mistake** | ■ Understand the data for ideal heart rate in permanent atrial fibrillation. The RACE-II study demonstrated no difference in major cardiovascular outcomes (including cardiovascular mortality, heart failure, stroke, and arrhythmic events) between strict (<80 bpm) versus lenient (<110 bpm) rate control. Notably, this study was investigating rate control in patients who were asymptomatic. However, in order to prevent tachycardia-induced cardiomyopathy, the general goal is to have resting heart rates well below 100 bpm, even if asymptomatic, although some studies suggest lenient rate control is no worse than strict control.<br>■ Develop comfort by individualizing the risks and benefits of any clinical action. For example, while there was no difference in major cardiovascular events, the strict rate control arm did have a nonsignificant but positive trend across the board for adverse events such as dizziness and hypotension. |

| Antidote | ■ Not applicable |
| --- | --- |
| Note(s) | ■ From a systems perspective, stricter rate control usually requires more hospital visits and higher medication dosages. |
| | ■ Though the heart rate threshold for tachycardia-mediated cardiomyopathy is unknown, any tachycardic rate (i.e., >100 bpm) is thought to have some risk. As such, it is reasonable to increase control to a threshold lower than 110 bpm in the RACE-II study. Interestingly, the mean heart rate achieved in RACE-II was 76 and 93 bpm for the strict and lenient control arms, respectively. |
| | ■ Remember that the RACE-II heart rate thresholds were for patients at rest. In the presence of moderate exercise, the heart rate maximum for the strict rate control arm was defined as <110 bpm. |
| | ■ If medications are limited due to side effects, other therapies like atrioventricular (AV) node ablation and pacing can be considered. |
| Further Reading | ■ The landmark RACE-II trial is worth a read to further understand the study's nuances: Van Gelder IC, et al. Lenient versus strict rate control in patients with atrial fibrillation. *N Engl J Med.* 2010;362(15):1363-1373. |

## MISTAKE: LENIENT RATE CONTROL IN SYMPTOMATIC ATRIAL FIBRILLATION

| Case Example | A 79-year-old female with permanent atrial fibrillation ($CHA_2DS_2$-VASC 6) presents to your office for a routine follow-up. Her heart rate is 106 bpm. She also brought her Apple watch with her, and you are able to see that her average heart rate is between 100–105 bpm. She reports significant palpitations and decreased exercise tolerance. Her transthoracic echocardiogram demonstrates normal heart function. You keep her on her current metoprolol succinate 100 mg. The patient becomes very irate and demands better control of her symptoms. |
| --- | --- |
| Reasoning Error(s) | ■ Incorrect application of the RACE-II trial data to all patients with atrial fibrillation |
| | ■ Lack of understanding of how heart rate influences hemodynamics in atrial fibrillation and heart failure |
| | ■ Lack of up-to-date information on patient's symptoms and comorbidities |
| | ■ Psychological bias that inaction is less consequential than acting |
| How to Avoid the Mistake | ■ Remember that the RACE-II trial investigated only patients who were asymptomatic. Control heart rates to provide symptomatic relief and based on the unique clinical circumstances for each patient (e.g., patients with HFrEF may be more symptomatic with higher heart rates). |
| | ■ Understand that faster heart rates lead to decreased ventricular filling due to less diastolic filling time. This leads to decreased cardiac output, which is further amplified by the lack of atrial kick in atrial fibrillation and poor left ventricular function in heart failure. The summation of this may be significant symptoms such as decreased exercise tolerance. |
| | ■ Always establish as comprehensive a handle on a patient's symptoms and comorbidities as possible prior to making a clinical action. |
| | ■ Understand that inaction can be a clinical error as much as an act of commission. |

**Antidote** ■ Not applicable

**Common Scenarios** ■ Symptomatic atrial fibrillation
■ Cardiac resynchronization therapy (CRT)
■ Heart failure (for hemodynamics)

**Note(s)** ■ Interestingly, a post hoc analysis of the RACE-II data did not demonstrate any difference in cardiovascular outcomes or quality of life between strict and lenient rate control in patients with both atrial fibrillation and heart failure. However, some experts do advocate for stricter rate control in patients with heart failure.
■ Stricter rate control is required for optimal benefit from CRT because the CRT device needs to pace the ventricles, meaning that high intrinsic ventricular rates preclude the CRT device from taking effect.

**Further Reading** ■ An older but great review on tachycardia-mediated cardiomyopathy: Umana E, et al. Tachycardia-induced cardiomyopathy. *Am J Med.* 2003:114(1):51–55.

## MISTAKE: RATE CONTROL OF COMPENSATORY RAPID VENTRICULAR RATES

**Case Example** A 79-year-old male with HFrecEF (EF = 55–60%), chronic atrial fibrillation on dabigatran and metoprolol, and recent stents to the mid-left anterior descending coronary artery presents with profound hypotension (SBP 60s) in the setting of hemorrhagic shock. The patient is in atrial fibrillation with rates in the 130s. You continue the patient's home metoprolol succinate to control the rates. You feel proud of reducing the rates to under 100 but are dismayed to see that the patient's blood pressure drops further to SBP 50s.

**Reasoning Error(s)** ■ Reliance on fast thinking and association of high ventricular rates to a need for rate control without thinking about each individual scenario
■ Continuing home medications (e.g., metoprolol) without thinking about individual cases

**How to Avoid the Mistake** ■ Always think about the driving factors behind any pathology such as rapid ventricular rate. For example, in a patient with chronic atrial fibrillation, the heart rate response may be due to overexcitability associated with the nature of atrial fibrillation, but it may also be in response to a stressor such as hypovolemia (akin to compensatory sinus tachycardia).
■ Reassess suitability of chronic therapies in the setting of acute clinical changes. For example, home metoprolol may be inappropriate in the setting of hypotension and/or hemorrhage.

**Antidote** ■ Decrease or withhold unnecessary rate control

**Common Scenarios** ■ Sepsis
■ Hypovolemic shock (e.g., hemorrhage)
■ Brief periods of sympathetic release (e.g., movement, emotion)

**Note(s)** ■ The ventricular rate can provide insight to whether the RVR is more compensatory or intrinsic excitability of the myocardium. For instance, jumping from a rate of 90–180 is likely not compensatory.

## MISTAKE: NOT CONSIDERING VAGAL MANEUVERS FOR ACUTE RATE CONTROL

| | |
|---|---|
| **Case Example** | A 23-year-old female with uncontrolled hyperthyroidism presents with dizziness and is found to be in AVNRT with rates up to the 180s. Blood pressure remains stable in the low 110s. You immediately proceed to administer IV metoprolol in an attempt to rate control the patient. |
| **Reasoning Error(s)** | ■ Subconscious bias favoring pharmacologic therapies as more effective<br>■ Lack of knowledge regarding effectiveness of nonpharmacologic therapies for acute rate control leading to dismissal as a viable option |
| **How to Avoid the Mistake** | ■ Always consider cost-effective and nonpharmacologic interventions in addition to more invasive and pharmacologic options.<br>■ Understand the proper technique to optimize the success of vagal maneuvers for acute rate and rhythm control. The REVERT trial demonstrated that a modified Valsalva maneuver is effective at terminating up to 44% of supraventricular tachycardias (SVTs). Given the minimal side effect profile, vagal maneuvers are an excellent choice for initial treatment of arrhythmias. |
| **Antidote** | ■ Not applicable |
| **Common Scenarios** | ■ Any supraventricular arrhythmia (though certain rhythms such as flutter are traditionally more difficult to control without electrical cardioversion) |
| **Note(s)** | ■ Be wary of using a carotid sinus massage in patients with significant carotid stenosis as the risk of stroke from dislodging a clot is approximately 1 in 1000 massages. You can consider auscultating over the carotids for bruits prior to performing a carotid massage. |
| **Further Reading** | ■ The REVERT trial is worth a read! It investigated the utility of a modified vagal maneuver for the acute termination of supraventricular arrhythmias: Appelboam A, et al. Postural Modification to the Standard Valsalva Manoeuvre for Emergency Treatment of Supraventricular Tachycardias (REVERT): a randomised controlled trial. *Lancet.* 2015;386(10005):1747–1753. |

## MISTAKE: USING NONDIHYDROPYRIDINE CALCIUM CHANNEL BLOCKERS FOR RATE CONTROL IN HFrEF

| | |
|---|---|
| **Case Example** | A 73-year-old female with HFrEF (EF = 30%) is admitted for decompensated heart failure. After aggressive diuresis, the patient is found to be in atrial fibrillation with rapid ventricular response. You give the patient diltiazem to try and control the heart rate. Unfortunately, the patient enters cardiogenic shock and is transferred to the cardiac intensive care unit. |
| **Reasoning Error(s)** | ■ Not routinely considering contraindications and adverse effects of a clinical action<br>■ Lack of knowledge regarding common contraindications for patients with HFrEF |

**How to Avoid the Mistake**

- Always think of not only the indication but also the contraindication to each clinical action (diagnostic or therapeutic).
- Understand that the negative inotropic effects of nondihydropyridine calcium channel blockers may cause decompensation in patients with systolic dysfunction. β-Blockers have counterintuitively been shown to be beneficial despite their negative inotropy, probably more related to autonomic effects. They should be initiated slowly.

**Antidote**

- Discontinue nondihydropyridine use.

**Common Scenarios**

- Diltiazem
- Verapamil

**Note(s)**

- Dihydropyridine calcium channel blockers such as amlodipine, felodipine, and nifedipine are generally safe for judicious use in HFrEF if needed based on small studies. However, heart failure specific medications (i.e., GDMT) should be prioritized for blood pressure control.
- While β-blockers are considered safer in the presence of systolic dysfunction, they should be used judiciously as they may also lead to cardiogenic shock.

## MISTAKE: USING β-BLOCKERS OR CALCIUM CHANNEL BLOCKERS IN SINUS NODE OR ATRIOVENTRICULAR NODE DYSFUNCTION

**Case Example**

A 78-year-old female with intermittent Mobitz I heart block presents to the emergency department with atrial fibrillation with RVR. You quickly administer 5 mg of metoprolol IV and repeat the dose 5 minutes later due to continued RVR. The patient's heart rhythm suddenly regularizes, and the rate drops to the 40s with subsequent ECG demonstrating complete heart block.

**Reasoning Error(s)**

- Not routinely considering contraindications and adverse effects of a clinical action
- Lack of knowledge of the mechanism of β-blockers

**How to Avoid the Mistake**

- Understand the mechanism by which β-blockers control heart rate. They slow not only the AV node but also the sinus node. Use of β-blockers (especially high doses) may lead to high-grade heart block, long conversion pauses, and/or further depression of sinus node dysfunction.
- Always think of not only the indication but also the contraindication to each clinical action (diagnostic or therapeutic).

**Antidote**

- Hold further β-blockers
- Apply cardioversion pads to patient for safety

**Common Scenarios**

- β-Blockers
- Calcium channel blockers
- Amiodarone

| | |
|---|---|
| **Note(s)** | ■ β-Blockers are not absolutely contraindicated in the presence of sinus node or AV node dysfunction (e.g., first-degree AV block), but extreme care should be exerted, and doses should be escalated gradually under monitoring. In high-degree heart block (second-degree or higher), β-Blockers are absolutely contraindicated. |
| | ■ Note that β-blockers affect AV nodal (and not infra-Hisian) conduction. Thus, for example, it would not be expected that a β-blocker necessarily worsens Mobitz II block though out of an abundance of caution they are typically avoided. |

## MISTAKE: ATRIOVENTRICULAR NODAL BLOCKADE IN PREEXCITED ATRIAL FIBRILLATION

| | |
|---|---|
| **Case Example** | A 24-year-old male presents with an irregularly irregular wide-complex rhythm. After a careful glance, you astutely diagnose preexcited atrial fibrillation. You immediately order metoprolol to control the rate. To your bewilderment, the patient's heart rates jump dramatically to the high 200s and then soon degenerates into ventricular fibrillation. |
| **Reasoning Error(s)** | ■ Lack of knowledge regarding contraindications to treatment of preexcited atrial fibrillation |
| | ■ Not thinking through preexcited atrial fibrillation mechanistically when considering contraindications |
| | ■ Fast thinking and relying on reflexes such as AV nodal blockade for atrial fibrillation |
| **How to Avoid the Mistake** | ■ Understand the rationale behind contraindication of AV nodal blockade in preexcited atrial fibrillation. Remember that electrical signals always travel the path of least resistance. The presence of a more refractory AV node diverts more signals to the accessory pathway that can conduct at extremely fast rates and potentially degenerate into ventricular tachycardia (VT) or fibrillation. |
| | ■ Especially for unfamiliar conditions, consider reasoning through the pathophysiology and interventions mechanistically to help elicit possible contraindications that are not commonly taught. |
| | ■ Remember that procainamide is safe for all types of wide-complex tachycardias, whether preexcited or aberrant or ventricular. |
| | ■ Practice slow thinking and ask for help managing unfamiliar scenarios. |
| **Antidote** | ■ Cardioversion |
| | ■ Procainamide |
| **Common Scenarios** | ■ β-Blockers |
| | ■ Calcium channel blockers |
| | ■ Amiodarone |
| | ■ Digoxin |
| | ■ Adenosine (though less dangerous given its short half-life) |

**Note(s)**

- The first-line treatment for preexcited atrial fibrillation is procainamide given its lack of effectiveness on the AV note while decreasing the excitability of the accessory pathway. Second-line treatment is ibutilide.
- Procainamide can induce hypotension if given too rapidly and has negative inotropic effects, so it's necessary to be careful in heart failure patients
- Preexcited atrial fibrillation may mimic monomorphic VT in several ways, such as precordial concordance. The key differentiating feature is the irregularity associated with preexcitation.

## Atrial Fibrillation/Flutter: Rhythm Control

### MISTAKE: ANTIARRHYTHMIC THERAPY AFTER A SINGLE EPISODE OF ATRIAL FIBRILLATION/FLUTTER

**Case Example**

A 39-year-old female with morbid obesity presents to your clinic for a preop evaluation prior to undergoing bariatric surgery. She is coincidentally noted to be in atrial fibrillation but remains asymptomatic. Happy to have identified atrial fibrillation, you eagerly start her on amiodarone and a Holter monitor. Two weeks later, the patient returns, and you beam at the Holter results that demonstrate no further atrial fibrillation.

**Reasoning Error(s)**

- Lack of careful assessment of a common condition, potentially due to viewing the disease in an oversimplified manner
- Forgetting to consider the etiology of the arrhythmia
- Lack of knowledge regarding the side effect profile of antiarrhythmic therapy

**How to Avoid the Mistake**

- Think carefully about antiarrhythmic therapy. Generally, it becomes a lifelong medication, though they do not have to be lifelong therapy. In fact, antiarrhythmic drugs are rarely effective for a patient's lifetime.
    - Does the patient actually require antiarrhythmic therapy (e.g., is the patient symptomatic or experiencing the arrhythmia often, especially in uncontrolled or dangerous ways)? What is the context in which the arrhythmia was discovered (e.g., post-cardiac surgery versus hospitalization)?
    - Is this the right time to start an antiarrhythmic (e.g., hemodynamically unstable)?
    - Do you have enough information about the arrhythmia to inform long-term care for the patient (e.g., does it occur once a year or persist for weeks at a time)?
    - Does the patient have comorbidities (e.g., heart failure) that would be better served with rhythm control?
- Understand that generally rhythm control agents possess a more significant short- and long-term side effect profile compared to rate control agents.
- Always assess for reversible causes of atrial fibrillation, including hypo/hyperthyroidism, electrolyte abnormalities, and ingestions (e.g., alcohol, recreational drugs).

**Antidote**

- Not applicable

**Common Scenarios**

- Not applicable

**Note(s)**
- Atrial fibrillation burden is a concept that strives to move away from thinking about atrial fibrillation in a binary manner (present or not). This is useful, since not all atrial fibrillation shares the same features such as duration and stroke risk.

## MISTAKE: DAILY ANTIARRHYTHMICS FOR INFREQUENT ATRIAL FIBRILLATION

**Case Example**
A 45-year-old male presents to your clinic for management of intermittent palpitations. He was recently on a long-term loop recorder and discovered to have brief episodes of atrial fibrillation a few times a week. You start the patient on amiodarone, and the patient's symptoms disappear. However, 5 years later, the patient is noted to have bluish sclera and hyperthyroidism.

**Reasoning Error(s)**
- Forgetting the option to use pill-in-the-pocket therapy
- Lack of understanding of the evidence behind pill-in-the-pocket therapy
- Institutional or training background–related unfamiliarity with pill-in-the-pocket therapy

**How to Avoid the Mistake**
- Remember that antiarrhythmic therapy may be used in several manners: one-time (e.g., cardioversion in the setting of rapid ventricular response), daily, and pill-in-the-pocket (as needed).
- Understand the evidence behind pill-in-the-pocket therapy for atrial fibrillation. Several studies, including a prominent study in *The New England Journal of Medicine* in 2004 by Alboni et al., have demonstrated effectiveness of the pill-in-the-pocket approach and decreased hospitalization or emergency visits. However, its overall efficacy is not high, and the approach is most reasonable for patients with rare atrial fibrillation.
- Learn how to effectively prescribe pill-in-the-pocket therapy. Patients should be reliable and able to recognize their symptoms and quickly consume the antiarrhythmic drug of choice. The two most common antiarrhythmics used for pill-in-the-pocket approach are flecainide and propafenone.

**Antidote**
- Not applicable

**Common Scenarios**
- Paroxysmal atrial fibrillation

**Note(s)**
- Be sure to rule out the presence of significant structural heart disease (e.g., systolic dysfunction, coronary artery disease, significant left ventricular hypertrophy) prior to using Class 1C antiarrhythmics, as there is a significant increase in mortality in those patients! Because many patients with atrial fibrillation possess structural heart disease, the use of the pill-in-the-pocket approach is limited.
- Natural history studies on paroxysmal atrial fibrillation have shown that most episodes self-terminate within 24–48 hours; however, the pill-in-the-pocket approach is useful for quicker termination of episodes that are symptomatic.
- Daily antiarrhythmic therapy can have additional undesirable consequences such as increasing pacing or defibrillation thresholds. Be judicious about use of antiarrhythmics!

**Further Reading**

- A wonderful review article on pill-in-the-pocket treatment of paroxysmal atrial fibrillation: Reiffel JA, et al. "Pill in the pocket" antiarrhythmic drugs for orally administered pharmacologic cardioversion of atrial fibrillation. *Am J Cardiol.* 2020;140:55–61.

## MISTAKE: ATTEMPTING RHYTHM CONTROL TOO LATE

**Case Example**

A 78-year-old female with palpitations is newly diagnosed with atrial fibrillation. You prescribe some metoprolol, and the patient's symptoms improve, but she remains in atrial fibrillation. Given decent rate control, the patient is continued on metoprolol for over a year. The patient returns citing worsening palpitations, and a Holter monitor demonstrates frequent periods of rapid ventricular response. You attempt rhythm control with amiodarone but are unable to convert the patient to sinus rhythm.

**Reasoning Error(s)**

- Lack of understanding that atrial fibrillation facilitates further atrial fibrillation
- Not knowing that the chronicity of atrial fibrillation affects the success rate of rhythm control
- Focusing on rate control despite lack of success given more familiarity and comfort
- Not considering a patient's future comorbidities that may impact wishes on rhythm control

**How to Avoid the Mistake**

- Understand that atrial fibrillation over time leads to structural changes that act as substrate for further atrial fibrillation—the basis for the common saying "atrial fibrillation begets atrial fibrillation." Most therapies for atrial fibrillation, whether antiarrhythmic drugs or ablation, have less efficacy the longer the patient is in persistent atrial fibrillation.
- Consider rate control as a viable option despite the general trend toward increased adverse effects with antiarrhythmic therapy.
- Think about the patient's future—are they likely to have significant cardiac comorbidities such as systolic dysfunction or valvular disease? Certain comorbidities may increase the desire to achieve rhythm control, and waiting too long (i.e., years) will significantly decrease the ability to maintain sinus rhythm due to years of atrial remodeling (i.e., substrate for maintaining the arrhythmia).

**Antidote**

- Not applicable

**Common Scenarios**

- Not applicable

**Note(s)**

- The most common structural effect of long-standing atrial fibrillation is dilation of the left atrium, which acts as further substrate for atrial fibrillation.
- One simple way to think about who benefits the most from being in sinus rhythm is the more cardiac issues one has, the greater is the benefit of sinus rhythm (though more difficult to maintain it).

| Further Reading | ■ Recent evidence suggests that rhythm control may be more effective in atrial fibrillation when attempted soon after initial diagnosis (i.e., within the first months to year): Kirchhof P, et al. Early rhythm-control therapy in patients with atrial fibrillation. *N Engl J Med.* 2020;383:1305–1316. |

## MISTAKE: OVERRELIANCE ON CHEMICAL CARDIOVERSION OF ATRIAL FLUTTER

| Case Example | A 45-year-old female presents in typical flutter. You attempt a flecainide push followed by increasing the dosages, and the patient develops a second-degree type I heart block. |
|---|---|
| Reasoning Error(s) | ■ Not realizing the low success rates of chemical cardioversion in atrial flutter<br>■ Not realizing the duration required after administration of medicine to see cardioversion<br>■ Lack of understanding the mechanism that underlies the increased difficulty of pharmacologically cardioverting atrial flutter<br>■ Hesitancy to electrically cardiovert given it is a more invasive intervention |
| How to Avoid the Mistake | ■ Understand that atrial flutter is uniquely difficult to cardiovert chemically.<br>■ Remember that the efficacy of chemical cardioversion for atrial flutter is not high and may take >1 hour to occur after drug administration.<br>■ Understand that atrial fibrillation is generally easier to chemically control than atrial flutter given a higher atrial rate (approximately 600 versus 300 bpm) that bombards the AV node, which is a rate-dependent brake. In other words, the faster the atrial rate, the more refractory is the AV node becomes, making pharmacologic control of the ventricular rate easier. |
| Antidote | ■ Electrical cardioversion |
| Common Scenarios | ■ Not applicable |
| Note(s) | ■ Typical atrial flutter is most commonly found around the cavotricuspid isthmus (CTI) as a macroreentrant circuit. Thus, CTI ablation is a highly effective (>90%) method of cardioverting typical flutter. On the other hand, atypical flutter is often due to scarring and fibrosis (e.g., from prior infarction or cardiac surgery) and much more difficult to locate and ablate definitively.<br>■ Contrary to popular belief, calcium channel blockers and β-blockers are primarily rate control agents. Conversion in response to a β-blocker should not be interpreted as the β-blocker causing cardioversion (it would have happened spontaneously anyways). Chemical cardioversion involves antiarrhythmic agents such as ibutilide IV or oral flecainide. |

## MISTAKE: TREATMENT OF FLUTTER WITH CLASS 1C ANTIARRHYTHMICS WITHOUT ATRIOVENTRICULAR NODAL BLOCKADE

**Case Example**

A 45-year-old female presents with typical 2:1 atrial flutter. You administer flecainide and are surprised to find that the flutter becomes 1:1, leading to significant hemodynamic deterioration.

**Reasoning Error(s)**

- Lack of knowledge regarding the complete physiology of Class 1 antiarrhythmics
- Focusing only on the benefits of a medication without considering the potential drawbacks
- Forgetting to be proactive rather than reactive about potential adverse effects of a therapy

**How to Avoid the Mistake**

- Understand that Class 1 antiarrhythmics (especially Class 1C) possess relatively significant ability to slow the atrial cycle length, which increases AV conduction (less refractoriness of the AV node). Thus, despite a decrease in atrial rate due to sodium channel blockade, the ventricular rate may increase due to the increase in AV conduction. Vagolytic effects are probably more minor (more typical of Type 1a agents such as disopyramide). To prevent this, use a concomitant AV nodal blocker such as a β-blocker.
- Always consider both risks and benefits to any clinical action.
- Focus on anticipating adverse events and being proactive rather than being reactive.

**Antidote**

- AV nodal blockers (e.g., β-blocker)

**Common Scenarios**

- Class 1C antiarrhythmics
  - Flecainide
  - Encainide
  - Propafenone
  - Moricizine
- Class 1A antiarrhythmics (less likely)
- Class 1B antiarrhythmics (less likely)

**Note(s)**

- The sodium channel–blocking potency of Class 1 antiarrhythmics are 1C > 1A > 1B.
- Class 1A antiarrhythmics (particularly disopyramide) possess the strongest anticholinergic properties among antiarrhythmics.
- Type Ic agents have a use-dependent effect where the faster the rates, the more they block, and hence have the most profound effect on conduction and slowing of cycle length.

## MISTAKE: USING FLECAINIDE, ENCAINIDE, MORICIZINE, PROPAFENONE, AND/OR DRONEDARONE IN STRUCTURAL HEART DISEASE

**Case Example**

A 62-year-old male with a recent anterior STEMI is noted to have paroxysmal atrial fibrillation. You start him on daily flecainide, and the patient appears content that his atrial fibrillation is less prevalent. However, a month later, the patient suddenly passes away without a clear explanation. On autopsy, the patient appears to have had no clear cause, suggesting that sudden death was most likely due to proarrhythmia in the setting of recent myocardial infarction.

**Reasoning Error(s)**

- Lack of knowledge regarding the safety of Class 1C antiarrhythmics and dronedarone in structural heart disease
- Misinterpreting what "structural heart disease" refers to in the setting of 1c antiarrhythmics
- Forgetting to consider contraindications to medications
- Lack of complete information regarding patient comorbidities prior to drug initiation

**How to Avoid the Mistake**

- Understand the evidence behind why flecainide, encainide, and propafenone are contraindicated in structural heart disease. In the CAST trials, an increase in mortality was seen in post–myocardial infarction patients treated with Class 1C antiarrhythmics. Dronedarone in the ANDROMEDA trial was associated with increased mortality in patients with systolic dysfunction.
- Remember that structural heart disease is a vague term that most directly refers to prior myocardial infarction as studied in the CAST trial, but their preclusion is often extended to any coronary artery disease, left ventricular dysfunction, and structural changes such as significant left ventricular hypertrophy and hypertrophic cardiomyopathy.
- Always consider contraindications in addition to indications for each clinical action.
- Do not start Class 1C antiarrhythmics without complete information regarding the presence of structural heart disease.

**Antidote**

- Stop the agent immediately.

**Common Scenarios**

- Flecainide
- Encainide
- Moricizine
- Propafenone
- Dronedarone

**Note(s)**

- When in doubt, amiodarone is the standard antiarrhythmic in lieu of Class 1C antiarrhythmics given it has no contraindications due to structural heart disease. However, the long-term toxicities of amiodarone are greater than those of Class 1C agents.
- Dronedarone is an alternative to amiodarone in the setting of significant thyroid disease (e.g., toxic multinodular goiter) due to its lack of an iodine moiety.

## MISTAKE: FORGETTING TO CONSIDER PHARMACOLOGIC PRETREATMENT PRIOR TO ELECTRICAL CARDIOVERSION

**Case Example**

A 66-year-old female presents to you for persistent palpitations in the setting of atrial fibrillation diagnosed 1 year ago. Despite rhythm control with various medications, the patient has remained in atrial fibrillation and is currently taking only metoprolol. You suggest trialing electrical cardioversion and she agrees. Unfortunately, the patient remains in atrial fibrillation after the cardioversion.

**Reasoning Error(s)**

- Lack of knowledge or experience regarding chemical pretreatment prior to electrical cardioversion
- Only thinking about cardioversion in distinct entities (pharmacologic versus electrical)

**How to Avoid the Mistake**

- Understand that some smaller studies support higher efficacy of electrical cardioversion with pharmacologic pretreatment compared to electrical cardioversion alone. However, electrical cardioversion is usually highly effective at terminating atrial fibrillation/flutter with or without antiarrhythmic agents. The main benefit of antiarrhythmic agent pretreatment is to help with maintenance of sinus rhythm.
- Consider pretreatment of electrical cardioversion with an antiarrhythmic such as amiodarone or ibutilide. Usual pretreatment duration is a few weeks prior to the scheduled cardioversion.

**Antidote**

- Not applicable

**Common Scenarios**

- Not applicable

**Note(s)**

- Ibutilide is a Class III antiarrhythmic that is not widely used given a general lack of knowledge regarding its efficacy and safety. Notably, the efficacy of ibutilide is greater than that of amiodarone for cardioverting atrial fibrillation. Careful QTc monitoring should be performed during the initiation of ibutilide.
- Similar to pretreatment of electrical cardioversion, antiarrhythmic drug therapy can be synergistically improved by adding sympatholytics such as a β-blocker. This is particularly true in cases where the atrial fibrillation is driven by surges in catecholamine such as in significant bursts of emotion.
- If the first episode of persistent atrial fibrillation, an antiarrhythmic agent is usually not used, which is reserved for recurrences after the first cardioversion.

## MISTAKE: LONG-TERM AMIODARONE IN YOUNG AND MIDDLE-AGED PATIENTS

**Case Example**

A 34-year-old female with morbid obesity and paroxysmal atrial fibrillation presents to you for management of persistent palpitations. You initiate 400 mg daily amiodarone, and her symptoms improve as a result of less time spent in atrial fibrillation. The patient is happy for 6 years but then returns with worsening shortness of breath and rapid weight gain. Labs demonstrate hypothyroidism, and chest imaging shows extensive pulmonary fibrosis.

| | |
|---|---|
| **Reasoning Error(s)** | ■ Lack of knowledge regarding the cumulative dose-dependent toxicities of amiodarone |
| | ■ Considering only relatively short-term outcomes |
| | ■ Lack of efforts to find the minimal effective dosage for each individual patient |
| **How to Avoid the Mistake** | ■ Understand that most toxicities of amiodarone such as pulmonary fibrosis and hyper/hypothyroidism are dose dependent. Thus, these side effects are more likely to become clinically relevant in younger patients on long-term amiodarone. |
| | ■ Use the lowest dose of amiodarone possible to achieve clinical outcomes. After starting amiodarone, it is worth trialing lower doses for chronic maintenance therapy. |
| | ■ Individualize all clinical decisions to the patient with both short-term and long-term considerations. |
| **Antidote** | ■ Not applicable |
| **Common Scenarios** | ■ Not applicable |
| **Note(s)** | ■ The use of amiodarone in younger patients in the acute setting (e.g., only a bolus in the setting of RVR) is usually safe and effective, since most amiodarone-induced toxicities are thought to be dependent on the cumulative dose exposure. |

## MISTAKE: AMIODARONE IN PROLONGED QTc

| | |
|---|---|
| **Case Example** | A 78-year-old female with HFrEF (EF = 30%) is admitted for decompensated heart failure. She soon goes into atrial fibrillation with rapid ventricular response. Her ECG also demonstrates a QTc of 510 ms. Given her soft blood pressures, you immediately start her on amiodarone. The patient's atrial fibrillation is controlled soon but she goes into torsade soon after. |
| **Reasoning Error(s)** | ■ Thinking of amiodarone as the antiarrhythmic of choice that can be used in almost any patient (the fewest contraindications) |
| | ■ Lack of knowledge regarding QTc prolonging effects of amiodarone |
| | ■ Historical assumptions that amiodarone |
| | ■ Fast thinking that only associates certain infamous, strongly QTc-prolonging medications with QTc prolongation |
| **How to Avoid the Mistake** | ■ Understand that amiodarone prolongs QTc in a dose-dependent manner and should be used cautiously in the setting of prolonged QTc. While it's QTc prolonging effects are less than that of other Class III antiarrhythmics such as dofetilide or sotalol, close attention to QTc is still required. |
| | ■ Understand the data for amiodarone-induced torsade. Despite historical assumption that the medication is not very pro-arrhythmic, large epidemiologic studies demonstrate that amiodarone is one of the most common causes of drug-induced torsade (perhaps due to the assumption that it does not cause torsade). The estimated risk of amiodarone-induced torsade is 1.5%. |
| | ■ Understand the main safety considerations for all medications prior to use. |

| | |
|---|---|
| **Antidote** | ▪ Stop amiodarone immediately. |
| **Common Scenarios** | ▪ Not applicable |
| **Note(s)** | ▪ Other risk factors for torsade due to amiodarone use include female sex, hypokalemia, hypomagnesemia, and poor left ventricular systolic function. |
| | ▪ Unfortunately, amiodarone is one of the most effective drugs at treating refractory arrhythmias such as VT or atrial fibrillation. In these cases, there is often no choice regardless of QTc. Fortunately, amiodarone has a relatively low torsade de pointes risk relative to other Class III agents. |

## MISTAKE: NOT ACTIVELY CHECKING FOR MEDICATION INTERACTIONS IN THE PRESENCE OF AMIODARONE

| | |
|---|---|
| **Case Example** | An 82-year-old male with a recent large anterior STEMI is diagnosed with a left ventricular apical thrombus. His medications include sacubitril-valsartan, metoprolol succinate, eplerenone, dapagliflozin, metformin, semaglutide, simvastatin, and amiodarone. You bridge the patient over to warfarin but are surprised that the patient's INR is much higher than expected for the warfarin doses used. |
| **Reasoning Error(s)** | ▪ Lack of knowledge regarding amiodarone's common drug interactions |
| | ▪ Prescribing medications without thinking about drug interactions |
| **How to Avoid the Mistake** | ▪ Remember common medications that interact with amiodarone in a clinically significant manner: |
| |   ▪ Warfarin (approximately 25% elevation in INR) |
| |   ▪ DOACs (especially dabigatran): variable, check factor Xa levels |
| |   ▪ Simvastatin (may increase simvastatin's potency by up to two fold) |
| |   ▪ Digoxin (approximately 50% elevation in digoxin's effects) |
| | ▪ Manually check for drug interactions especially when using medications known to interact widely with medications; use pharmacists as part of multidisciplinary care! |
| **Antidote** | ▪ Not applicable |
| **Common Scenarios** | ▪ Warfarin |
| | ▪ DOACs |
| | ▪ Simvastatin |
| | ▪ Digoxin |
| **Note(s)** | ▪ Amiodarone is metabolized by the cytochrome P450 system (CYP 3A4 and CYP2C8). |
| | ▪ The half-life of amiodarone is very long (ranging from 30 to 180 days) due to its accumulation in adipose tissue. Thus, interactions may persistent for a while after continuation of amiodarone. |
| | ▪ Generally, cut the warfarin dose in half when starting amiodarone or digoxin and follow the INR closely. It can rise very rapidly. |

## MISTAKE: INITIATING IBUTILIDE OR SOTALOL WITHOUT CLOSE QTc MONITORING

| | |
|---|---|
| **Case Example** | A 70-year-old female presents to your outpatient clinic with persistent atrial fibrillation. The patient has been symptomatic despite trials of multiple medications. An in-office ECG reveals a QTc of 478 ms. You prescribe sotalol and plan for a 1-week follow-up. The patient never makes it to the follow-up visit, and you check her chart to realize that she died of cardiac arrest soon after starting the sotalol. |
| **Reasoning Error(s)** | ■ Thinking that a baseline acceptable QTc is enough for initiation of sotalol or ibutilide<br>■ Lack of knowledge regarding the QTc-prolonging effects of sotalol or ibutilide |
| **How to Avoid the Mistake** | ■ Understand that sotalol and ibutilide possess strong QTc-prolonging effects and require close in-hospital monitoring during initiation. Furthermore, the risk of torsade is twice as high from sotalol in females.<br>■ Remember that QTc prolongation is monitored with serial ECG's and that a normal baseline QTc does not indicate the inability of a QTc to prolong significantly. |
| **Antidote** | ■ Not applicable |
| **Common Scenarios** | ■ Sotalol<br>■ Ibutilide<br>■ Dofetilide |
| **Note(s)** | ■ The Class III antiarrhythmic effects of sotalol generally do not begin until reaching doses of 80 mg twice daily. Lower doses of sotalol impose β-blocker effects only.<br>■ Not all QTc-prolonging medications pose the same risk of inducing torsade. Class III antiarrhythmics such as sotalol and dofetilide prolong cardiac repolarization and thus carry a higher risk than Class 1C agents, which prolong the QTc via widening of the QRS.<br>■ Type 1C agents are potent sodium channel blockers and primarily widen the QRS with less effects on repolarization. Although they will therefore prolong QT, they have much less of a risk in causing torsade de pointes.<br>■ Torsade is more likely in a prolonged QTc in the presence of bradycardia. |

## MISTAKE: LACK OF CONSIDERATION FOR ABLATION THERAPY

| | |
|---|---|
| **Case Example** | A 74-year-old female with HFrEF (EF = 30%) and persistent atrial fibrillation presents seeking advice for ongoing palpitations. The patient is "sick" of dealing with her palpitations despite having tried numerous antiarrhythmic medications and even electrical cardioversion. You tell the patient that unfortunately there are no options left, but she notes that she saw a television advertisement recently about something called "ablation therapy" for atrial fibrillation. |

| | |
|---|---|
| **Reasoning Error(s)** | ■ Cognitive bias toward the most common methods of treating atrial fibrillation/flutter—pharmacologic and electrical rate and rhythm control<br>■ Lack of knowledge on the evidence behind ablative therapy |
| **How to Avoid the Mistake** | ■ Remember that ablation therapy (either catheter based or surgical) is a well-established and important method of rhythm control for atrial fibrillation/flutter, particularly typical (cavotricuspid isthmus–dependent flutter). Ablation is first-line therapy for recurrent typical atrial flutter because antiarrhythmic drugs work poorly, and the ablation procedure is very effective and safe. Ablation can also be considered early in atrial fibrillation in experienced centers, as most head-to-head trials show ablation to be superior in efficacy and quality of life compared to antiarrhythmic drug therapy.<br>■ Understand that ablation in atrial fibrillation and typical flutter may be effective in reducing recurrence and atrial fibrillation burden and improving quality of life beyond that observed with pharmacologic therapy alone. Furthermore, in specific cases such as systolic dysfunction (e.g., CASTLE-AF Trial), ablation therapy may potentially hold benefits over other methods.<br>   ■ The EARLY-AF Trial (*N Engl J Med.* 2021) is a recent trial that is among the first to provide interesting evidence to support catheter ablation as a potential first-line therapy. Other studies include a subset of the EAST-AFNET and STOP-AF First trials. |
| **Antidote** | ■ Not applicable |
| **Common Scenarios** | ■ Atrial fibrillation<br>■ Atrial flutter<br>■ Almost any other arrhythmia, though techniques and success rates vary |
| **Note(s)** | ■ Currently, ablation therapy is generally reserved for patients who fail appropriate control with antiarrhythmic medication. However, more evidence such as the EAST-AFNET trial suggests that early rhythm control (e.g., with ablation as first-line therapy) may improve cardiovascular outcomes.<br>■ Remember that ablation therapy does not obviate the need for long-term anticoagulation! |
| **Further Reading** | ■ An excellent summary of clinical trials for ablation in atrial fibrillation: Amuthan R, et al. What clinical trials of ablation for atrial fibrillation tell us – and what they do not. *Heart Rhythm.* 2021;2(2):174-186. |

## Supraventricular Tachycardia

### MISTAKE: OVERRELIANCE ON AGE-PREDICTED MAXIMUM HEART RATE TO DIAGNOSE SUPRAVENTRICULAR TACHYCARDIA

| | |
|---|---|
| **Case Example** | An 89-year-old female without prior cardiac history is admitted for *Escherichia coli* bacteremia and is discovered to have borderline blood pressures in the setting of a heart rate of 155. The ECG is notable for a tachyarrhythmia that appears sinus rhythm given its regularity despite an inability to discern clear P waves given the fast rate. However, you remember that the age-calculated maximum heart rate for the patient would be 220 – 89 = 131, suggesting that this is actually an arrhythmia. |

**Reasoning Error(s)**
- Reliance on a commonly taught concept without understanding the evidence
- Overreliance on a single piece of evidence without good cause
- Not realizing the multitude of formulas for age-predicted maximum heart rate

**How to Avoid the Mistake**
- Learn the most common formulas for age-predicted maximum heart rate.
  - Fox formula: HR = 220 − age
  - Tanaka formula: HR = 208 − (0.7 × age)
- Understand the evidence behind the various age-calculated maximum heart rate formulas. Notably, all formulas were based on health subjects. Many cardiac patients are chronotropically incompetent (e.g., in the setting of chronic heart failure) and/or are on AV nodal blockers that decrease the maximum heart rate.
  - The Fox formula was created in 1971 based on a convenience sample. Notably, the vast majority of participants off which the formula was derived were <55 years old and without cardiac comorbidities. Since its release, it has been noted to have a wide standard deviation that increases at extremes of age.
  - The Tanaka formula was derived in 2001 from a meta-analysis that was then validated in a study of health adults that notably included more older subjects.
- In the absence of a pathognomonic clinical finding, synthesize decisions based on a multitude of clinical data.

**Antidote**
- Not applicable

**Common Scenarios**
- Not applicable

**Note(s)**
- Checking the heart rate's rate of change (slope) on telemetry can be very helpful for detecting tachyarrhythmias. A sudden jump (depicted as a steplike increase in heart rate rather than a gradual slope upwards) favors arrhythmia.
- Most sinus tachycardia does not stay "fixed" at one rate. For example, the heart rate over the course of a minute may read 134, 137, 130, and so forth. Certain arrhythmias, particularly re-entrant circuits such as atrial flutter, may sustain a very consistent rate for extended periods.
- One formula (without robust evidence) for the predicted maximum heart rate for patients on β-blockers is HR = 164 − (0.7 × age).

**Further Reading**
- The original papers behind the Fox and Tanaka formulas for age-predicted maximum heart rates:
  - Fox SM, et al. Physical activity and the prevention of coronary heart disease. *Ann Clin Res.* 1971;3(6):404-432.
  - Tanaka H, et al. Age-predicted maximal heart rate revisited. *JACC.* 2001;37(1):153-156.

## MISTAKE: ADENOSINE IN THE SETTING OF RECENT CAFFEINE INGESTION

**Case Example**
A 42-year-old male presents in the afternoon with palpitations and is found in an undifferentiated supraventricular rhythm. In a diagnostic and potentially therapeutic action, you decide to administer adenosine. Despite three attempts at 6 mg, 12 mg, and 12 mg, you are unable to elicit any effect of adenosine. Upon asking the patient, he reveals that he drank two cups of coffee that morning.

**Reasoning Error(s)**
- Lack of understanding the mechanism(s) of adenosine and/or caffeine
- Forgetting to screen and warn patients of avoiding methylxanthine intake

**How to Avoid the Mistake**
- Understand the mechanism of adenosine and methylxanthines. Methylxanthines such as caffeine block the adenosine receptors, thus inhibiting the effect of adenosine.
- Warn patients prior to use of adenosine regarding what foods to avoid; in the acute setting, screen for ingestion of the most common methylxanthine, which is caffeine.

**Antidote**
- Not applicable

**Common Scenarios**
- Caffeine
- Theophylline
- Pentoxifylline
- Carbamazepine

**Note(s)**
- Some clinicians prefer to avoid adenosine due to its relatively increased difficulty of use and brief but unpleasant side effects. However, adenosine is still technically the drug of choice for terminating narrow-complex tachycardia because it is a simple bolus and the side effects are transient.

## MISTAKE: ADENOSINE IN THE SETTING OF SEVERE REACTIVE AIRWAY DISEASE OR HEART BLOCK

**Case Example**
A 46-year-old female with moderate asthma presents with palpitations. ECG reveals likely slow-fast AVNRT. You administer adenosine as a therapeutic and potentially diagnostic aid. The patient becomes wheezy and short of breath within seconds of administration.

**Reasoning Error(s)**
- Lack of awareness regarding common contraindications to adenosine use
- Thinking about therapeutic benefits without potential adverse effects and contraindications

**How to Avoid the Mistake**
- Understand common contraindications to adenosine use: significant reactive airway disease (e.g., COPD, asthma) and heart block. However, understand that adenosine will almost always cause transient heart block, and that a patient with underlying AV conduction disease or asthma will usually tolerate adenosine because its half-life is so short. The severity of these contraindications should be balanced against the benefits.
- Make it a habit to consider indications and contraindications when prescribing medications.

| | |
|---|---|
| **Antidote** | ■ Not applicable |
| **Common Scenarios** | ■ Reactive airway disease |
| | ■ Heart block |
| **Note(s)** | ■ Adenosine also has a dilator effect and can lead to a coronary steal phenomenon, which diverts blood from areas of fixed stenoses to healthier regions, exacerbating supply-demand mismatch. |

## MISTAKE: PUSHING ADENOSINE WITHOUT A SALINE FLUSH AND/OR THREE-WAY STOPCOCK

| | |
|---|---|
| **Case Example** | A 50-year-old male presents with palpitations and dizziness. He is found to be in an undifferentiated SVT to the 160s. You decide to administer adenosine to help diagnose the rhythm and perhaps terminate it. Despite repeated pushes of adenosine at increasing dosages (6 mg, 12 mg, 12 mg), there is no response whatsoever recorded on the ECG tracing during administration. |
| **Reasoning Error(s)** | ■ Forgetting the short duration of adenosine |
| | ■ Not taking into consideration the total time taken to administer the medication and flush it effectively |
| | ■ Not using a large-bore IV line |
| **How to Avoid the Mistake** | ■ Understand that the half-life of adenosine is approximately a mere 10 seconds. Thus, the duration of action (including side effects) usually last <1 minute. |
| | ■ Carefully plan out (and practice if needed) the steps to successfully administer adenosine given its short duration of action. Ensure that the plan includes use of a large-bore IV line, a saline flush, and a three-way stopcock. |
| **Antidote** | ■ Readminister adenosine using a saline flush. |
| **Common Scenarios** | ■ Slow administration (physical pushing) of medication |
| | ■ Lack of a saline flush |
| | ■ Delay in switching syringes (lack of a preloaded three-way stopcock) |
| | ■ Using a small-gauge IV line |
| **Note(s)** | ■ Elevation of the arm receiving adenosine in a lever-like fashion may expedite the transit of adenosine toward the central vasculature. |

## MISTAKE: USING THE SAME VOLTAGES FOR ELECTRICAL CARDIOVERSION/DEFIBRILLATION IN ALL PATIENTS

| | |
|---|---|
| **Case Example** | A 75-year-old female admitted for heart failure decompensation is discovered to be in a stable slow atrial flutter. You charge up the defibrillator to 200 J as you have seen during multiple prior rapids and arrests. Despite some light sedation, the patient complains vehemently that the shock was excruciatingly painful! |
| **Reasoning Error(s)** | ■ Not realizing that the required energy for electrical cardioversion depends on the clinical scenario |
| | ■ Lack of knowledge regarding the energy required for cardioverting in different scenarios |
| | ■ Forgetting that voltages may be increased in a stepwise fashion in most scenarios |

**How to Avoid the Mistake**

- Understand that the success of electrical cardioversion differs based on many factors.
  - The rhythm matters: atrial fibrillation requires greater energy (usually at least 100 J) than atrial flutter or other SVTs (50 J may be sufficient). Monomorphic VT should be shocked with at least 100 J, whereas ventricular fibrillation and polymorphic VT demands 200 J.
  - Medications such as antiarrhythmics may change the defibrillation threshold (e.g., amiodarone increases the threshold, whereas sotalol lowers it). There are many other factors such as the specific machine, location of the pads, and so forth.
  - Studies have shown that using a maximum shock first will result in overall less voltage applied than sequentially higher shocks that are initially unsuccessful. If the patient is completely sedated, usually give maximum shock for atrial fibrillation.
- Assess the urgency of the clinical situation. For instance, is the patient hypotensive and crashing? Realize that most cardioversions can be achieved.

**Antidote**

- Not applicable

**Common Scenarios**

- Not applicable

**Note(s)**

- Note that there is a difference between cardioversion and defibrillation. Cardioversion is used to convert non–life-threatening arrhythmias and is synchronized with the QRS complex. Defibrillation is delivered without consideration to the part of the cardiac cycle and usually for life-threatening arrhythmias. In short, synchronize the shock for any organized rhythm to avoid the small but tangible risk of precipitating ventricular fibrillation.

# Ventricular Tachycardia

## MISTAKE: TREATING AN UNDIFFERENTIATED WIDE-COMPLEX TACHYCARDIA AS SUPRAVENTRICULAR

**Case Example**

A 50-year-old male presents with a hemodynamically stable wide-complex tachyarrhythmia. Looking at the ECG, you run through several criteria for assessing wide-complex tachycardias and conclude that the patient likely has a supraventricular tachyarrhythmia with a left bundle-branch block. You subsequently administer a β-blocker, but the arrhythmia persists, and the patient suddenly becomes hypotensive.

**Reasoning Error(s)**

- Focusing too much on the academics of differentiating wide-complex tachycardia
- Not comparing the current arrhythmia to prior ECGs and arrhythmia episodes
- Interpreting the ECG in isolation without considering clinical context
- Lack of knowledge on how to differentiate between ventricular and wide-complex SVTs
- Disbelief that an arrhythmia can be ventricular in origin given the patient's current stability

| | |
|---|---|
| **How to Avoid the Mistake** | ■ Remember that the pretest probability of a wide-complex tachycardia being ventricular in origin exceeds 80%. Therefore, any wide-complex tachycardia should be treated as ventricular until definitively proven otherwise. It is not worth putting a patient's life in danger over academic zeal. |
| | ■ Compare arrhythmias to prior recorded ECGs to assess for preexisting conduction defects that may lead to a wide-complex tachycardia of supraventricular origin. |
| | ■ Always integrate clinical context into ECG interpretation. A teenager without prior cardiac history is less likely to experience VT; on the other hand, a geriatric patient with multiple prior myocardial infarctions is at high risk for VT. Hemodynamic stability does not help differentiate between supraventricular versus ventricular origin. |
| | ■ Learn the key conceptual signs that suggest a ventricular wide-complex tachycardia. You may also apply one or more of several criteria such as Brugada or Vereckei. The following factors favor VT: |
| | ■ AV dissociation (presence of more P waves than QRSs, capture, or fusion beats) |
| | ■ Precordial concordance of QRS (either all positive or negative) |
| | ■ QRS width (VT is usually much wider than aberrant conduction; >150 ms) |
| | ■ Initial dominant R in aVR |
| **Antidote** | ■ Not applicable |
| **Common Scenarios** | ■ Not applicable |
| **Note(s)** | ■ The main differentiating factor in whether a wide-complex tachycardia is SVT or VT is the presence of structural heart disease, in which case the diagnosis is VT >90% of the time. |
| | ■ The QRS calculated by the ECG machine is often wrong, especially in the presence of QRS fragmentation. Thus, it is often helpful to manually calculate the QRS duration, which can significantly change the diagnosis. |
| | ■ Severe hyperkalemia may lead to widening of the QRS that mimics VT. |

## MISTAKE: DIAGNOSING SUPRAVENTRICULAR TACHYCARDIA WITH ABERRANCY BASED ON TERMINATION OF A WIDE-COMPLEX TACHYCARDIA WITH ADENOSINE

| | |
|---|---|
| **Case Example** | A 40-year-old female with no prior medical history presents with what appears to be an SVT with aberrancy based on a prior ECG demonstrating a bundle-block morphology at fast ventricular rates (i.e., a rate-related block). You administer adenosine, which terminates the arrhythmia, and excitedly diagnose the patient with SVT with aberrancy. A month later, the patient represents with a wide-complex tachycardia and is managed by another team, who continues to attempt control with vagal maneuvers and metoprolol pushes given your diagnosis of wide-complex tachycardia responsive to adenosine. The patient degenerates into ventricular fibrillation, and the autopsy reveals a large anterior STEMI in the setting of spontaneous coronary artery dissection. On review of the wide-complex tachycardia, it appears different from the adenosine-responsive wide-complex tachycardia in the past. |

**Reasoning Error(s)**
- Lack of knowledge or experience with types of VT that are sensitive to adenosine
- Well-intentioned reasoning that correlates adenosine use with supraventricular arrhythmias
- Not understanding why incorrectly diagnosing an SVT may be consequential

**How to Avoid the Mistake**
- Learn about adenosine-sensitive VT, which often originates from the (usually right) ventricular outflow tract. This type of VT often occurs in patients without structural heart disease and may account for up to 10% of monomorphic VT.
- Make clinical decisions based on a multitude of data and evidence rather than solely well-intentioned logic, which may not bear out empirically given the complexity and unknowns of human physiology.
- Think of patient management in terms of the acute setting as well as the future. An incorrect diagnosis of SVT may be lethal for a patient in the future as diagnoses are often taken for granted once added to a patient's medical history.

**Antidote**
- Not applicable

**Common Scenarios**
- Not applicable

**Note(s)**
- Outflow tract VTs seem to be result from an overactivity of cAMP, which is inhibited by adenosine.
- There is no clear danger to the use of adenosine during VT; thus, it is reasonable to trial adenosine if the patient is stable and an outflow tract VT is suspected.

## MISTAKE: FORGETTING TO ASSESS FOR REVERSIBLE CAUSES OF VENTRICULAR TACHYCARDIA

**Case Example**
A 64-year-old male is admitted to the cardiac intensive care unit for recurrent monomorphic VT. Each occurrence results in high doses of amiodarone and lidocaine, as well as occasional electrical cardioversions. Bloodwork has been limited in the setting of malfunctioning laboratory instruments. You push for use of the point-of-care blood analyzer, which demonstrates a potassium level of 2.3 mEq/L.

**Reasoning Error(s)**
- Tunnel vision (perhaps due to unfamiliarity or acuity of the situation) on medical treatment of VT
- Lack of knowledge regarding common triggers of VT

**How to Avoid the Mistake**
- Always think about the underlying etiologies (particularly reversible causes) of any pathology. Fixing the underlying problem may be more effective than using other means.
- Understand the common triggers of VT. Monomorphic VT most commonly occurs in the setting of myocardial scars which form the basis for reentry; these scars may be caused by a prior infarct, surgical scar, or cardiomyopathy. Polymorphic VT is often found in the setting of active ischemia.

**Antidote**
- Not applicable

| Common Scenarios | ■ Electrolyte abnormalities (hypokalemia, hypomagnesemia) |
|---|---|
| | ■ Severe hyperthyroidism (thyroid storm) |
| | ■ Ischemia |
| | ■ Prior myocardial scar/fibrosis (infarct, surgery, cardiomyopathy) |
| | ■ Sympathetic discharge/storming |
| Note(s) | ■ Sustained VT is defined as that lasting a minimum of 30 seconds or that causing hemodynamic compromise (including in <30 seconds) |
| | ■ The three most common antiarrhythmics for monomorphic VT are amiodarone, lidocaine, and procainamide. Lidocaine generally has the least effect on blood pressure and the quickest onset of action. The first choice of antiarrhythmic is often institutional, though lidocaine is a poor drug for monomorphic VT. Procainamide or amiodarone are better because of their effect on conduction and refractoriness. |

## MISTAKE: ELECTRICALLY CARDIOVERTING ALL STABLE VENTRICULAR TACHYCARDIA

| Case Example | A 55-year-old male with a large anterior STEMI complicated by ischemic cardiomyopathy (EF = 20%) presents with palpitations and is found to be in stable sustained VT. You become acutely scared because you have never independently managed VT before. You proceed to emergently shock the patient, which resolves the arrhythmia but causes the patient long-lasting posttraumatic stress disorder. |
|---|---|
| Reasoning Error(s) | ■ High-pressure situation with classically taught association that VT is extremely dangerous leading to immediate focus on most definitive therapy (i.e., electrical cardioversion) |
| | ■ Lack of understanding the reason why VT is considered so dangerous (more so than SVT) |
| How to Avoid the Mistake | ■ Understand that VT is dangerous for two key reasons: (1) decreased diastolic filling time leading to inadequate cardiac output; and (2) as an unstable arrhythmia, VT carries a higher risk of degenerating into ventricular fibrillation or asystole. |
| | ■ Assess hemodynamic stability and triage patients to pharmacologic versus electrical cardioversion similar to most other arrhythmias. Pads should be placed on all patients regardless and shocks can be delivered immediately if necessary, decreasing the risk of trialing medications initially. |
| | ■ Always give sedation if you have the opportunity (based on hemodynamic stability). |
| Antidote | ■ Not applicable |
| Common Scenarios | ■ Not applicable |
| Note(s) | ■ Patients who have a VT on ECG but have no pulse should NOT be treated as pulseless electrical activity. Pulseless VT should be treated with immediate cardioversion. Note that PEA refers to rhythms with a normal rate that do not perfuse. |
| | ■ Idiopathic VT (not associated with structural heart disease) is usually not dangerous and does not degenerate to ventricular fibrillation. |

## MISTAKE: WITHHOLDING MAGNESIUM IN TORSADE DUE TO NORMAL MAGNESIUM LEVELS

**Case Example**      A 65-year-old female on methadone suddenly goes into torsade de pointes. Her blood pressure is stable, and she is mentating well. You check a STAT basic metabolic panel to find that the magnesium level is 2.4 mEq/L and defer further administration of magnesium. The patient's torsade does not break and she rapidly deteriorates into ventricular fibrillation and dies despite an attempted electrical cardioversion.

**Reasoning Error(s)**
- Well-intentioned and logical thinking that normal magnesium levels preclude benefit of magnesium infusion during torsade
- Lack of knowledge or unfounded fear of hypermagnesemia and its adverse effects

**How to Avoid the Mistake**
- Understand the evidence behind magnesium supplementation in torsade. The benefit in treating and reducing recurrence of torsade was seen even in patients with normal magnesium levels (though an old study based on only 12 patients; Tzivoni D, et al, *Circulation*. 1988).
- Remember that hypermagnesemia rarely results in adverse effects unless extreme. Despite the evidence being not very robust, the benefits of empiric magnesium administration likely outweigh the risks.

**Antidote**
- Give magnesium!

**Common Scenarios**
- Not applicable

**Note(s)**
- It is important to note that torsade almost always results from medications, though the risk of torsade is increased by electrolyte derangement (hypokalemia, hypomagnesemia) and bradycardia.
- Isoproterenol is another treatment consideration that may be used to shorten the QT interval and speed up heart rates (because long QT and torsade de pointes are heightened by bradycardia). Temporary pacing (at higher rates) can also be helpful.

## MISTAKE: OVERLY RAPID MAGNESIUM ADMINISTRATION IN TORSADE

**Case Example**      A 65-year-old female on methadone suddenly goes into torsade de pointes. Her blood pressure is stable, and she is mentating well. You check a STAT basic metabolic panel to find that the magnesium level is 2.4 mEq/L and astutely order magnesium despite the normal serum levels. The bolus is administered as fast as possible over a minute. The patient becomes hypotensive and then soon asystolic.

**Reasoning Error(s)**
- Lack of knowledge or experience with administering magnesium boluses
- Lack of knowledge regarding the adverse effects of rapid magnesium infusion
- Perception that magnesium should be administered as fast as possible given the presence of an uncommon and infamously dangerous arrhythmia (a very high-pressure situation)

| How to Avoid the Mistake | ■ Understand that rapid magnesium infusion may lead to hypotension and, rarely, asystole. |
| | ■ Decide the speed of magnesium administration based on the stability of the patient. When stable, administration over 15 minutes is considered safe. In unstable patients (e.g., without a pulse), magnesium may be administered as fast as over 2 minutes. |
| Antidote | ■ Not applicable |
| Common Scenarios | ■ Not applicable |
| Note(s) | ■ Repeat doses of magnesium may be administered if the torsades does not resolve. Generally, experts recommend no more than 4–6 grams of magnesium over 1 hour. |
| | ■ Symptoms of hypermagnesemia primarily occur at severely elevated levels (>7 mg/dL). Most commonly, the symptoms are nonspecific (nausea, GI upset, generalized weakness, mental status changes). New decreased reflexes are perhaps the most recognizable feature of magnesium toxicity. |

## MISTAKE: FORGETTING TO TREAT SYMPATHETIC DISCHARGE IN VENTRICULAR TACHYCARDIA

| Case Example | A 62-year-old male with incessant VT is transferred to the cardiac intensive care unit. Despite the use of amiodarone, lidocaine, and procainamide, the patient's VT does not subside. Electrical cardioversion with 200 J is also attempted multiple times to no avail. You cannot think of any further measures and watch in horror as the patient deteriorates hemodynamically and soon arrests. |
| Reasoning Error(s) | ■ Lack of knowledge that monomorphic VT may be facilitated by sympathetic activation, particularly in the setting of VT storm |
| How to Avoid the Mistake | ■ Understand that monomorphic VT is often found in patients with prior myocardial scars but that the scars serve as substrate rather than an initiation trigger. One such trigger is sympathetic overactivity. |
| | ■ Remember that β-blockers not only possess rate-control properties (or even antiarrhythmic properties in the case of sotalol) but also decrease sympathetic tone. |
| | ■ Most cardiac conditions including CAD, CHF, and arrhythmias are worsened by excess sympathetic tone. Use β-blockers as much as possible. The effect of many antiarrhythmic drugs, including amiodarone, is improved by adding β-blockers. |
| Antidote | ■ Consider use of β-blockers (e.g., metoprolol, sotalol). |
| | ■ Consider intubation/sedation as a last-line resort if refractory to electrical and pharmacologic cardioversion. |
| Common Scenarios | ■ Not applicable |
| Note(s) | ■ VT storm is defined loosely but refers to multiple (generally more than three, and at least two) episodes of monomorphic VT within 24 hours. |
| | ■ Intubation/sedation is often effective. |

# Miscellaneous

## MISTAKE: NOT STAT CONSULTING CARDIOLOGY FOR INAPPROPRIATE IMPLANTABLE CARDIOVERTER-DEFIBRILLATOR SHOCKS

**Case Example**

A 52-year-old male with HFrEF (EF = 20%) and recent implantable cardioverter-defibrillator (ICD) implantation presents with inappropriate shocks for the past 2 days. On assessment, the patient is comfortable and in normal sinus rhythm at 70–80 bpm.

**Reasoning Error(s)**

- Assuming that all ICD shocks are appropriate
- Lack of understanding the mechanism by which ICDs decide to shock or not
- Thinking that the ICD shock is an "event of the past" and that the patient is now stable without further shocks

**How to Avoid the Mistake**

- Investigate whether an ICD shock is appropriate or not. This is done via interrogation of the device to ascertain whether the shock was fired appropriately (in response to VT or VF), inappropriately (for SVT), or due to device malfunction. Other clues depending on the setting include review of telemetry or ECG during the arrhythmia. Note: every shock (not just a few) should be investigated.
- Understand the mechanism of ICD shocks. Each device has a conditional shock zone and a shock done. The conditional shock zone has a series of calculations (e.g., comparing the rhythm to a stored copy of the patient's baseline rhythm) performed by the device to try and discriminate SVT versus VT. The shock zone operates solely based off the heart rate (which is higher than that of the conditional shock zone). For most newer ICDs, antitachycardia pacing (ATP) is used to attempt and break the arrhythmia prior to deployment of shocks.
- Remember that shocks may occur when the patient's heart rate exceeds that of the defibrillation threshold, regardless of the actual rhythm such as during a paroxysmal SVT. In other words, the patient is at the mercy of the tachyarrhythmia, and the ICD should be deactivated or modified immediately.

**Antidote**

- Deactivate or reprogram the ICD immediately.

**Common Scenarios**

- Not applicable

**Note(s)**

- In simple terms, the most common default conditional shock and shock thresholds are 170 and 200 bpm, though thresholds are customized to each patient. More specifically, ICD programming can be quite sophisticated for patients with VT and other arrhythmias. For primary prevention devices, often there is just one zone at a very high rate and a monitor zone at a lower rate with no therapy.
- While ICD shocks are lifesaving, they are very painful and associated with emotional distress (up to posttraumatic stress disorder), especially after receiving more than five shocks (the evidence is mixed for a single shock, but it is certainly unpleasant).

# Valvular Disease

Richard John Sekerak III

Mistake: Forgetting Medical Hemodynamic Optimization of Mitral Stenosis

**Infective Endocarditis**

Mistake: Forgetting to Prescribe Preprocedural Antibiotic Prophylaxis in High-Risk Patients

Mistake: Delay in Onboarding the Surgical Team

Mistake: Overlooking Culture-Negative Endocarditis

Mistake: Overvaluing Transthoracic Echocardiography for Ruling-Out Infective Endocarditis

Mistake: Routine Use of Oral Antibiotics for Infective Endocarditis

# Aortic Stenosis

## MISTAKE: FORGETTING TO SCREEN FOR BICUSPID AORTIC VALVE IN FIRST-DEGREE RELATIVES

**Case Example**

A 38-year-old male is referred for a transthoracic echocardiogram (TTE) given a "clicking" murmur at an annual physical. TTE reveals a bicuspid aortic valve (BAV) without leaflet calcification or restriction. You reassure the patient that BAV is a common finding that requires serial surveillance every 3–5 years. The patient feels better and strolls happily out of your office. At the next follow-up visit in 3 years, the patient tells you that his sister had rupture of an aortic root aneurysm.

**Reasoning Error(s)**

- Not knowing the genetics of BAV
- Lack of understanding the clinical implication of a BAV
- Only focusing clinical care on the immediate patient at hand

**How to Avoid the Mistake**

- Understand that BAV is the most common congenital heart anomaly, occurring in approximately 1 in 100 people. While the anomaly is likely polygenic, the *NOTCH1* gene, which is involved in cell differentiation, has been linked. Though BAV may result sporadically, BAV is usually inherited in an autosomal dominant manner.
- Learn why knowledge of a BAV matters. Compared to a trileaflet aortic valve, BAV is prone to earlier and heavier calcification (due to increased turbulence) and hence aortic stenosis (AS). It may also be more prone to aortic insufficiency. Furthermore, BAV may be associated with other connective tissue disorders such as aortic dilation and systemic conditions (e.g., Marfan's, Turner's).
- Remember to screen all first-degree family members when a BAV is discovered in your patient.

**Antidote**

- Screen all first-degree relatives for BAV.

**Common Scenarios**

- Not applicable

**Note(s)**

- Some trileaflet aortic valves may be difficult to differentiate from bicuspid valves using TTE in the setting of heavy calcification. Further characterization may be done with transesophageal echocardiography (TEE), computed tomography (CT), or magnetic resonance imaging (MRI).

## MISTAKE: MEASUREMENT OF AORTIC VALVE INDICES WITHOUT HEMODYNAMIC OPTIMIZATION

**Case Example**   You are evaluating a patient with suspected AS. You note on the TTE that the patient's transaortic pressure gradient does not meet criteria for severe AS. You conclude that the patient has moderate AS. On repeat TTE months later, the patient's hemodynamic parameters are consistent with severe AS. The patient is confused at the discrepancy. You examine the reports closer and realize that the patient had been severely hypertensive during the original TTE and normotensive on the follow-up.

**Reasoning Error(s)**
- Clinical rigidity that focuses exclusively on criteria without contextualization
- Lack of knowledge or forgetting that aortic valve hemodynamic parameters depend on overall body hemodynamics
- Not thinking through the physiology of how common vital signs and hemodynamic states affect indices of aortic valve severity

**How to Avoid the Mistake**
- Understand that all key indices of AS are flow dependent. This means that any significant alteration in hemodynamics (e.g., severe hypertension leading to a significant increase in afterload) may confound the severity of AS.
- Interpret each clinical criterion with context. Strive to understand the circumstances in which clinical criteria are defined and what influences each clinical criterion. In particular, all echocardiogram findings should be interpreted in the context of the heart rate and blood pressure due to their flow-dependence.
- Ensure that patients undergoing evaluation for AS are hemodynamically optimized (e.g., normotensive, not tachycardic, not in an unusual output state such as sepsis).

**Antidote**
- Repeat study when the patient is hemodynamically optimized.

**Common Scenarios**
- Uncontrolled hypertension or tachycardia
- High-output states (e.g., anemia, hyperthyroidism, sepsis)
- Reduced cardiac output (e.g., systolic dysfunction)

**Note(s)**
- Currently, there are no medical (noninvasive) treatments that are proved to slow the progression of AS.

**Further Reading**
- An excellent refresher on the pathophysiology of AS (and many more cardiovascular diseases!): Lilly LS. *Pathophysiology of Heart Disease: An Introduction to Cardiovascular Medicine.* 17th ed. Wolters Kluwer; 2021.

## MISTAKE: FORGETTING TO ASSESS FOR LOW-FLOW, LOW-GRADIENT AORTIC STENOSIS

**Case Example**   An 82-year-old male with nonischemic cardiomyopathy (ejection fraction [EF] = 20%) and known AS presents for an echocardiogram due to new dyspnea and angina on exertion. You note that the patient meets criteria for severe AS by valve area (<1 cm²); however, you are surprised to see an aortic valve mean gradient of 30 mmHg and a peak velocity of 3.1 m/s. You conclude that the patient does not have severe AS and set up a follow-up in 1 year. A few months later, you are distressed to hear that the patient passed from a subdural hemorrhage after experienced syncope while running up a flight of stairs.

| | |
|---|---|
| **Reasoning Error(s)** | ■ Clinical rigidity that focuses exclusively on criteria without contextualization<br>■ Lack of knowledge or forgetting that aortic valve hemodynamic parameters depend on overall body hemodynamics<br>■ Lack of knowledge regarding the impact of systolic dysfunction on aortic valve indices (i.e., that the indices are flow dependent)<br>■ Incorrectly thinking of low-flow low-gradient AS as a binary entity (either severe or not). |
| **How to Avoid the Mistake** | ■ Understand that all key indices of AS are flow dependent. Without the generation of proper forward stroke volume, the standard aortic valve severity indices may not be reached.<br>■ Explore the possibility of low-flow, low-gradient AS with a dobutamine stress echo. Patients with true severe AS often have an increase in the mean gradient to appropriate thresholds (e.g., >40 mmHg). However, a proportion of patients with severe systolic dysfunction may not sufficiently augment their cardiac output with dobutamine to determine stenosis severity. In these patients, aortic valve calcium quantification by CT is very helpful.<br>■ Understand that low-flow, low-gradient AS is not a binary entity and that severity may be underestimated (e.g., moderate rather than severe AS). |
| **Antidote** | ■ Dobutamine stress echo |
| **Common Scenarios** | ■ Systolic dysfunction (heart failure with reduced EF [HFrEF])<br>■ Diastolic dysfunction (heart failure with preserved EF [HFpEF])<br>■ Other causes of poor forward stroke volume (e.g., arrhythmias without atrial kick, severe tachyarrhythmias, severe mitral regurgitation [MR]) |
| **Note(s)** | ■ In addition to low-flow, low-gradient AS in reduced left ventricular EF (LVEF) (classic), there is low-flow, low-gradient AS with preserved LVEF (paradoxical). The low gradient in these patients is due to decreased forward stroke volume causing inadequate flow across the aortic valve to unmask severe gradients and need not be from systolic dysfunction.<br>■ Consider the differences in diagnosis for low-flow, low-gradient AS in regard to aortic valve replacement (AVR). |
| **Further Reading** | ■ Excellent easy-to-read summary of paradoxical low-flow, low-gradient AS: Pibarot P, Dumesnil JG. Low-flow, low-gradient aortic stenosis with normal and depressed left ventricular ejection fraction. *J Am Coll Cardiol.* 2012;60:1845–1853. |

# MISTAKE: LACK OF CLOSE FOLLOW-UP IN SEVERE ASYMPTOMATIC AORTIC STENOSIS

**Case Example**   You are caring for a patient in your outpatient clinic who you have worked-up for AS. You have correctly identified your patient as having severe AS due to meeting all three criteria: velocity, gradient, and valve area parameters. On questioning, your patient does not report any symptoms of exertional dyspnea, decreased exercise tolerance, exertional angina, presyncope, or syncope. You perform an exercise treadmill test in which the patient remains asymptomatic and appropriately augments their blood pressure with exertion. You conclude that your patient has severe asymptomatic AS. You decide on follow-up with your patient as needed. Unfortunately, your patient dies 1.5 years later.

**Reasoning Error(s)**
- Lack of understanding of the trajectory and prognosis of AS
- False reassurance from the lack of presence of any symptoms due to AS

**How to Avoid the Mistake**
- Understand that the rate of progression of symptoms is high: progression from asymptomatic to symptomatic severe AS is estimated to be 30%–50% at 2 years.
- Understand that the morbidity and mortality of AS in relation to its severity are often described as "falling off a cliff." This refers to the often asymptomatic nature of AS, which is followed by a very abrupt decline once symptoms present. The average survival for patients with symptomatic AS is 2–3 years in the absence of mechanical intervention.
- Frequent monitoring of patients with severe AS, even when asymptomatic, as symptom onset may trail hemodynamic compromise, and may be difficult for the patient to identify. Current guidelines suggest serial echocardiographic evaluation every 6–12 months.

**Antidote**
- TTE monitoring q6–12 months

**Common Scenarios**
- Not applicable

**Note(s)**
- Many patients with severe asymptomatic AS will go on to develop indications for intervention within a few years (some estimates approach 50% within 2 years of diagnosis).
- Currently, guidelines do not recommend routine valve intervention for asymptomatic severe AS unless one of the following criteria is met. However, several ongoing studies are investigating the use of earlier valve intervention as the procedural morbidity and mortality have dramatically decreased over time.
    - Critical stenosis (defined as a peak velocity >5 m/s or peak gradient >60 mmHg)
    - Accompanied by systolic dysfunction
    - Symptoms are elicited on exercise testing.
    - Alternate indication for cardiac surgery

**Further Reading**
- An excellent article reviewing the natural history of AS: Gahl B, et al. Natural history of asymptomatic severe aortic stenosis and the association of early intervention with outcomes: a systematic review and meta-analysis. *JAMA Cardiol.* 2020;5(10):1102–1112.

## MISTAKE: FORGETTING TO USE THE DIMENSIONLESS INDEX FOR DETERMINING AORTIC STENOSIS SEVERITY

**Case Example**

An 83-year-old male with prior asymptomatic severe AS presents to your clinic for new-onset shortness of breath. TTE demonstrates preserved LV function with the following aortic valve indices: AVA 0.7 cm², peak velocity of 3.8 m/s, mean gradient of 37 mmHg, and dimensionless index (DI) 0.20. Though the aortic valve area is compatible with severe AS, you decide against intervention in the setting of the peak velocity and mean gradient falling under moderate AS. The interventional attending frowns and notes that the dimensionless index (DI) is 0.20, which signifies severe AS.

**Reasoning Error(s)**
- Not realizing the limitations and pitfalls in calculating AS indices
- Lack of knowledge of the DI and/or its value
- Reliance on classic medical school teaching that focuses on the velocity, valve area, and gradient, usually without introduction of the concept of DI

**How to Avoid the Mistake**
- Realize that the aortic valve area is calculated from the continuity equation based on measurement of the LV outflow tract (LVOT) cross-sectional area, which is notoriously difficult to measure accurately (human errors as well as the LVOT being more elliptical rather than circular). Many equations within echocardiography rely on squaring the LVOT area, and thus even small inaccuracies can become significant.
- Understand that the DI is a measurement that is independent of the LVOT cross-sectional area, avoiding potential measurement errors. It is calculated by dividing the LVOT time-velocity integral (TVI) (also known as the velocity-time integral [VTI]) with that of the aortic valve. Furthermore, the DI is largely independent of hemodynamic loading conditions and the incident angle of the Doppler. This provides a higher-fidelity measurement for determining AS severity. A DI <0.25, which corresponds to an aortic valve area of approximately 0.8 cm², suggests severe AS.
- As you progress through clinical training, resist the urge to feel comfortable with your knowledge from medical school. Verify, build on the foundational teaching, and expect that much of the foundational teaching may have been overly simplified.

**Antidote**
- Not applicable

**Common Scenarios**
- Not applicable

**Note(s)**
- The TVI represents the distance traveled by blood during a unit of time. It is used to calculate stroke volume and cardiac output.

# MISTAKE: FORGETTING TO VERIFY ASYMPTOMATIC SEVERE AORTIC STENOSIS WITH EXERCISE STRESS TESTING

**Case Example**   You are evaluating a 76-year-old male patient in your outpatient clinic, who has a known history of hypertension and hyperlipidemia. On physical exam, you auscultate a crescendo-decrescendo murmur at the right upper sternal border; you are concerned that your patient has AS and you order a TTE for your patient. On his TTE report, your patient meets criteria for severe AS based on his valve area (0.6 cm²), mean gradient (68 mmHg), and peak velocity (4.2 m/s). Your patient denies any syncope or presyncope events, angina at rest or with exertion, exertional dyspnea, or any change in exercise tolerance. You conclude that your patient has asymptomatic severe AS because of his reported lack of symptoms. You decide to continue medical management and plan to follow-up with your patient in 6 months. You are surprised when you are notified that your patient experienced syncope while shoveling snow on a cold winter day 2 months later.

**Reasoning Error(s)**
- False reassurance based on patient's history
- Lack of understanding the importance of determining whether a patient is truly asymptomatic
- Lack of knowledge of further confirmatory testing in asymptomatic severe AS
- Incorrect belief that exercise stress testing is contraindicated in all types of AS

**How to Avoid the Mistake**
- Understanding the natural history of severe AS criteria based on symptomology. The average length of survival for patients with symptomatic AS is merely 2–3 years in the absence of mechanical intervention. Furthermore, there are fewer indications for valve replacement when asymptomatic irrespective of severity. Thus, it is incredibly important to correctly categorize whether a patient is symptomatic.
- For patients with asymptomatic severe AS, it is recommended to confirm the absence of symptoms with exercise stress test to rule out symptomatic severe AS and to further classify hemodynamic changes with known valve stenosis.
- Understand that, under close supervision of an experienced clinician, exercise stress testing for asymptomatic severe AS is safe and can provide further information in terms of patient's exercise tolerance and functional capacity, thus offering further prognostic information. Some studies estimate that up to 20% of reported asymptomatic severe AS patients will have symptoms with exercise stress testing.

**Antidote**
- Exercise stress testing

**Common Scenarios**
- Not applicable

**Note(s)**
- Similar to heart failure, the American Heart Association has defined four stages of AS:
  - Stage A: At risk but with normal hemodynamics
  - Stage B: Progressive AS with mild to moderate hemodynamic compromise
  - Stage C: Asymptomatic severe AS
  - Stage D: Symptomatic severe AS

**Further Reading**
- Excellent article evaluating the use of exercise stress testing to stratify asymptomatic AS: Maréchaux S, et al. Usefulness of exercise-stress echocardiography for risk stratification of true asymptomatic patients with aortic valve stenosis. *Eur Heart J*. 2010;31(11):1390–1397.

## MISTAKE: EXERCISE STRESS TESTING IN SEVERE SYMPTOMATIC AORTIC STENOSIS

**Case Example:**
You are caring for a 79-year-old male with a history of coronary artery disease (CAD), chronic obstructive pulmonary disease (COPD), hyperlipidemia (HLD), and severe symptomatic AS. Today, he reports 2 months of mild exertional dyspnea and angina with exertion. Recent pulmonary function tests and TTE argue against worsening COPD and AS, and you think perhaps the CAD is worsening. You send this patient for an exercise stress test to further classify his CAD to try to identify any reversible ischemia. During the stress test, your patient's blood pressure falls precipitously and he experiences syncope.

**Reasoning Error(s)**
- Not knowing the harms of exercise stress testing in severe symptomatic AS
- Inability to correlate symptoms to a specific disease (e.g., worsening dyspnea and AS)
- Lack of attention that results in prolonged exposure of exercise testing in the presence of newly aware symptomatic AS

**How to Avoid the Mistake**
- Understand that exercise testing iatrogenically creates an exaggerated state of supply-demand mismatch in severe AS. In older studies, symptomatic severe AS patients most commonly experienced hemodynamic collapse (abrupt falls in blood pressure) during exercise testing. This can be very dangerous, often leading to syncope. Other complications include supraventricular and ventricular tachyarrhythmias as well as, very rarely, asystole.
- Explore the patient's symptom history carefully and try your best to correlate with objective tests that may suggest whether worsening symptoms correlate to one disease process or another. Remember, the symptoms of severe AS worsen gradually and are related to inadequate cardiac output (syncope, angina, dyspnea).
- Avoid all exercise stress testing in severe AS with symptoms due to possibility of hemodynamic collapse. If a patient undergoes stress testing without knowledge of symptoms (e.g., stress testing in severe AS to determine whether a patient is truly asymptomatic), terminate the testing as soon as symptoms arise.

**Antidote**
- Terminate exercise stress testing immediately.
- AVR

**Common Scenarios**
- Not applicable

**Note(s)**
- Nonexercise stress tests are not contraindicated in symptomatic severe AS because the cardiac output can match the overall demand of the body (i.e., noncardiac muscles require a constantly oxygen supply since they are no more active during the stress test than at baseline).

**Further Reading**
- Excellent prospective study evaluating complications in exercise stress testing, including AS: Atterhög JH, et al. Exercise testing: a prospective study of complication rates. *Am Heart J*. 1979;98(5):572–579.

## MISTAKE: INADEQUATE CONTROL OF CHRONIC HYPERTENSION IN SEVERE AORTIC STENOSIS

| | |
|---|---|
| **Case Example** | A 73-year-old male with hypertension (HTN), hyperlipidemia (HLD), chronic kidney disease (CKD), HFpEF, and severe AS presents to your outpatient clinic for routine follow-up. You notice that his home systolic blood pressures are consistently >140 mmHg. |
| **Reasoning Error(s)** | ■ Lack of awareness of the prognostic implication of uncontrolled hypertension in AS<br>■ Lack of knowledge of pathophysiologic mechanisms contributing to increased LV stress in patients with AS and HTN<br>■ Incorrect choice of antihypertensives in patients with AS |
| **How to Avoid the Mistake** | ■ Understand that patients with mild to moderate AS who have concomitant untreated HTN had a 56% greater rate of ischemic cardiovascular events and twice the mortality than patients without HTN. Hence, an integral part of managing any patient with AS is to control their blood pressure to standard targets of <130/80.<br>■ Understand that uncontrolled HTN accelerates LV remodeling in AS, with significant hemodynamic implications while also potentially accelerating the stenosis.<br>■ Consider HTN treatment with angiotensin-converting enzyme (ACE) inhibitors, as they have the added benefit of reducing pathologic LV remodeling. |
| **Antidote** | ■ Not applicable |
| **Common Scenarios** | ■ Not applicable |
| **Note(s)** | ■ Thiazide diuretics may worsen stroke volume (especially if the LV cavity is small) and be less beneficial, although future studies are needed to discern this. Be careful when diuresing patients with severe AS since they are very preload dependent.<br>■ Uncontrolled hypertension in severe AS predisposes patients to flash pulmonary edema. |
| **Further Reading** | ■ Excellent retrospective study evaluating the relationship between BP and AS: Nielsen OW, et al. Assessing optimal blood pressure in patients with asymptomatic aortic valve stenosis: the Simvastatin Ezetimibe in Aortic Stenosis Study (SEAS). *Circulation.* 2016;134(6):455–468. |

## MISTAKE: LACK OF VALVE INTERVENTION FOR SEVERE SYMPTOMATIC AORTIC STENOSIS

| | |
|---|---|
| **Case Example** | A 74-year-old male with HTN, CKD, and anemia is admitted to the hospital for exertional angina. As part of his workup, he receives a TTE, which reveals severe AS. He is discharged from the hospital and follows up with his primary care provider, who focuses on possible CAD as the primary cause of his angina. Two months after his PCP visit, the patient has a syncopal event where he hits his head and has a fatal brain hemorrhage. |

**Reasoning Error(s)**
- Lack of knowledge of indications for AVR
- Not knowing that valve intervention in the setting of symptomatic severe AS applies to both high-gradient and low-flow, low-gradient AS
- Clinical equipoise regarding most likely cause of symptoms
- Thinking that symptoms must occur at rest
- Incorrect belief that a valve replacement is indicated only after a clinical event

**How to Avoid the Mistake**
- Understand the indications for AVR in symptomatic AS:
  - Severe symptomatic high-gradient AS
  - Severe symptomatic low-flow, low-gradient AS
- Remember that symptoms are defined as exertional syncope (or presyncope), angina, or dyspnea that is elicited from either history or exercise testing. The patient need not be symptomatic only by history as their exertional levels at baseline are often limited.
- Determine the likelihood of symptoms being attributable to severe AS. This can be challenging in patients with multiple comorbidities that overlap in symptomology (e.g., COPD and heart failure). Remember that AS symptoms are exertional and are almost never at rest, whereas severe COPD and heart failure may present with symptoms at rest. Certain physical exam findings may also sway you toward or away from AS as the most likely culprit. However, if there is uncertainty, valve replacement is likely indicated as it will at least clarify the situation while fixing a problem that will soon need to be fixed.
- Coronary angiography is routinely performed in anticipation of AVR and helps delineate the contribution of coronary disease to the patient's symptoms.

**Antidote**
- AVR

**Common Scenarios**
- Not applicable

**Note(s)**
- AVR is indicated in all symptomatic patients with high-gradient AS. Notably, patients with low-flow, low-gradient AS are considered to have symptomatic severe AS. Regardless of whether the low-flow, low-gradient AS is classic (reduced LVEF) or paradoxical (preserved LVEF), AVR is indicated.
- Limited evidence suggests an improved 1-year mortality benefit when using an ACE inhibitor or ARB after AVR.

## MISTAKE: LACK OF VALVE INTERVENTION FOR SEVERE ASYMPTOMATIC AORTIC STENOSIS

**Case Example**
An 83-year-old female with HTN, T2DM, and CKD presents for follow-up. On your last visit with her, you auscultated a III/VI, crescendo-decrescendo murmur at the right upper sternal border; you also noted that her carotid upstroke was weak. You referred this patient for TTE, which revealed severe AS (AVA 0.8 cm², mean gradient of 44 mmHg, and a peak velocity of 4.4 m/s); her LVEF is additionally measured to be 45%. However, both at this current visit and at the previous visit she denies any episodes of syncope, exertional angina, or changes in exercise tolerance. You classify her severe AS as asymptomatic and do not refer for valve replacement. You are upset to learn that she died 7 months later.

| | |
|---|---|
| **Reasoning Error(s)** | ■ False sense of reassurance given the asymptomatic nature (symptom-triggered treatment mindset)<br>■ Lack of knowledge of indications for valve replacement for patients with asymptomatic but severe AS<br>■ Forgetting the poor prognosis in patients with asymptomatic severe AS and benefits of valve intervention in these patients |
| **How to Avoid the Mistake** | ■ Understand the indications and rationale for AVR in severe asymptomatic AS:<br> ■ LVEF <50%<br>■ To help with cardiac output and prevent worsening heart failure<br> ■ Worsening LVEF on three or more serial imaging studies<br>■ Potential heart failure (myocyte exhaustion) due to high afterload<br> ■ Critical AS (aortic velocity ≥5 m/s)<br>■ Significantly higher risk of poor outcomes<br> ■ Rapid progression (aortic velocity increasing by ≥3 m/s yearly)<br>■ Inevitable need for replacement and high risk for late valve intervention given rapid progression<br> ■ Concomitant open-heart surgery<br>■ To minimize complications of multiple operations<br>■ Think beyond simply symptoms when determining clinical action. For example, prevention of downstream consequences is just as important as curing a disease state. |
| **Antidote** | ■ AVR |
| **Common Scenarios** | ■ Not applicable |
| **Note(s)** | ■ For patients with asymptomatic severe AS but with LVEF >50%, check whether the LVEF may be overestimated in the setting of significant MR, which increases LVEF (albeit the stroke volume is not all forward). Often, fixing the aortic valve may also improve the MR due to decreasing the afterload.<br>■ Most patients with asymptomatic severe AS develop symptoms within 5 years. |
| **Further Reading** | ■ Longitudinal follow-up of patients with asymptomatic severe AS: Pellikka PA, et al. Outcome of 622 adults with asymptomatic, hemodynamically significant severe aortic stenosis during prolonged follow-up. *Circulation.* 2005;111(24):3290–3295. |

## MISTAKE: USING TRANSCATHETER AORTIC VALVE REPLACEMENT IN BICUSPID AORTIC VALVE STENOSIS

| | |
|---|---|
| **Case Example** | A 60-year-old male presents to your office for evaluation of aortic valve intervention in the setting of severe symptomatic AS. You astutely suspect a BAV given the patient's relatively young age. TTE and CT transcatheter AVR (TAVR) protocol confirm a BAV though it reveals an above average sized aortic annulus. You eagerly refer the patient to your interventionalist colleague for a TAVR who refuses to place a TAVR, noting that a balloon expandable valve often leads to an incomplete seal and substantive valvular leak for bicuspids. |

| | |
|---|---|
| **Reasoning Error(s)** | ■ Assuming that TAVR applies to any type of aortic valve anatomy |
| | ■ Not having considered the anatomical implications for TAVR of BAV |
| | ■ Lack of familiarity with valvular intervention strategies for BAV |
| | ■ Not knowing the evidence for TAVR in bicuspid AS |
| **How to Avoid the Mistake** | ■ Understand that BAVs possess a different anatomy compared to tricuspid aortic valves that may influence compatibility with TAVR models, which are currently designed for tricuspid aortic valves. For instance, fusion of two cusps in a bicuspid valve leads to a narrow orifice area that may cause improper and asymmetric expansion of the valve leaflets using a TAVR valve. Furthermore, the constrained aortic orifice may lead to improper sealing and leak, especially with a balloon expandable valve. Hence, TAVR is avoided in bicuspids but can be considered in higher-risk surgical patients. |
| | ■ Realize that all large TAVR trials have mostly excluded patients with BAVs. Thus, while use of TAVR in BAV is not an absolute contraindication, remember that it is an off-label indication done in extenuating circumstances such as patients with prohibitive surgical risk or in ongoing clinical trials. |
| | ■ Remember that international guidelines currently recommend surgical AVR for BAV. However, this recommendation should be taken in context based on the patient's surgical risk, institutional experience using TAVR in BAV, and patient preferences. |
| **Antidote** | ■ Not applicable |
| **Common Scenarios** | ■ Not applicable |
| **Note(s)** | ■ BAV is the most common congenital cardiac abnormality, occurring in approximately 1 in 100 patients. Early-onset AS (e.g., <70 years old) should prompt suspicion for BAVs, which are more prone to calcification and at an earlier age. However, you may be surprised to find that up to 1 in 4 severely stenotic aortic valves in patients 80 years or older are bicuspid. |
| | ■ In contrast to international guidelines, the US Food and Drug Administration has recently formally approved TAVR use in aortic valves regardless of anatomy. |
| | ■ Given the association of aortic root dilation with BAVs, evaluation of the aortic arch should be performed in all patients noted to have a BAV. |
| **Further Reading** | ■ Excellent review article on the role of TAVR in bicuspid AS: Vincent F, et al. Transcatheter aortic valve replacement in bicuspid aortic valve stenosis. *Circulation.* 2021;143(10):1043–1061. |

## MISTAKE: FORGETTING TO CUSTOMIZE THE TRANSCATHETER AORTIC VALVE REPLACEMENT VALVE TO PATIENT CHARACTERISTICS

| | |
|---|---|
| **Case Example** | A 75-year-old female with severe symptomatic AS and two-vessel CAD undergoes TAVR with a supra-annular the self-expanding valve. The patient tolerates the procedure well without complications. Three months later, the patient is admitted with crushing substernal chest pain during an inferior STEMI. In the cath lab, you have significant difficulty cannulating the right coronary artery given the presence of a supra-annular self-expanding valve. |

| | |
|---|---|
| **Reasoning Error(s)** | ▪ Lack of knowledge of the various TAVR valve types and their unique features |
| | ▪ Not knowing the range of sizes for each TAVR valve type |
| | ▪ Foregoing meticulous planning of valve anatomy and most compatible valve preop (e.g., based on CT TAVR studies) |
| **How to Avoid the Mistake** | ▪ Learn the two major TAVR valve types and their key distinctive features: |
| |     ▪ CoreValve Evolut: self-expanding (higher risk for conduction block); supra-annular (difficult to access the coronaries afterward); repositionable if not fully deployed |
| |     ▪ Edwards Sapien: balloon-expandable (lower risk for conduction block); intra-annular; outer skirt that reduces paravalvular leak; more common for valve-in-valve interventions |
| | ▪ Remember that each valve type possesses several different sizes. The CoreValve ranges from 23 to 34 mm, whereas the Sapien is between 20 and 29 mm. An especially large annulus may require the CoreValve due to the wider size range. A CoreValve may also be useful in small annuli given the supra-annular design, which creates a slightly larger effective orifice compared to an intra-annular design for any given valve size. Always plan meticulously prior to operating to ensure the best outcomes. Obtain CT studies gated on the aortic valve and extended to the iliofemoral arteries to obtain insight into the patient's unique anatomy and compatibility with TAVR valve types. Consider other workup such as a left heart catheterization for potential coronary intervention prior to TAVR since it may be more difficult to access the coronaries after TAVR (particularly for CoreValve). |
| **Antidote** | ▪ Not applicable |
| **Common Scenarios** | ▪ Not applicable |
| **Note(s)** | ▪ Among patients with AS, up to 40% possess significant coronary artery disease that may require intervention either before or after TAVR. Depending on the TAVR valve choice (particularly CoreValve Evolut), it may be easier to revascularize prior to valve deployment. |
| | ▪ In the RE-ACCESS study, almost all cases of unsuccessful coronary cannulation post-TAVR were in the CoreValve Evolut and specifically of the right coronary artery (RCA). Furthermore, cannulation time and contrast medium used were greater for the RCA. |
| **Further Reading** | ▪ The RE-ACCESS study that investigated ability to access the coronaries after TAVR: Barbanti M, et al. Coronary cannulation after transcatheter aortic valve replacement: the RE-ACCESS Study. *JACC Cardiovasc Interv.* 2020;13(21):2542–2555. |

## MISTAKE: ROUTINE BALLOON VALVULOPLASTY FOR AORTIC STENOSIS

| | |
|---|---|
| **Case Example** | A 75-year-old female with severe symptomatic AS presents to your valve clinic. She inquiries about the various options for valve intervention. As a first-year fellow, you describe the range of options from surgical valve replacement to transcatheter valve replacement and balloon valvuloplasty. The patient exclaims "Well, I don't want a new object in my heart! Let's do the balloon valvuloplasty." You agree and eagerly inform the attending about your knack at patient-centered decision-making. |

**Reasoning Error(s)**
- Lack of understanding the consequences of aortic balloon valvuloplasty
- Forgetting the short longevity of balloon valvuloplasty for calcific AS
- Not knowing the modern indications for aortic balloon valvuloplasty

**How to Avoid the Mistake**
- Understand the complications of balloon valvuloplasty. As you may imagine with the mechanism of a balloon valvuloplasty, a balloon is expanded to literally crack apart the calcifications that are restricting leaflet movement. As the calcium cracks, pieces may detach and embolize distally, causing complications such as stroke.
- Remember that the average duration of improved AS after aortic balloon valvuloplasty is only 6–12 months. In one study (Dawson et al, 2020), the mean aortic valve area after balloon valvuloplasty went from 0.79 cm² at 1 month to 0.73 cm² at 6 months and 0.66 cm² at 12 months. Mean preprocedure aortic valve area was 0.65 cm².
- Remember that isolated aortic balloon valvuloplasty is rarely performed nowadays, mainly in patients who are so critically ill (e.g., infection) that they may not tolerate a valve replacement or may introduce risk to the valve prosthesis.

**Antidote**
- Not applicable

**Common Scenarios**
- Not applicable

**Note(s)**
- The mortality rate for balloon aortic valvuloplasty severe symptomatic AS is very high at 1, 6, and 12 months: approximately 10%, 21%, and 28%, respectively (Klecyznski et al, 2021).

## MISTAKE: FORGETTING TO CONSIDER RENIN-ANGIOTENSIN-ALDOSTERONE SYSTEM BLOCKADE AFTER TRANSCATHETER AORTIC VALVE IMPLANTATION

**Case Example**

A 75-year-old female with severe symptomatic AS undergoes valve replacement with a 23-mm Edwards Sapien 3. She tolerates the procedure well without complications and is discharged with follow-up in a week. When you are seeing her in clinic a week later, you are surprised that the patient was not started on an ACE inhibitor prior to discharge.

**Reasoning Error(s)**
- Not knowing the preliminary evidence for a role of renin-angiotensin-aldosterone system (RAAS) blockade post transcatheter aortic valve implantation (TAVI)
- Lack of patient-centered decision-making

**How to Avoid the Mistake**
- Understand that RAAS blockade (i.e., ACE inhibitors or ARBs) currently have weak to moderate evidence to suggest potential decreased mortality post-TAVI. Hypothesized mechanisms include increasing positive LV remodeling once the high afterload state has been removed and positive changes to endothelial function.
- Whether you believe in the utility of RAAS blockade post-TAVI, the patient should be informed of the potential benefit. Ultimately, the patient may decide that they want to try an ACE inhibitor or ARB (perhaps in lieu of another medication) given the potential benefit and low risk.

**Antidote**
- Not applicable

**Common Scenarios**
- Not applicable

| | |
|---|---|
| **Note(s)** | ■ Be conscientious about starting an ACE inhibitor or ARB in patients post-TAVR who may be especially prone to contrast-induced acute kidney injury, such as those with borderline renal function. |
| **Further Reading** | ■ Retrospective study of RAAS blockade post-TAVI: Inohara T, et al. Association of renin-angiotensin inhibitor treatment with mortality and heart failure readmission in patients with transcatheter aortic valve replacement. *JAMA*. 2018;320(21):2231-2241. |

## MISTAKE: AVOIDING TRANSCATHETER AORTIC VALVE REPLACEMENT DUE TO ANTICIPATED DUAL ANTIPLATELET THERAPY IN HEYDE SYNDROME

| | |
|---|---|
| **Case Example** | A 75-year-old female with known severe asymptomatic AS presents to the emergency department with significant melena. Initial endoscopy is unrevealing, and a video capsule endoscopy is undertaken that reveals numerous AVMs. Her bleeding resolves and she is sent home but re-presents with melena several times over the next few months. Understandably, the patient is very frustrated but informed that there is no easy solution to fixing her bleeding issue. She mentions seeing on Google the possibility of her bleeding due to shearing of the von Willebrand factor (vWF) dimers in the setting of her severe AS. You tell her that while this could be the case, a TAVR is not an option given her risk of GI bleeding and the necessity for antiplatelet therapy in the initial months after TAVR. The patient continues to present for recurrent bleeding and eventually dies due to a massive bleeding event from her AVMs. |
| **Reasoning Error(s)** | ■ Lack of familiarity with Heyde syndrome<br>■ Lack of understanding the mechanism of severe AS facilitating GI bleeding<br>■ Not recognizing the curative solution for GI bleeding secondary to Heyde syndrome |
| **How to Avoid the Mistake** | ■ Recognize GI bleeding that is potentially due to severe AS. Heyde syndrome is upper GI bleeding caused by formation of AVMs in the setting of disrupted integrity of vWF multimers due to shearing forces caused by the narrowed aortic orifice. Specifically, vWF is critical to preventing angiogenesis (i.e., formation of AVMs).<br>■ Understand that the solution to Heyde syndrome is relieving the narrowed aortic orifice. This is most often done via TAVR since most patients with Heyde syndrome are older and at higher surgical risk.<br>■ Remember that while antiplatelet(s) are recommended post-TAVR for the first 3–6 months, the increase in bleeding risk due to the antiplatelets is offset by the relatively fast resolution of AVMs in the presence of intact vWF multimers. Furthermore, while still under investigation, DAPT has been associated with increased bleeding with little to no improvement in ischemic outcomes. Thus, antiplatelet monotherapy can further decrease bleeding risk post-TAVR in patients with Heyde syndrome. |
| **Antidote** | ■ Not applicable |
| **Common Scenarios** | ■ Not applicable |

| | |
|---|---|
| **Note(s)** | ■ Stroke rates post-TAVR are similar to those post-SAVR, approximately 7%. Approximately 10% of patients undergoing TAVR are newly diagnosed with atrial fibrillation, which may partly explain stroke further out from the TAVR date. |
| | ■ The major bleeding risk within the first 30 days of TAVR was approximately 10% in the PARTNER-II trial, which demonstrated noninferiority of TAVR (versus SAVR) in intermediate-risk surgical patients with severe symptomatic AS. |
| **Further Reading** | ■ Excellent review on antithrombotic therapy post-TAVR: Guedeney P, et al. Antithrombotic therapy after transcatheter aortic valve replacement. *Circulation*. 2019;12(1):e007411. |

# Aortic Insufficiency

## MISTAKE: β-BLOCKERS IN AORTIC REGURGITATION

| | |
|---|---|
| **Case Example** | A 62-year-old female with a history of polysubstance use disorder and CAD is being evaluated after presenting to the hospital with fevers and altered mental status. Initial TTE demonstrates an echodensity concerning for infective endocarditis of the aortic valve. A few days later, she is found newly dyspneic with a new III/VI diastolic murmur at the left, third intercostal space with a widened pulse pressure. Repeat TTE reveals acute aortic insufficiency likely from valvular perforation. As a part of her treatment, the patient is continued on metoprolol as it is a home medication. Her pulmonary edema worsens, and she is transferred to the CCU for cardiogenic shock. |
| **Reasoning Error(s)** | ■ Continuing chronic medications without appropriate evaluation of the current clinical context |
| | ■ Limited understanding of physiologic effect of β-blockers on aortic regurgitation (AR) pathology |
| **How to Avoid the Mistake** | ■ Understand the relationship between β-blockers and heart rate in the context of aortic insufficiency: β-blockers block the compensatory tachycardia often needed in acute aortic insufficiency; lengthen diastolic time, which increases the regurgitant flow (as aortic insufficiency occurs during diastole); and decrease cardiac output (and potentially worsening venous congestion). β-Blockers are less detrimental (though should be avoided if possible) in chronic AR. |
| | ■ Continuously reevaluate the need for each medication as a patient's clinical situation evolves. This is especially important for chronic medications from the home medication list or long-term medications started inpatient. |
| **Antidote** | ■ Afterload reduction |
| **Common Scenarios** | ■ Not applicable |
| **Note(s)** | ■ While the principles of avoiding β-blockers still holds true in acute aortic insufficiency, the treatment is generally urgent surgery, especially when complicated by cardiogenic shock. |
| | ■ β-Blockers are cautiously used in patients with aortic dissection complicated by AR due to the need to strike a fine balance between maintaining compensatory tachycardia for the aortic insufficiency but also minimizing aortic wall stress. |

# MISTAKE: INADEQUATE MANAGEMENT OF HYPERTENSION IN AORTIC REGURGITATION

**Case Example**

A 67-year-old male with HTN, HLD, T2DM, CAD, and COPD was just discharged from the hospital. He immigrated to the United States nearly a decade ago but has had limited medical follow-up. He presented to a hospital after new dyspnea on exertion. During his hospital admission, he was noted to be volume overloaded and received a TTE, which revealed severe AR without indication for intervention. You are evaluating him in your clinic and focus your attention on his new heart failure symptoms, optimizing his diuretic dosage. You notice the patient's blood pressure is elevated to the 150s but defer hypertension management to his PCP.

**Reasoning Error(s)**

- Lack of understanding the pathophysiologic mechanisms behind aortic insufficiency
- Lack of knowledge of beneficial effect of vasodilators in aortic insufficiency
- Deferring management of a common disease to another provider despite it being an integral part of care for a cardiac condition

**How to Avoid the Mistake**

- Learn the maladaptive pathophysiology of AR: LV volume overload (specifically, diastolic volume) leading to LV dilation and eccentric hypertrophy.
- Understand that the primary goal of medical therapy for patients with chronic AR is to control systolic hypertension to improve cardiac output, reduce progression of AR and pathologic remodeling of the LV, and minimize LV wall stress. Good choices include vasodilators such as ACE inhibitors, ARBs, and dihydropyridine (DHP) calcium channel blockers.
- Remember that long-term vasodilator therapy decreases and delays the need for AVR in severe asymptomatic AR and normal LVEF.
- For medical conditions that heavily influence the condition you are caring for, establish open communication with whoever manages those conditions or manage them yourself. Do not simply assume that those conditions (e.g., hypertension) will be managed (let alone optimally).

**Antidote**

- Hypertension management

**Common Scenarios**

- Not applicable

**Note(s)**

- Based on the Framingham study, the presence of systolic hypertension seems to be the main predictor of adverse outcomes in patients with asymptomatic chronic AR.
- The most common causes of aortic insufficiency are idiopathic, aortic root dilation (most common in developed countries), and valve degeneration.

**Further Reading**

- Landmark trial evaluating the benefit of blood pressure control with vasodilator therapy in patients with AR: Scognamiglio R, et al. Nifedipine in asymptomatic patients with severe aortic regurgitation and normal left ventricular function. *N Engl J Med*. 1994;331:689–694.

## MISTAKE: FORGETTING TO USE RENIN-ANGIOTENSIN-ALDOSTERONE SYSTEM BLOCKADE IN SEVERE AORTIC REGURGITATION

**Case Example**
A 72-year-old female is transferred to your care on the cardiology floor due to severe chronic AR with clinical signs and symptoms of heart failure and significantly elevated systolic blood pressure. Due to her hypertension, you start her on a regimen of hydrochlorothiazide and amlodipine. She symptomatically improves over the hospital stay, and you discharge her with follow-up, which she does not attend. The patient continues to have multiple episodes of decompensation over the next year.

**Reasoning Error(s)**
- Assuming all hypertensive medications are equal when treating AR
- Incomplete understanding of the mechanism by which RAAS blockade is beneficial in AR
- Lack of reflex for GDMT for AR similar to heart failure

**How to Avoid the Mistake**
- Understand the mechanism by which RAAS blockade benefits AR. RAAS inhibition reduces LV afterload, decreases LV wall stress, and reduces LV remodeling by limiting dilatation and hypertrophy. In fact, ACE inhibitors have been shown in studies to significantly reduce all-cause and cardiovascular mortality in patients with AR.
  - Consider the specific mechanistic targets of antihypertensives and how your choice relates to the pathophysiology of a patient's disease. ACE inhibitors and ARBs not only have antihypertensive effects but also improve LV remodeling in aortic insufficiency similar to their role in systolic heart failure.

**Antidote**
- ACE inhibitor or ARB

**Common Scenarios**
- Not applicable

**Note(s)**
- In chronic aortic insufficiency, increased LV end-diastolic diameter (LVEDD) and LV end-systolic diameter (LVESD) are markers of LV volume overload. Furthermore, an increased LVESD often correlates with systolic dysfunction (if not a high risk for impending systolic dysfunction).

**Further Reading**
- Large, retrospective study indicating the beneficial implications of RAAS blockade in AR: Elder DH, et al. The impact of renin-angiotensin-aldosterone system blockade on heart failure outcomes and mortality in patients identified to have AR: a large population cohort study. *JACC*. 2011;58(20):2084–2091.

## MISTAKE: LACK OF VALVE INTERVENTION FOR ASYMPTOMATIC AORTIC REGURGITATION WITH LEFT VENTRICULAR EJECTION FRACTION ≤55%

**Case Example**
A 64-year-old female with HTN, T2DM, and long-standing rheumatoid arthritis receives a TTE after a murmur was auscultated during a new patient visit. Per the TTE report, the patient has severe AR with an LVEF of 50%. The report does not note any other valvular abnormalities or any obvious wall motion abnormalities. The patient does not have any symptoms such as shortness of breath, fatigue, syncope, or chest pain. You continue to care for her over several years. You are startled when you receive a message that she has been admitted to the CCU with cardiogenic shock due to heart failure secondary to AR.

| | |
|---|---|
| **Reasoning Error(s)** | ■ Assuming systolic dysfunction in severe AR is reflected by typical LVEF values |
| | ■ Lack of understanding of indications of valve intervention in asymptomatic AR |
| | ■ False reassurance by lack of symptoms |
| **How to Avoid the Mistake** | ■ Understand the indications for AVR in asymptomatic severe AR: |
| | ■ LVEF ≤55% |
| | ■ LVESD >50 mm |
| | ■ Worsening LVEF to ≤55% or increase in LVEDD >65 mm on three or more serial imaging studies |
| | ■ Concomitant open-heart surgery |
| | ■ Avoid the assumption that LVEF is an equal assessment of systolic function across all types of heart disease. Due to the regurgitant blood flow, an LVEF ≤55% reflects significant LV dysfunction and reduced forward cardiac output. |
| | ■ Think beyond simply symptoms when determining clinical action. For example prevention of downstream consequences is just as important as curing a disease state. |
| **Antidote** | ■ AVR |
| **Common Scenarios** | ■ Not applicable |
| **Note(s)** | ■ LV dilatation corresponds with severity of AR disease and reflects LV systolic dysfunction (whether subclinical or apparent). |
| **Further Reading** | ■ One of the original studies evaluating the effects of AVR on patients with chronic AR with regard to changes in LV function: Bonow RO, et al. Long-term serial changes in left ventricular function and reversal of ventricular dilatation after valve replacement for chronic aortic regurgitation. *Circulation*. 1988;78(5):1108–1120. |

# Mitral Regurgitation

## MISTAKE: FORGETTING TO OPTIMIZE AFTERLOAD REDUCTION IN MITRAL REGURGITATION

| | |
|---|---|
| **Case Example** | You are following a 71-year-old male with HTN, HLD, and severe primary MR in cardiology clinic. On today's visit, he tells you that his exercise tolerance has gradually decreased over the past few months to a mere two city blocks. His BP is 128/90 on hydrochlorothiazide. You note that this may be due to age-related deconditioning and reassure him that his blood pressure is stellar. |
| **Reasoning Error(s)** | ■ Lack of understanding the relationship between afterload and regurgitant flow in MR due to inadequate understanding of the pathophysiology of MR |
| | ■ Not optimizing chronic medications with evolving clinical context |
| | ■ False reassurance by a normal blood pressure |

| | |
|---|---|
| **How to Avoid the Mistake** | ■ Understand that the degree of MR is a function of afterload. Hence, afterload reduction is crucial in treating MR, particularly those with chronic MR that appears functional. Reducing afterload will increase cardiac output by decreasing flow from the left ventricle to the left atrium (the regurgitation) and improve symptoms such as exertional dyspnea. |
| | ■ Remember that while vasodilator therapy for afterload reduction has no benefit in asymptomatic normotensive patients with severe primary MR, the above patient has symptoms and thus would benefit from an attempt at optimizing medical therapy. |
| | ■ Always verify that chronic medications are necessary and/or optimal for a patient's evolving clinical status. Though the above patient has well-controlled hypertension, switching out an afterload reducing agent such as losartan would be better than hydrochlorothiazide for optimizing forward flow. |
| **Antidote** | ■ Afterload reduction |
| **Common Scenarios** | ■ Not applicable |
| **Note(s)** | ■ Acute MR may be a deadly complication of STEMI with papillary muscle rupture. A mainstay of treatment in acute MR is afterload reduction, often with intravenous sodium nitroprusside or nicardipine. These, however, may cause systemic hypotension and mechanical support with an intra-aortic balloon bump can be used to reduce afterload while also increasing diastolic blood pressure and systemic perfusion. |

## MISTAKE: OVERLOOKING SYSTOLIC DYSFUNCTION IN SEVERE MITRAL REGURGITATION WITH NORMAL EJECTION FRACTION

| | |
|---|---|
| **Case Example** | You are reviewing the TTE of one of your clinic patients. She recently had a hospitalization after developing shortness of breath, orthopnea, and reduced exercise tolerance. She was treated with IV diuresis and discharged without a diuretic given a normal LVEF and no history of heart failure. When reviewing the TTE report, you notice that the patient has severe MR but are reassured to see an LVEF of 55%. You later find out your patient is readmitted back to the hospital one week later for similar symptoms. |
| **Reasoning Error(s)** | ■ Equating LVEF as an equal marker of systolic dysfunction across a spectrum of disease |
| | ■ Limited knowledge on relationship between LVEF and MR |
| | ■ Lack of pathophysiologic knowledge that facilitates understanding of LVEF in severe MR |

| How to Avoid the Mistake | ■ Understand the pathophysiology of MR. With significant backward flow, the left atrial volume (and hence pressure) increase, which leads to increased preload and LV end-diastolic volume (and pressure). Over time, this volume overload leads to ventricular dilation, which may worsen MR due to mitral annular dilation and maladaptation of the leaflets. A vicious cycle begins that eventually leads to heart failure due to overdilation that impairs contractility. |
|---|---|
| | ■ Understand that the EF is simply a measure of how much overall blood leaves the ventricle (not necessarily forward out of the heart). In the case of MR, a significant amount of blood leaves retrograde due to decreased afterload from the faulty mitral valve. Furthermore, the LV end-diastolic volume is larger to begin with due to increased preload. Since more blood leaves the ventricle overall due to less afterload, the EF increases. In severe MR, the EF may increase significantly, not uncommonly by approximately 10% or more (a normal LVEF is probably around 70%). Hence, an LVEF <60% with severe MR likely signals systolic dysfunction. |
| | ■ Always interpret data in context. For example, EF should be interpreted in the context of stroke volume and afterload. |
| Antidote | ■ Not applicable |
| Common Scenarios | ■ Not applicable |
| Note(s) | ■ Patients with severe MR and LVEF <60% should have routine systolic heart failure guideline-directed medical therapy (GDMT) initiated. |
| | ■ Since the LVEF in severe MR may be difficult to interpret, ongoing work is looking into the utility of a "forward" EF that considers only the amount of blood pushed forward. One study in 2017 demonstrated that this may improve patient selection and timing for mitral valve intervention. |
| Further Reading | ■ Study that evaluated forward EF compared to total LVEF in regard to outcomes in patients with MR: Dupuis M, et al. Forward left ventricular ejection fraction: a simple risk marker in patients with primary mitral regurgitation. *J Am Heart Assoc.* 2017;6(11): e006309. |

## MISTAKE: FORGETTING SERIAL TRANSTHORACIC ECHOCARDIOGRAPHIC MONITORING FOR ASYMPTOMATIC SEVERE PRIMARY MITRAL REGURGITATION

| Case Example | A 70-year-old female was referred to your clinic for follow-up of incidentally discovered severe MR with a normal LVEF (70%). She has no symptoms. You reassure her that there is nothing to do now because she is asymptomatic without other comorbidities. The patient is pleased and disappears for a few years, after which you see her hospitalized for heart failure exacerbation. |
|---|---|
| Reasoning Error(s) | ■ Reassurance based on the lack of symptoms |
| | ■ Lack of understanding the natural trajectory of severe primary MR |
| | ■ Lack of adequate follow-up |
| | ■ Not knowing the ideal time for valve intervention in primary MR |

**How to Avoid the Mistake**

- Understand that the average risk of developing symptoms in severe primary MR is approximately 10% per year. Virtually all patients with severe primary MR will have developed symptoms within 10 years of diagnosis. Furthermore, compensatory and eventually maladaptive changes of the LV occur that may require valve intervention despite the lack of symptoms. Thus, these patients should be monitored every 6–12 months with TTE.
- Understand that the ideal time to intervene on asymptomatic severe primary MR is prior to the development of systolic dysfunction. Frequent monitoring will provide valuable information such as changes in LVEF and/or LVESD over time.
- Ensure that patients with asymptomatic severe primary MR are plugged in with good follow-up, such as through a comprehensive valve center. This may also involve working with social work and care coordination for patients who are frequently lost to follow-up.

**Antidote**

- Not applicable

**Common Scenarios**

- Not applicable

**Note(s)**

- If a TTE is unable to adequately characterize the MR, TEE is recommended. Discrepancies between TTE and TEE may be investigated with CMR. However, TTE is usually adequate for routine surveillance to monitor changes in LVEF and LVESD once severe MR is established.

## MISTAKE: OVERLOOKING MITRAL VALVE INTERVENTION IN SYMPTOMATIC SEVERE PRIMARY MITRAL REGURGITATION WITH NORMAL LEFT VENTRICULAR FUNCTION

**Case Example**

A 54-year-old female with mitral valve prolapse presents to the hospital because of increasing shortness of breath and dyspnea on exertion. On transthoracic echocardiogram, she is noted to meet criteria for severe MR; her LVEF is 70%. She is discharged from the hospital after resolution of symptoms. You see her in your outpatient clinic and continue to manage her symptomatically and with medical therapy. Unfortunately, she has multiple hospital admissions over the next few months.

**Reasoning Error(s)**

- Being falsely reassured by normal LVEF
- Being falsely reassured by mild symptoms (lack of severity)
- Confusing the indications for intervention between primary and secondary MR
- Lack of knowledge of the indications for intervention in MR
- Hoping that medical therapy can slow or reverse the symptoms or degree of MR

**How to Avoid the Mistake**

- Understand that the onset of symptoms in chronic MR marks the beginning failures of compensatory adaptive mechanisms. Furthermore, prognosis worsens when primary MR becomes symptomatic, irrespective of symptom severity. Thus, symptomatic primary MR is a clear indication for mitral valve intervention.
- Recognize that MR is a mechanical problem that requires a mechanical solution. Optimized medical therapy has not been shown to reverse symptoms or to cause enough remodeling to avoid surgery.
- Learn other indications for valve intervention in primary MR. In asymptomatic primary MR, the primary determinant for intervention is prognosis and trajectory. For example, if the LVEF is reduced (≤ 60%), that suggests that despite the absence of symptoms, the LV is already in the maladaptive phase and requires prompt salvage. If the LVEF is preserved (e.g., ~70%) but the LV is dilating at a noticeable rate, then valve intervention is recommended proactively.

**Antidote**

- Mitral valve repair or replacement

**Common Scenarios**

- Symptomatic severe primary MR (regardless of LVEF)
- Asymptomatic severe primary MR with LVEF ≤60% or LVESD ≥40 mm
- Asymptomatic severe primary MR with LVEF >60% but progressive increase in LV size or decrease in LVEF

**Note(s)**

- Mitral valve repair is typically preferred to replacement due to lower operative mortality, lower postoperative valvular complications (e.g., thromboembolism), and great durability that seems at least comparable to replacement.

**Further Reading**

- Excellent review on mitral valve repair versus replacement: Mick SL, et al. Mitral valve repair versus replacement. *Ann Cardiothorac Surg.* 2015;4(3):230–237.

## MISTAKE: MITRAL VALVE REPLACEMENT FOR PRIMARY MITRAL REGURGITATION

**Case Example**

A 50-year-old female with severe primary MR secondary to degenerative disease presents to your clinic for an opinion on fixing the MR. You recommend mitral valve replacement, which has recently been shown to have excellent outcomes with lower operative risk.

**Reasoning Error(s)**

- Electing for the technically less difficult treatment due to local experience/limitations
- Lack of familiarity with evidence on mitral valve repair versus replacement in primary MR
- Following referral patterns of local practices without understanding outcomes data

| | |
|---|---|
| **How to Avoid the Mistake** | ■ Understand that mitral valve repair has superior outcomes (operative mortality, valve-related complications, and long-term outcomes including survival) compared to mitral valve replacement. Though mitral repair is technically more challenging, given the superior outcomes particularly in lower-risk surgical patients, referral for repair at an experienced surgical center should be considered rather than electing for replacement (or sometimes MitraClip) given the limited experience of the local surgeons.<br>■ Offer patients the option for a second opinion when local experience is limited. This is not a sign of weakness but rather good judgment and superior clinical skills to recognize the limitations of a center. |
| **Antidote** | ■ Not applicable |
| **Common Scenarios** | ■ Not applicable |
| **Note(s)** | ■ Mitral valve repair avoids the increased thrombogenicity associated with a mitral valve replacement, which is even more thrombogenic than AVRs.<br>■ The evidence for the superiority of mitral valve repair over replacement in primary MR is strongest for degenerative MR. |

## MISTAKE: FAILURE TO RECOGNIZE ACUTE MITRAL REGURGITATION OR AORTIC INSUFFICIENCY AS A SURGICAL EMERGENCY

| | |
|---|---|
| **Case Example** | A 55-year-old female with no known past medical history presents in acute hypoxic respiratory failure secondary to flash pulmonary edema. An emergent bedside TTE demonstrates severe spontaneous mitral chordal rupture; troponin and ECG rule out ischemic papillary muscle rupture. You astutely recall that MR is treated with afterload reduction and immediately start IV nitroprusside. The patient's blood pressure and oxygenation improve somewhat over the next few hours and you feel ecstatic that you managed acute MR. When the case is staffed the next morning on rounds, your attending frowns and declares that the patient should have been referred for surgery immediately. |
| **Reasoning Error(s)** | ■ Assuming that acute MR is treated similarly to chronic MR<br>■ Bias toward medical management (lack of experience with referring patients for emergent surgical management) |
| **How to Avoid the Mistake** | ■ Understand that hemodynamically significant acute MR and aortic insufficiency are surgical emergencies. While acute management does include medical management such as afterload reduction, the key is surgical correction of the anatomic disruptions.<br>■ While much of cardiology revolves around medical management, there are many cases that require invasive management. In particular, always consider a mechanical (surgical) solution for mechanical pathology. |
| **Antidote** | ■ Not applicable |
| **Common Scenarios** | ■ Not applicable |
| **Note(s)** | ■ Common causes of acute MR include spontaneous chordal rupture, ischemic posteromedial papillary muscle rupture (single blood supply), degenerative disease/mitral valve prolapse, and infective endocarditis.<br>■ Common causes of acute aortic insufficiency include infective endocarditis, aortic dissection, and iatrogenic complications (e.g., TAVI, balloon valvuloplasty). |

## MISTAKE: FIXING SECONDARY MITRAL REGURGITATION IN LEFT VENTRICULAR EJECTION FRACTION <20%

**Case Example**

A 73-year-old male with distant ischemic cardiomyopathy is evaluated for new gradual-onset dyspnea. The patient appears profoundly volume overloaded and a TTE was done, which demonstrated an LVEF 10%–15% and severe functional MR. You refer the patient for transcatheter edge-to-edge repair (MitraClip); shortly after the procedure, the patient is admitted to the ICU with cardiogenic shock.

**Reasoning Error(s)**

- Assuming that all patients with severe MR improve with valve intervention
- Not considering the mechanism of LV function after mitral valve intervention
- Lack of knowledge on indications for mitral valve intervention for patients with severe secondary MR

**How to Avoid the Mistake**

- Understand that fixing the MR suddenly leads to an unaccustomed increase in afterload for the LV. In patients with a severely reduced systolic function (e.g., LVEF <20%), the ventricle is weak and cannot handle the additional afterload postsurgery. This means that fixing the mitral valve may induce cardiogenic shock.
- Always consider the consequences of all clinical actions, no matter how big or small. Thinking through the mechanism related to the intervention and disease process may help identify consequences with which you are not familiar.

**Antidote**

- Not applicable

**Common Scenarios**

- LVEF ≤20%
- LVESD ≥70 mm
- PASP >70 mmHg

**Note(s)**

- The COAPT Study in 2018 demonstrated the feasibility and safety of using MitraClip for severe functional MR in the setting of HFrEF (specifically, ischemic cardiomyopathy). Additionally, MitraClip compared to medical therapy resulted in a 32% reduction in heart failure hospitalizations and 17% all-cause mortality benefit at 2 years.

**Further Reading**

- The COAPT Study: Stone GW, et al. Transcatheter mitral-valve repair in patients with heart failure. *N Engl J Med*. 2018;379:2307–2318.

## MISTAKE: CONCOMITANT REPLACEMENT OF AORTIC AND MITRAL VALVES IN SEVERE AORTIC STENOSIS/MITRAL REGURGITATION

**Case Example**

A 75-year-old female presents with acute hypoxic respiratory failure in the setting of flash pulmonary edema. The patient has had numerous similar presentations over the past year. A TTE demonstrates an LVEF of 40%, severe AS, and severe MR. You recommend simultaneous aortic and mitral valve replacement.

**Reasoning Error(s)**

- Assuming that all concomitant valve issues should be intervened upon simultaneously
- Lack of reasoning through the pathophysiology of MR in concomitant AS
- Forgetting that mitral valve interventions are not without additional risks/consequences

| | |
|---|---|
| **How to Avoid the Mistake** | ■ Understand that MR is affected by any condition, including AS, that increases afterload. Concomitant severe AS contributes significant afterload and may significantly increase the degree of observed MR. Fixing the AS first may improve the MR to the point where intervention on the mitral valve is unnecessary.<br><br>■ Remember that the mitral valve position is more thrombogenic when prosthetic valve replacements are used. Similarly, use of a MitraClip to reduce the MR may iatrogenically induce mitral stenosis (MS) if baseline afterload is significantly decreased with correction of a narrowed aortic orifice. |
| **Antidote** | ■ Not applicable |
| **Common Scenarios** | ■ Not applicable |
| **Note(s)** | ■ Concomitant severe AS/MR represents a very preload-dependent state. Take extra caution with maneuvers such as diuresis and Valsalva as they may lead to hemodynamic collapse and syncope. |

# Mitral Stenosis

## MISTAKE: NOT VERIFYING, CONTINUING, OR INITIATING SECONDARY PROPHYLAXIS FOR RHEUMATIC HEART DISEASE

| | |
|---|---|
| **Case Example** | A 37-year-old female with rheumatic fever as a child presents to your clinic to establish care. She is in good health without any symptoms. You review her recent transthoracic echocardiogram and note moderate MS. You reassure her that she is healthy, and schedule follow-up in a year to monitor the MS. Seven months later, you learn that she was hospitalized for acute rheumatic fever. |
| **Reasoning Error(s)** | ■ False reassurance by current good health of patients with prior rheumatic heart disease<br><br>■ Thinking recurrent rheumatic fever occurs only in the presence of a repeat infection<br><br>■ Thinking recurrent rheumatic fever does not occur after mitral valve replacement<br><br>■ Associating rheumatic fever only with developing countries and only prescribing prophylaxis accordingly<br><br>■ Lack of knowledge of secondary prophylaxis guidelines for rheumatic heart disease<br><br>■ Deferring secondary prophylaxis to another doctor (deferring responsibility) |

| | |
|---|---|
| **How to Avoid the Mistake** | ■ Understand that rheumatic fever may occur after initial infection even without a repeat symptomatic infection. This means that patients who immigrate from a developing country to a developed country do not lose their risk of recurrent infection. Furthermore, prior rheumatic fever imposes a higher risk for recurrent rheumatic fever. |
| | ■ Realize that recurrent rheumatic fever may occur despite prior resolution of infection and/or mitral valve replacement. Thus, patients require prophylactic medication for at least 10 years after the initial infection or until age 40, whichever is longer. In patients with particularly high risk for Group A streptococcal exposure, lifelong prophylaxis may be considered. |
| | ■ Learn the common antibiotic regimen for secondary prophylaxis of rheumatic fever: IM penicillin G every 4 weeks, oral penicillin V twice daily, oral sulfadiazine 1 g daily, or macrolides (in the case of intolerance to penicillin). |
| | ■ Given the potentially life-changing impact of secondary prophylaxis, ensure that the patient has someone managing the secondary prophylaxis. If nobody is, then you should lead the initiative as the consequences tie directly to the patient's valvular health. |
| **Antidote** | ■ Secondary prophylaxis for rheumatic heart disease |
| **Common Scenarios** | ■ Not applicable |
| **Note(s)** | ■ Primary prevention of rheumatic fever involves early detection of streptococcal (Group A) pharyngitis and treatment with penicillin or amoxicillin. Interestingly, there has never been a strain of Group A strep that has been resistant to penicillins. Alternatives in the case of intolerance include clindamycin or erythromycin. |
| | ■ Interestingly, four of five cases of rheumatic MS occur in women. |

## MISTAKE: LACK OF EXERCISE TESTING IN SEVERE ASYMPTOMATIC MITRAL STENOSIS

| | |
|---|---|
| **Case Example** | A 43-year-old female with hypertension and rheumatic heart disease from India presents to your clinic for follow-up. Recent TTE reveals severe MS. She denies all symptoms including dyspnea on exertion, decreased exercise tolerance, and chest pain. Given her good health, you advise her to follow-up in 1 year. Before this follow-up appointment, your patient is hospitalized with flash pulmonary edema. |
| **Reasoning Error(s)** | ■ False reassurance for patients with asymptomatic MS |
| | ■ Lack of knowledge regarding the role of exercise testing in patients with asymptomatic severe MS |
| | ■ Taking echocardiographic findings for granted without thinking about whether the findings make sense (are compatible with the clinical presentation) |

**How to Avoid the Mistake**

- Understand that the asymptomatic nature of MS depends on many factors such as the patient's activity levels and level of symptom tolerance. However, eliciting the presence of symptoms is essential to determining prognosis and optimal timing of valve intervention. In these cases, an exercise stress test may help elicit symptoms and better contextualize the imaging findings.
- Develop a habit of not only interpreting test results but also contextualizing them for each patient. For example, if echocardiography demonstrates severe MS but the patient is asymptomatic (or vice versa), further investigation is likely warranted.

**Antidote**

- Exercise stress testing

**Common Scenarios**

- Not applicable

**Note(s)**

- Rheumatic MS presents primarily with fusion of the commissures as opposed to leaflets and/or subvalvular (mitral annulus) calcification. Notably, there is usually a long latent period in between initial infection and development of MS. Since the latency period is shorter in developing countries, it is hypothesized that recurrent bouts of rheumatic fever may hasten progression.
- Once MS becomes symptomatic, the prognosis is very poor (<15% 1-year survival rate). This is in stark contrast to a >80% 10-year survival rate in asymptomatic patients.

## MISTAKE: FORGETTING MEDICAL HEMODYNAMIC OPTIMIZATION OF MITRAL STENOSIS

**Case Example:**

A 65-year-old male presents with worsening dyspnea on exertion over the past year. He becomes short of breath when he walks his usual mile a day on a flat surface. A transthoracic echocardiogram demonstrates a normal ejection fraction with a mean mitral valve gradient of 8 mm Hg, mitral valve area of 1.2 cm, and pulmonary artery systolic pressure of 35 mm Hg in the setting of likely rheumatic heart disease. The left atrium is mildly dilated. He has never had palpitations nor been discovered to have atrial fibrillation. The patient inquires regarding the potential therapeutic options, and you tell him that he will continue to be followed for now with serial echocardiograms every year. In response, the patient asks whether there are any medications that can help, and you tell him that a mechanical problem must have a mechanical solution. The patient continues to live his life with significant limitations to his walking ability.

**Reasoning Error(s)**

- Assuming that MS is managed exclusively surgically
- Lack of familiarity with managing MS given its relatively rare incidence
- Not reasoning through the pathophysiology of MS

**How to Avoid the Mistake**

- Understand the pathophysiology of MS. Hemodynamic consequences from MS arise due to inadequate LV filling and increased left atrial pressures due to increased afterload. Thus, medical management targets heart rate (the lower, the more diastolic filling time) and preload reduction (thus decreasing left-sided pressures transmitted to the pulmonary vasculature).
- Consider diuretics, salt restriction, and β-blockers as tolerated in all patients with moderate to severe MS. While these therapies do not improve the actual mitral stenosis, it can improve the left-sided pressures that lead to dyspnea.

| | |
|---|---|
| **Antidote** | ■ Not applicable |
| **Common Scenarios** | ■ Not applicable |
| **Note(s)** | ■ Severe MS on TTE is defined as a mitral valve area ≤1.0 cm² with mean mitral valve gradient >10 mmHg. Associated findings include TR velocity >3 m/s, pressure half-time >220 msec, and systolic pulmonary artery pressure >50 mmHg. |

# Infective Endocarditis

## MISTAKE: FORGETTING TO PRESCRIBE PREPROCEDURAL ANTIBIOTIC PROPHYLAXIS IN HIGH-RISK PATIENTS

| | |
|---|---|
| **Case Example** | A 71-year-old male with CAD and T2DM presents to your clinic. He has a prior bioprosthetic mitral valve replacement for severe mitral valve prolapse. He currently denies any symptoms and appears well on exam. He has no prior history of infective endocarditis. He is planned for a tooth extraction next week and you note that the patient is medically optimized. The patient is admitted to the hospital two weeks later with fever and malaise and found with a moderate-sized vegetation on the mitral valve on TTE. |
| **Reasoning Error(s)** | ■ Inadequate knowledge of indications for antibiotic prophylaxis for endocarditis |
| | ■ Lack of awareness of comorbidities that influence clinical decisions (e.g., prosthetic valve) |
| | ■ Lack of knowledge on endocarditis prophylaxis regimen(s) |
| **How to Avoid the Mistake** | ■ Understand that antibiotic prophylaxis of infective endocarditis is desired for procedures that lead to a large inoculation of bacteria in patients at increased risk for development of endocarditis (usually related to structural anomalies and/or immunocompromise). These are primarily dental procedures such as removal of molars and gingival manipulation. |
| | ■ Learn the main indications for antibiotic prophylaxis of endocarditis: |
| | ■ Prosthetic valve(s) or apparatus (e.g., clips, chords) |
| | ■ Prior infective endocarditis |
| | ■ Congenital heart disease |
| | ■ Heart transplant with abnormal valve(s) |
| | ■ Perform a thorough history, physical, and diagnostic evaluation as applicable to fully appreciate your patient's risk for endocarditis. |
| | ■ Remember that the most commonly recommended antibiotic for prophylaxis is amoxicillin |
| **Antidote** | ■ Antibiotic prophylaxis |
| **Common Scenarios** | ■ Not applicable |
| **Note(s)** | ■ While antibiotic prophylaxis is recommended as above, there is limited actual evidence to determine the risk reduction for infective endocarditis with preprocedure antibiotic prophylaxis. Therefore, prophylaxis is only recommended for those with the highest risk of infective endocarditis. |

# MISTAKE: DELAY IN ONBOARDING THE SURGICAL TEAM

**Case Example**

A 45-year-old female with polysubstance use disorder presents to the hospital with fevers, joint pains, and worsening dyspnea on exertion. Exam reveals scattered Janeway lesions and chest imaging reveals numerous septic emboli to the lungs. TTE demonstrates a 3-cm tricuspid vegetation and blood cultures grow methicillin-resistant *S. aureus* (MRSA). You continue vancomycin over the next week, but the patient's condition continues to deteriorate. The infectious diseases team recommends adding ceftaroline for double MRSA coverage. Despite that, the patient continues to worsen and develops an infectious glomerulonephritis, thrombocytopenia (thought due to severe bone marrow suppression in the setting of critical illness), and hyponatremia. The cardiothoracic team is consulted for valve intervention but note that the operation is not possible in the setting of the thrombocytopenia and hyponatremia (given significant intravascular fluid shifts during the bypass that is required intraoperatively). The patient dies a few days later.

**Reasoning Error(s)**

- Relying too heavily on medical therapy to treat a complicated problem
- Sequential thinking rather than working in parallel and contingency planning
- Limited knowledge on the overlap of medical and surgical management of patients with infective endocarditis

**How to Avoid the Mistake**

- Recognize that infective endocarditis is best managed through a multidisciplinary team that includes internists, cardiologist, infectious disease specialists, and cardiac surgeons; do not be afraid to consult your surgical colleagues early on in the patient's management. Early consultation allows for all parties to follow along and offer their perspective longitudinally, such as if clinical course is headed in the wrong direction and may preclude intervention (missed window).
- Understand that working on multiple clinical strategies simultaneously as part of contingency planning may reduce morbidity and mortality associated with complex and often unpredictable diseases such as infective endocarditis.

**Antidote**

- Early consultation to cardiothoracic surgery

**Common Scenarios**

- Not applicable

**Note(s)**

- Indications for surgical intervention in left-sided infective endocarditis include:
  - Large vegetation (cutoffs vary by society, minimum 10 mm)
  - New-onset heart failure due to valve dysfunction
  - New conduction abnormalities suggestive of infiltration (heart block)
  - Paravalvular or root abscess
  - Refractory bacteremia (failure to clear blood cultures) after 5 days of appropriate antibiotics
  - Persistent signs of infections including complications of endocarditis after clearance of bacteremia
  - High-risk organisms (e.g., *S. aureus*, fungal, multidrug-resistant organisms)
- Any intracardiac devices should be considered carefully for removal.

| | |
|---|---|
| **Further Reading** | ■ Excellent comparative study evaluating the impact of multidisciplinary management of patients with native valve endocarditis: Chirillo F, et al. Impact of a multidisciplinary management strategy on the outcome of patients with native valve infective endocarditis. *Am J Cardiol.* 2013;112(8):1171–1176. |

## MISTAKE: OVERLOOKING CULTURE-NEGATIVE ENDOCARDITIS

| | |
|---|---|
| **Case Example** | A 37-year-old male with IV drug use presents to the emergency department with 3 days of fever and malaise. Initial physical exam is unrevealing beyond a blood pressure of 95/60. Initial labs are notable for a leukocytosis and an elevated ESR and CRP. You begin empiric coverage with vancomycin and piperacillin-tazobactam while awaiting pan-culture results. Several days later, the blood cultures have all been negative to date, yet the patient has not improved clinically. Your exam now reveals a new systolic murmur at the left lower sternal border, some mild pain with joint movement, and a few scattered hyperpigmented nodules on the fat pads of his hands. You suspect endocarditis but defer further workup with a TTE because the blood cultures were negative. The patient suffers an embolic stroke hours later, and a TTE demonstrates a large vegetation on the aortic valve. |
| **Reasoning Error(s)** | ■ Lack of recognition or suspicion for culture-negative endocarditis<br>■ Incorrect definition of culture-negative endocarditis<br>■ Disregarding your own clinical acumen and pre-test probability based on the patient presentation |
| **How to Avoid the Mistake** | ■ Understand that culture-negative endocarditis does not specifically refer to organisms that are not cultured easily, such as the HACEK organisms (*Haemophilus, Aggregatibacter, Cardiobacterium, Eikenella,* and *Kingella*). Instead, culture-negative endocarditis quite literally means any endocarditis where the blood cultures remain negative. The most common cause of culture-negative endocarditis is antibiotic therapy prior to obtaining blood cultures.<br>■ Remember, endocarditis is diagnosed based on the Duke Criteria. You need not have a positive blood culture to make the diagnosis. Continue working up infective endocarditis (e.g., with a TTE) if the clinical presentation is suggestive, even if cultures come back negative.<br>■ If at all possible, defer antibiotic initiation prior to blood culture collection. |
| **Antidote** | ■ Not applicable |
| **Common Scenarios** | ■ Not applicable |
| **Note(s)** | ■ Culture-negative endocarditis is more common than you may think—about 10% of all endocarditis cases.<br>■ Molecular testing (such as polymerase chain reaction) of serum samples may be useful in culture-negative endocarditis and most frequently identifies streptococci, staphylococci, and enterococci. |

## MISTAKE: OVERVALUING TRANSTHORACIC ECHOCARDIOGRAPHY FOR RULING-OUT INFECTIVE ENDOCARDITIS

**Case Example**

A 56-year-old female with mitral valve prolapse presents to the emergency department with fevers and general malaise over the past week. While examining her, you auscultate a murmur at the cardiac apex but are unsure whether it is new. Suspecting endocarditis, you order a transthoracic echocardiogram in addition to a standard infectious workup. The TTE demonstrates no valvular vegetations and you rule out infective endocarditis.

**Reasoning Error(s)**

- Lack of knowledge on the sensitivity of TTE for detecting valvular vegetations
- High activation energy barrier for obtaining a TEE (logistical barriers)
- Overreliance on one piece of data

**How to Avoid the Mistake**

- Understand that while TTE is the initial imaging modality to obtain in patients with suspected infective endocarditis but does not constitute a definitive means of ruling out endocarditis given its wide-ranging sensitivity between 40% and 80% depending on the study.
- Recognize that TEE has a higher sensitivity (>90%) in identifying infective endocarditis and provides more detailed information to assess potential valve structure and dysfunction, RV and LV function, and complications such as abscesses or perforations. The logistical energy required to obtain a TEE should never be a consideration for whether a patient receives a TEE.
- Pursue clinical management based on overall clinical picture without overemphasizing a single piece of data. Look for concordance and discordance equally between data.

**Antidote**

- TEE

**Common Scenarios**

- Not applicable

**Note(s)**

- Perivalvular abscesses are most commonly seen in the setting of prosthetic valves because the annulus is the typical site of infection.

## MISTAKE: ROUTINE USE OF ORAL ANTIBIOTICS FOR INFECTIVE ENDOCARDITIS

**Case Example**

A 23-year-old male with a history of IV drug use comes to the hospital due to fevers and chills. He also describes mild chest pain with breathing. On exam, you auscultate a murmur at the cardiac apex, but he is hemodynamically stable. You suspect endocarditis and astutely hold off on antibiotics prior to obtaining blood cultures. You then start empiric vancomycin and cefepime. As you had suspected, blood cultures are positive for viridians streptococci and TTE reveals a large vegetation on the atrial side of the mitral valve that is flopping in and out of the LV. You narrow antibiotics to ceftriaxone with remarkable clinical improvement over the subsequent week. Given his quick improvement, you transition to oral amoxicillin-clavulanate and discharge the patient. Unfortunately, the patient represents 3 weeks later in septic shock, with a repeat TTE demonstrating new abscess formation.

| | |
|---|---|
| **Reasoning Error(s)** | ■ Inadequate understanding of the POET study and misapplication of data |
| |    ■ Generalizing the study to all infectious endocarditis |
| |    ■ Believing that MRSA was included in the study population |
| |    ■ Limited IV antibiotic course (<10 days) |
| | ■ False reassurance of patient symptoms, while not considering possible long-term complications of shorter duration IV antibiotic therapy |
| | ■ Lack of understanding standard treatment in infective endocarditis |
| **How to Avoid the Mistake** | ■ Understand the POET study enough to base clinical decisions. The study investigated the safety and efficacy of transitioning to oral antibiotics specifically in left-sided endocarditis from three species (*Staphylococcus aureus*, coagulase-negative *Staphylococcus*, various streptococcal species, and *E faecalis*). Notably, all *S. aureus* was methicillin-susceptible and almost no patients who use IV drugs were included. All patients received a minimum of 10 days of IV antibiotics and had a TEE that confirmed improving endocarditis prior to transition to oral antibiotics. Last, the patients were highly selected for a very adherent group with good outpatient follow-up. It is not uncommon for patients with challenges to adherence and contraindications to discharge with IV access (e.g., chronic IV drug user) to remain in the hospital for the ensure duration of antibiotics. |
| | ■ Understand that standard treatment of uncomplicated infective endocarditis involves a minimum of 6 weeks of IV antibiotics from the date of clear blood cultures. Adjunct medical therapy may be considered such as gentamicin or rifampin, but their use is now discouraged except in very specific situations given lack of data on improved outcomes and easy development of resistance. |
| | ■ Regardless of any guidelines or data, always tailor clinical decisions to the individual patient. Always consult with your infectious diseases specialists on determining antibiotic regimen for infective endocarditis. |
| **Antidote** | ■ Not applicable |
| **Common Scenarios** | ■ Not applicable |
| **Note(s)** | ■ Distinct from the POET study, there are two studies from the 1990s evaluating a shorter (4-week) course of oral antibiotics in uncomplicated right-sided methicillin-susceptible *S. aureus* endocarditis. These two studies demonstrated a relatively high success rate (>90% cure) using a combination of ciprofloxacin and rifampin. However, depending on the local resistance profiles, ciprofloxacin may be inadequate coverage for *S. aureus*. Rifampin should never be used as monotherapy given its high susceptibility to resistance development. Thus, in practice, right-sided endocarditis is currently almost always treated with IV antibiotics albeit sometimes for <6 weeks. |
| **Further Reading** | ■ The POET study: Iversen K, et al. Partial oral versus intravenous antibiotic treatment of endocarditis. *N Engl J Med* 2019; 380:415–424. |

# Pulmonary Hypertension

Bliss J. Chang

## Diagnosis

### MISTAKE: DELAYED DIAGNOSIS OF PULMONARY HYPERTENSION

**Case Example**     A 57-year-old female with obesity presents to your clinic for follow-up of subacute dyspnea on exertion. Over the past 6 months, her exercise tolerance has decreased from 10 flat city blocks to a mere 2 city blocks. Her resting peripheral oxygen saturation is 95%. You examine her and think that you hear a prominent P2 and observe mild clubbing of her nails. However, you chalk it up to a variation of normal and continue assessing for common causes of dyspnea, such as pulmonary embolism, left-sided heart failure, chronic obstructive pulmonary disease (COPD), and anxiety, to no avail. You tell your patient that the dyspnea may be due to deconditioning and encourage daily exercise prior to the next follow-up in 6 months. The patient does not show up for the next follow-up, and you hear that she went to see your colleague, who astutely obtained a transthoracic echocardiogram (TTE) that demonstrated a normal left heart but elevated pulmonary systolic pressures. Your colleague then proceeded to diagnose the patient with group 1 pulmonary hypertension (PH) based on a right heart catheterization.

| | |
|---|---|
| **Reasoning Error(s)** | ■ Not realizing the average delay in diagnosis for PH |
| | ■ Dismissal of symptoms or physical exam findings that are abnormal but do not have a clear diagnostic correlation |
| | ■ Not routinely considering a diagnosis of PH on the differential |
| **How to Avoid the Mistake** | ■ Understand that PH is a significantly delayed diagnosis with a median delay to diagnosis of up to 2.5 years in some registries. Unsurprisingly, patients with delayed diagnosis have poorer outcomes, such as an 11% increase in mortality if the delay in diagnosis extends beyond 2 years. |
| | ■ Familiarize yourself with physical exam signs that may subtly suggest PH (or another condition that also merits diagnosis): |
| | ▪ Signs of pulmonary dysfunction: low peripheral oxygen saturation, clubbing (a sign of tissue hypoxia) |
| | ▪ Signs of elevated right heart pressures: prominent P2 (a sign of increased pulmonary pressures), holosystolic murmur over the left lower sternal border (a sign of tricuspid regurgitation, sometimes secondary to PH), right ventricular (RV) heave (a sign of an enlarged RV). |
| | ■ Familiarize yourself with evidence of right heart failure: elevated jugular venous pulse (JVP) (a sign of increased right atrial pressure), hepatojugular reflex (an additional sign of elevated right atrial and central venous pressure), ascites, and lower extremity edema (rare unless the PH is severe and long-standing). |
| | ■ Understand that the symptoms of PH are very nonspecific, but that the unifying quality is the long-standing and progressive nature (e.g., of dyspnea, decreased exercise tolerance, angina). |
| | ■ A high degree of suspicion is required for timely diagnosis. For patients with nonspecific symptoms, monitor carefully and frequently. If symptoms such as dyspnea on exertion do not resolve or have no clear explanation, have a low threshold for starting a noninvasive workup such as a TTE to begin ruling out PH. Take into consideration risk factors for PH, such as family history, congenital heart disease, autoimmune disorders, and a history of hypercoagulability (causing chronic pulmonary emboli). |
| **Antidote** | ■ Not applicable |
| **Common Scenarios** | ■ Not applicable |
| **Note(s)** | ■ Colloquially, the term "pulmonary hypertension" is used to refer to patients with PH that is intrinsic to the pulmonary arteries (i.e., not due to left-sided heart disease or group 2 PH). However, to be precise, it is often more useful to talk about the major site of issue: pulmonary ARTERIAL hypertension (group 1, due to arteriolar scarring) versus pulmonary VENOUS hypertension (group 2, due to left heart disease). |
| | ■ The most common cause of PH is left-sided heart disease (World Health Organization [WHO] group 2). These patients often do not need invasive testing unless there is suspicion that the degree of left heart disease is not sufficient to explain the PH. |
| | ■ A dilated left atrium usually reflects chronically elevated left-sided heart pressures and supports the diagnosis of group 2 PH. |

**Further Reading**
- Excellent review article that discusses PH underdiagnosis in middle- and low-income areas of the world where leading causes differ from that found in the US: Hasan B, et al. Challenges and special aspects of pulmonary hypertension in middle to low income regions: JACC state-of-the-art review. *JACC*. 2020;75(19):2463–2477.

## MISTAKE: DIAGNOSING PULMONARY HYPERTENSION BASED ON ECHOCARDIOGRAPHIC ESTIMATION OF RIGHT-SIDED PRESSURES

**Case Example**

A 50-year-old female with systemic sclerosis presents for evaluation of worsening exercise tolerance. Examination reveals a prominent P2 and an elevated JVP though the lungs are clear. Suspecting PH, a TTE is obtained which demonstrates an estimated pulmonary artery systolic pressure of 35 mmHg. You proceed to inform the patient of her new diagnosis of PH. The patient becomes alarmed and seeks a second opinion from your colleague who performs a right heart catheterization that reveals a mean pulmonary artery pressure of 16 mmHg.

**Reasoning Error(s)**
- Lack of understanding the method by which pulmonary artery pressure is calculated via echocardiography
- Forgetting scenarios that preclude the use of the TR jet for determination of right ventricular systolic pressure (RVSP)
- Incorrectly assuming that echocardiographic estimation of pulmonary arterial systolic pressure (PASP) correlates well with invasive measurements
- Forgetting that certain physiologic conditions such as anemia or sepsis can result in increased TR velocity until the condition is treated

**How to Avoid the Mistake**
- Understand that the pulmonary artery systolic pressure is calculated using the Bernoulli equation using the tricuspid regurgitation (TR) jet velocity. Thus, echocardiographic measures of PASP depend on the fidelity of the TR jet, which may vary significantly based on probe angulation and windows. A small error in measurement can lead to significant errors given the squaring of the TR velocity in the Bernoulli equation.
- Remember that not all patients have a visible or measurable TR jet. Even if a jet is visible, a TR jet that is especially severe or torrential may have little correlation with the RVSP off which the PASP is based.
- When using echocardiography as a screening test for PH, know that echocardiography can be thought of as providing the probability that the patient has PH rather than a diagnosis. Higher probability is reflected in a PASP >40 mmHg and/or TR velocity >3.4 m/s.

**Antidote**
- Right heart catheterization

**Common Scenarios**
- Not applicable

**Note(s)**
- Echocardiographic signs that increase the probability of PH include evidence of pressure overload (flattening of the interventricular septum during systole, an enlarged RV and/or right atrium, and a plethoric inferior vena cava).

## MISTAKE: FORGETTING THAT PULMONARY HYPERTENSION MAY BE OF MIXED ETIOLOGIES

| | |
|---|---|
| **Case Example** | A 55-year-old female with moderate COPD presents for dyspnea that is progressive over the past 3 months. Pulmonary function testing has remained stable. Right heart catheterization confirms that the diagnosis of PH, and in light of the severe COPD, the patient is labeled as having group 3 PH. No vasoreactivity testing, additional imaging, or treatment is initiated. Two months later, the patient presents to the emergency department with acute chest pain and shortness of breath. Chest CT PE protocol reveals a new pulmonary embolism and several chronic emboli. You and your colleagues ultimately diagnose the patient with both group 3 PH but also group 4 (chronic thromboembolic PH). |
| **Reasoning Error(s)** | ■ Incorrect belief that PH falls into only single classes<br>■ Lack of suspicion for additional etiologies of PH and stopping a thorough workup<br>■ Not considering the expected and actual severity of PH for a particular cause |
| **How to Avoid the Mistake** | ■ Understand that different classes of PH may coexist. For example, a patient with severe COPD may have both group 4 and group 3 PH. Treatment of patients with mixed etiologies follows that of the recommended strategies for individual groups of PH.<br>■ Any patient who is diagnosed with PH should have a full and thorough workup that checks for and excludes alternate classes of PH. Knowledge of all contributors to the PH can significantly change the treatment course.<br>■ Consider whether the severity of PH matches that commonly seen for a particular etiology. For example, isolated moderate COPD or ILD most often present with mild (rarely moderate) PH. Thus, severe PH would be out of proportion to that expected from a purely group 3 etiology. Note that it is possible for severe COPD to cause severe PAH. |
| **Antidote** | ■ Thorough workup for all classes of PH |
| **Common Scenarios** | ■ Not applicable |
| **Note(s)** | ■ PH can also be classified as precapillary, meaning due to elevated pressures intrinsic to the pulmonary arteries, or postcapillary meaning due to elevated pressures of the pulmonary veins. Precapillary PH may result from WHO groups 1, 3, 4, or 5, whereas postcapillary PH results from either group 2 or group 5.<br>■ PH due to systemic sclerosis is arterial and hence group 1. It behaves similarly to PAH that is idiopathic or from other rarer causes such as HIV infection.<br>■ As of 2020, several more drugs have been added to the list of drugs that definitely cause PH: benfluorex (now withdrawn from the market; formerly used for treatment of type 2 diabetes), methamphetamines, and dasatinib (a tyrosine kinase inhibitor treatment for leukemia). |

## MISTAKE: SINGLE PULMONARY CAPILLARY WEDGE PRESSURE TO EXCLUDE GROUP 2 PULMONARY HYPERTENSION

**Case Example**

A 75-year-old male with ischemic cardiomyopathy presents for worsening dyspnea on exertion over the past few months. The patient appears euvolemic; the patient is taken for a left heart catheterization to check for worsening obstructive coronary artery disease (CAD). At the same time, a right heart catheterization is performed to check for PH. Although the mean pulmonary artery pressure is 23 mmHg, the wedge pressure is 12 mmHg and group 2 PH is ruled out. The patient undergoes further tests, all of which are unremarkable, and is diagnosed with idiopathic PAH. He is started on ambrisentan and presents 1 month later with worsening heart failure. Upon further questioning, you discover that the patient took a double dose of his diuretic before being NPO for his original cath. His right atrium pressure was 1 mmHg at the time of the cath and his blood pressure was 80/50 mmHg. A careful review of his last echo shows a severely dilated left atrium and signs of diastolic dysfunction. Repeat cath at the time of this admission shows right atrium 8, pulmonary artery 50/30, and PCWP of 23 mmHg. Ambrisentan is stopped.

**Reasoning Error(s)**

- Not realizing that left-sided heart disease may present with a normal PCWP when under optimized conditions (e.g., volume)
- Thinking that PH cannot be a mix of more than one class

**How to Avoid the Mistake**

- Understand that the PCWP depends on multiple factors, including the health of the left ventricular myocardium but also the current hemodynamics optimization such as fluid status. Thus, the presence of PH may be masked either altogether or of the relative contribution from left-sided heart disease. This is particularly true of PH resulted from HFpEF.
- Given the potential to miss PH from left-sided heart disease, provocative maneuvers such as a fluid or exercise challenge can be used during the right heart catheterization to unmask a high PCWP. For instance, a 500-mL bolus of normal saline has been shown to unmask group 2 PH in 6% of patients thought to have isolated precapillary PH and 8% of patients without a diagnosis of any type of PH. The cutoff used for a fluid challenge by D'Alto et al (*Chest*, 2013) was a PCWP ≥18 mmHg in their study on standardizing the fluid challenge in PH diagnosis.
- Realize that PH may be mixed and of multiple classes. Thus, even if a patient clearly has a precapillary PH, they may also have postcapillary contribution which should be investigated.

**Antidote**

- Fluid and/or exercise challenge

**Common Scenarios**

- HFpEF
- Volume-optimized HFrEF

| | |
|---|---|
| **Note(s)** | ■ Institutional protocols likely vary on how to perform a fluid and/or exercise challenge. However, keep in mind that both the volume and the rate of fluid infusion affect the threshold PCWP that you are measuring against. |
| | ■ A quick method to determine whether PH has a precapillary component is to compute the transpulmonary gradient (TPG) or the diastolic pressure gradient (DPG). Both are similar concepts that focus on subtracting away the post–capillary pressure contribution. An elevated TPG or DPG suggests disease intrinsic to the pulmonary vasculature. Furthermore, the pulmonary vascular resistance (PVR) is elevated in precapillary PH. |

- ■ $TPG = mPAP - PCWP$, normal <12 mmHg
- ■ $DPG = dPAP - PCWP$, normal <7 mmHg
- ■ $PVR = \dfrac{TPG}{CO} = \dfrac{mPAP - PCWP}{CO}$ , normal ≤3 Woods units

## MISTAKE: CONTRAINDICATIONS TO VASOREACTIVITY TESTING

| | |
|---|---|
| **Case Example** | A 55-year-old female undergoes right heart catheterization for a presumptive diagnosis of PH based on an RVSP on TTE of 63 mmHg. The mean pulmonary artery pressure is calculated to be 41 mmHg and a PCWP of 18 mmHg is obtained that demonstrates a group 2 component in addition to likely pulmonary arterial hypertension. In order to check for responsiveness to calcium channel blockers (CCBs), a vasoreactivity testing is performed with 20 ppm of nitric oxide. The patient is noted to suddenly desaturate with presumed diagnosis of acute pulmonary edema. |
| **Reasoning Error(s)** | ■ Forgetting to consider the mechanism of vasoreactivity testing |
| | ■ Lack of knowledge on indications versus contraindications to vasoreactivity testing |
| | ■ Not integrating data real-time |
| **How to Avoid the Mistake** | ■ Understand that vasoreactivity testing reduces the existing (baseline) tone of the pulmonary arterioles as well as any vasoconstrictive component in pulmonary arterial hypertension. Acute decrease in vascular resistance will result in increased blood flow from the right to the left heart. In group 2 PH, this sudden increase in blood flow to the left may overwhelm the left ventricle (if it has little diastolic filling reserve) and lead to acute pulmonary edema. Patients are at risk for this in the setting of isolated HFpEF, severe mitral or aortic stenosis, and pulmonary veno-occlusive disease. |
| | ■ Remember that the purpose of vasoreactivity testing is to determine potential therapeutic response to high-dose CCBs. Thus, testing is indicated in patients with likely pulmonary arterial hypertension (PAH) (group 1). Patients with connective tissue disorders driving the PH are a notable exception where vasoreactivity testing may be positive but the long-term efficacy of CCBs has been shown to be minimal. |
| | ■ Integration of clinical data is needed in real time. Consideration for the possibility that a new finding will change a preformed plan is an important part of care. Additionally, one should think about the potential adverse effects for each clinical action, particularly for clinical actions that are less common. This will help avoid consequences that may not be obvious or routinely considered. |

| | |
|---|---|
| **Antidote** | ■ Termination of vasoreactivity testing |
| | ■ Diuresis |
| | ■ Oxygen therapy as needed (with consideration for noninvasive positive-pressure ventilation if severe) |
| **Common Scenarios** | ■ Left-sided heart failure |
| | ■ Severe aortic or mitral stenosis |
| | ■ Pulmonary veno-occlusive disease (PVOD) |
| | ■ Connective tissue disorders (positive vasoreactivity test but likely ineffective) |
| **Note(s)** | ■ The exact choice of vasoreactive agent and cutoff for trial is stylistic. Medication options include inhaled nitric oxide, IV epoprostenol, and IV adenosine. |
| | ■ Vasodilator responders, with the exception of patients with connective tissue disorders, should be started on high-dose CCBs. Notably, these doses are higher than the typical maximums used in hypertension (e.g., 20 mg daily amlodipine). |

## MISTAKE: OVERLOOKING LEFT MAIN COMPRESSION SYNDROME IN LONG-STANDING PULMONARY HYPERTENSION

| | |
|---|---|
| **Case Example** | A 57-year-old female with systemic sclerosis complicated by PH presents to your clinic for follow-up. She has done rather remarkably well and defied the odds, with minimal progression of her disease 5 years after diagnosis. Today, she remarks that she has been experiencing mild to moderate chest pain over the past few weeks. You reassure her that this is an expected part of long-standing PH and that the likelihood of her having coronary blockages is minimal. No workup is performed. The patient feels somewhat reassured and agrees to return for follow-up in 3 months. |
| **Reasoning Error(s)** | ■ Forgetting or lack of knowledge regarding a relatively common complication (LMCS) of long-standing PH |
| | ■ Not knowing the prevalence of left main compression syndrome (LMCS) to aid forming a pragmatic differential diagnosis |
| | ■ Not considering a differential diagnosis for a relatively common symptom in PAH |
| **How to Avoid the Mistake** | ■ Learn about left main compression syndrome. With long-standing severe PH, the left main coronary artery may dilate to the point where it compresses the left main coronary artery extrinsically, causing a supply-demand mismatch as if there were an intraluminal blockage. |
| | ■ Although the estimates of LMCS prevalence are based on small case series, they have ranged from 20% to 50% of patients with long-standing PAH who present with angina. Thus, LMCS may merit a more prominent spot on the differential for chest pain in patients with long-standing PAH. |
| | ■ Always consider a differential diagnosis for all clinical presentations no matter how routine they may be. In this case, angina is relatively common symptom in PAH classically attributed to a supply-demand mismatch of the RV. However, alternate diagnoses such as CAD and LMCS should be considered. |

| | |
|---|---|
| **Antidote** | ■ Coronary CT angiogram |
| **Common Scenarios** | ■ Not applicable |
| **Note(s)** | One treatment for LMCS is stenting of the left main coronary artery to help withstand the extrinsic force compressing the artery. However, more advanced therapies or strategies may ultimately need to be considered. |
| **Further Reading** | ■ Excellent contemporary study investigating the incidence of LMCS: Galie N, et al. Left main coronary artery compression in patients with pulmonary arterial hypertension and angina. *JACC*. 2017;2808–2817. |

## Treatment

### MISTAKE: LACK OF REFERRAL TO A PULMONARY HYPERTENSION SPECIALIST

| | |
|---|---|
| **Case Example** | A 58-year-old female musician on an international concert tour is newly diagnosed with idiopathic PAH by his private physician. The physician requests an additional consultation, but the patient feels anxious about her health information getting released and the inconvenience of having to cancel a publicity event and part of the tour. The physician starts with the online resources and prescribes amlodipine. Unfortunately, her symptoms continue to worsen. |
| **Reasoning Error(s)** | ■ Lack of interdisciplinary support from a wide range of experts (e.g., obstetrics, anesthesia) who manage PH patients<br>■ Focusing on patient-centered decision-making despite conflict with standards of care |
| **How to Avoid the Mistake** | ■ Recognize that PH is a very complicated and nuanced disease that is most effectively managed at centers with specialists that see high volumes of PH patients. Though management may be sufficient by a nonspecialist with help from various reference sources, there are many practical aspects to management that may not be available in those resources. Furthermore, the latest therapies may not be available outside of specialized treatment centers.<br>■ Specialty centers may be able to help with management of PH in various scenarios such as pregnancy and surgery (anesthesia, high-risk intubation).<br>■ Discuss the possibility of referral to a PH specialist with the patient. This may be difficult in very rural areas and may face numerous logistical barriers; however, the patient should be aware of the option to pursue more specialized care. |
| **Antidote** | ■ Refer to a PH specialist |
| **Common Scenarios** | ■ Not applicable |

**Note(s)**
- Studies such as that by Pi et al (*Chest*, 2020) from the University of Pittsburg Medical Center have demonstrated improved mortality and clinical outcomes (e.g., hospitalization rates) in patients who are managed by PH specialists. In particular, vasodilator therapy was more common and disease monitoring was closer.
- Patients with PH may often miss home therapies or experience delays in therapy in the emergency room setting. One way to reduce the likelihood of this is to immediately notify the patient's or institution's PH specialist when a patient with significant PH presents to the emergency department.

## MISTAKE: FORGETTING TO ENSURE REGULAR BOWEL MOVEMENTS

**Case Example**

A 58-year-old female with PAH and chronic constipation follows with you in clinic. Her symptoms have been stable, and she is optimized on medical therapy. She notes that her constipation is worse recently, requiring significant straining. You reassure the patient and advise her to eat foods with higher fiber. A week later, the patient arrests and dies while straining very hard on the toilet.

**Reasoning Error(s)**
- Lack of understanding the physiologic impact of constipation and straining on PH hemodynamics
- Forgetting to screen for common pitfalls that patients may encounter in their daily lives

**How to Avoid the Mistake**
- Understand the impact of straining (i.e., Valsalva) on PH hemodynamics. Constipation and other maneuvers such as heavy lifting lead to the Valsalva effect, which decreases the preload via an increase in intrathoracic pressure. Severe PH results in very minimal RV systolic function and low cardiac output. Any decrease in preload together with a relative increase in pulmonary pressures can cause hemodynamic collapse. There are also studies that suggest potential autonomic dysfunction related to Valsalva maneuvers in PH.
- Advise patients with PH to avoid movements that lead to a Valsalva effect due to increased risk of hemodynamic collapse and sudden cardiac death. Constipation is a common modifiable risk factor (with laxatives).

**Antidote**
- Laxatives

**Common Scenarios**
- Constipation
- Heavy lifting

**Note(s)**
- Iron supplements for anemia (common in PH) often lead to constipation. Be sure to provide a concurrent bowel regimen if a patient is on oral iron supplementation.

## MISTAKE: CONTRACEPTIVE MONOTHERAPY IN PULMONARY HYPERTENSION

**Case Example**     A 35-year-old female with severe PAH seeks pregnancy counseling. For her PH, the patient is on bosentan and sildenafil. You thoroughly explain the risks associated with pregnancy with PH and the patient agrees to start a progesterone-only oral contraceptive to avoid an increased risk of thromboembolism. Three months later, the patient experiences significant nausea and vomiting and is discovered to be pregnant. She is fearful of the news articles of people in her state who have had pregnancy termination and so proceeds with the very high-risk pregnancy. She subsequently develops severe heart failure in her third trimester and requires an emergent C-section. The baby is born prematurely at 28 weeks. The mother is recovering post C-section and dies from a sudden cardiac arrest 2 days later.

**Reasoning Error(s)**
- Not knowing the potential risks associated with pregnancy in severe PH
- Overlooking drug–drug interactions between contraceptives and PH medications
- Limited options for care of maternal risk

**How to Avoid the Mistake**
- Understand that pregnancy is associated with significant hemodynamic changes in all stages (pregnancy, labor, delivery, and postpartum). Patients with PH have significant morbidity and mortality associated with pregnancy, up to 30–50% in some studies. Furthermore, certain therapeutics such as endothelin receptor antagonists and riociguat are teratogenic. As such, expert recommendation is to avoid pregnancy and effective contraception is imperative. Given the potentially life-changing (or life-ending) impact of pregnancy in PH, dual contraceptive therapy should be a strong consideration.
- Be aware that hormonal contraceptives are less effective in the presence of certain medications such as bosentan (though not ambrisentan) due to their enzyme inducer effects. Specifically, the progesterone-only pill requires perfect adherence and has a higher risk for failure than combination oral contraceptive pills. For such patients, dual contraceptive therapy (including one barrier method) is more strongly recommended.
- Some patients may not desire dual contraceptive therapy (if at all). However, patients should be informed of the possibility of dual therapy as well as the very high risks associated with pregnancy and PH.

**Antidote**
- Dual contraception (preferably one barrier method)

**Common Scenarios**
- Not applicable

**Note(s)**
- Estrogen-containing contraceptives are disfavored in PAH due to concern that estrogen could promote worsening disease and increases the risk for pulmonary embolism and thrombosis.
- Current guidelines recommend consideration of pregnancy termination in patients who present pregnant or are unknowingly pregnant. This is obviously a very traumatic discussion and should be undertaken with the help of a multidisciplinary team that includes obstetric, pediatric, and anesthesia experts.

**Further Reading**
- An excellent review of pregnancy in PH: Olsson KM, et al. Pregnancy in pulmonary arterial hypertension. *Eur Respir Rev.* 2016;25:431–437.

## MISTAKE: ADMINISTERING TOO MUCH INTRAVENOUS FLUIDS IN PULMONARY HYPERTENSION

**Case Example**
A 30-year-old female with severe PH is admitted to the cardiology service in the setting of nausea and dyspnea on exertion. On physical exam she has no crackles. JVP is not checked, and moderate abdominal distention is noted. She is NPO for an abdominal ultrasound in the morning. Overnight, her blood pressure is 86/60 and you order a 1-L bolus of lactated ringers. To your dismay, her hypotension worsens to 70/55. A STAT TTE is obtained and demonstrates systolic and diastolic septal flattening with leading to significant underfilling of the LV.

**Reasoning Error(s)**
- Fast thinking that results in IV fluids for common scenarios (e.g., hypotension, acute kidney injury)
- Forgetting the tenuous fluid balance in PH patients and the pathophysiology of excess fluids (i.e. ventricular interdependence)
- Difficulty determining volume status by physical exam in right heart failure.

**How to Avoid the Mistake**
- Understand that PH strikes a tight fluid balance. This patient has presented in isolated right heart failure. IV fluids are not beneficial in this scenario as her blood pressure is low due to decreased forward flow, not dehydration. A JVP assessment in this patient would likely reveal a pressure >14–16 cmH$_2$O and thus no benefit in MORE fluid. Excess intravascular volume leads to dilation and impingement of the RV into the LV (a phenomenon called ventricular interdependence) that worsens diastolic LV filling and cardiac output. If needed, consider small boluses of fluid (e.g., 250 mL) with frequent clinical reassessment to determine further fluid need. Alternative therapy such as a peripherally acting pressor (vasopressin) would likely improve blood pressure without the risk of worsening the decreased LV filling.
- Be aware of common scenarios that often result in use of IV fluids that should be approached with caution in PH patients: hypotension, acute kidney injury, prehydration prior to contrast loads, and excessive continuous drip medications.
- Right and left heart failure patients have varied exams. JVP elevation alone is not sufficient as JVP assessment is difficult with long-standing right heart failure or severe tricuspid regurgitation. An echo is useful to determine increasing RV/LV ratio suggestive of volume overload that is leading to ventricular interdependence. A pulmonary artery catheter may also be considered to facilitate a safe fluid balance.
- The lack of "left" heart failure symptoms does not exclude fluid overload. Pulmonary hypertension patients often present with isolated ascites or edema in the absence of pulmonary edema or orthopnea.

**Antidote**
- Careful volume removal (likely with the aid of a pulmonary artery catheter)

| | |
|---|---|
| **Common Scenarios** | ■ Hypotension |
| | ■ Acute kidney injury |
| | ■ Prehydration before contrast loads |
| | ■ Continuous IV drip medications |
| **Note(s)** | ■ On echocardiography, septal flattening during diastole indicates volume overload whereas flattening during systole indicates pressure overload. |

## MISTAKE: DIURESING WITH STANDARD NET NEGATIVE GOALS IN SEVERE PULMONARY HYPERTENSION

| | |
|---|---|
| **Case Example** | A patient with severe group IV PH complicated by RV failure is admitted to you for volume management. You diurese aggressively with Lasix for a net negative 2 L/day. Half a day later, the patient's blood pressure falls drastically with an extremely narrow pulse pressure. At morbidity and mortality conference, you are told that the patient likely had hemodynamic collapse from taking off volume too quickly in the setting of severe PH. |
| **Reasoning Error(s)** | ■ Not considering the presence of a preload-dependent physiology |
| | ■ Forgetting to consider the synergistic effect of multiple preload-dependent pathologies |
| | ■ Memorizing buzz words such as "aortic stenosis" as associations for preload dependence without understanding the physiology and applicability of this concept to other preload-dependent states |
| | ■ Lack of recognition that the diuresis goal is not a fixed and/or memorized value |
| | ■ Lack of recognition that diuresis goals can be spread over time, including shorter intervals, rather than over the course of an entire day |
| **How to Avoid the Mistake** | ■ Consider preload every time you diurese. |
| | ■ If preload dependent, diurese gently (lower net negative goal such as 0.25–1.0 L/day or equivalent hourly rate). |
| | ■ Diurese more frequently as needed: start slow and uptitrate as needed. |
| **Antidote** | ■ Give back intravascular volume (e.g., lactated Ringer's, normal saline, albumin). |
| **Common Scenarios** | ■ Severe PH |
| | ■ Severe aortic stenosis |
| | ■ Severe diastolic dysfunction (e.g., heart failure with preserved ejection fraction, amyloid) |
| | ■ RV failure |
| | ■ Severe tricuspid regurgitation |
| | ■ Submassive/massive pulmonary embolism |
| | ■ Inferior myocardial infarction |
| | ■ Significant vasodilator therapy (e.g., nitroglycerin drip) |
| | ■ Constrictive pericarditis |
| | ■ Extreme tachycardia |
| | ■ Atrial fibrillation/flutter |

**Note(s)**

- The degree of preload dependence varies between patients with the same pathology such as severe PH. It is often difficult without invasive hemodynamic monitoring to determine the degree to which a patient is preload dependent. The ideal net negative diuresis goal should be determined via careful uptitration based on hemodynamic stability (e.g., blood pressure response, perfusion of extremities, strength of palpable pulse). Particularly high-risk and difficult patients should have invasive monitoring (e.g., a Swan-Ganz catheter).
- For patient comfort, in the absence of a Foley, diurese earlier in the day when the patient is awake, so they are not constantly awakening during the night.

## MISTAKE: CALCIUM CHANNEL BLOCKERS INDISCRIMINATE OF PULMONARY HYPERTENSION CLASS AND VASOREACTIVITY

**Case Example**

A 47-year-old female with recently diagnosed group 3 PH presents to your clinic for follow-up. You notice that the patient is not on any PH medications and initiate her on amlodipine, which is gradually uptitrated. Three weeks later, the patient develops worsening oxygenation and pulmonary edema despite a TTE demonstrating normal LV function.

**Reasoning Error(s)**

- Forgetting the specific population of PH patients who benefit from CCBs
- Lack of knowledge regarding the evidence for use of CCBs in PH
- Assuming a lack of downside to prescribing CCBs to all PH patients
- Overlooking contraindications to CCB therapy in PAH patients

**How to Avoid the Mistake**

- Understand that CCBs are only recommended in idiopathic PAH (IPAH) patients with positive vasoreactivity tests, excluding patients with connective tissue disease (who often have positive vasoreactivity tests). This is based on a small number of studies, including the landmark study in 1992 by Stuart Rich and colleagues in *N Engl J Med* that demonstrated a mortality benefit to high-dose CCBs in idiopathic PAH (group 1 PH; referred to as primary PH at the time). Notably, long-term CCB responders (meaning improvement for at least 1 year) compose a minority (~7%) of patients among those with IPAH; thus, vasoreactivity testing is performed as an attempt to determine who would benefit from CCB therapy. In particular, a positive response is defined as a decrease in mPAP of 10 mmHg to an mPAP of <40 mmHg.
- Patients with PH on high-dose CCBs may experience hypotension, worsening V/Q mismatch (due to loss of hypoxic vasoconstriction), and fluid retention. In the absence of data supporting a benefit from high-dose CCB therapy, patients without IPAH and a positive vasoreactivity test should not be prescribed CCBs.
- Remember that patients with IPAH complicated by RV failure or hemodynamic stability should not be initiated on high-dose CCBs as it will worsen hemodynamics. These patients should also avoid vasodilator testing, which may lead to hemodynamic collapse.
- The majority of patients do not benefit from CCBs alone.

**Antidote**

- Discontinue CCB therapy if not indicated

**Common Scenarios**

- Not applicable

| Note(s) | ■ "High-dose" CCB refers to higher doses than you may be accustomed to with hypertension treatment. For example, it is not uncommon to uptitrate to 20 mg of amlodipine (usual max dose 10 mg) or 200 mg of nifedipine (usually no higher than 120–180 mg). |
| --- | --- |
| | ■ Vasodilator testing is also important for its prognostic implications. Patients with a positive test have a better prognosis than their counterparts. |
| | ■ Patients with PAH that is not idiopathic (e.g., due to HIV infection) may be considered for a vasodilator test on a case-by-case basis. However, it is very rare for non-IPAH patients to be CCB responders. |
| | ■ Verapamil should be avoided as long-term high-dose CCB therapy due to its greater negative inotropic effects than diltiazem, nifedipine, and amlodipine. |
| Further Reading | ■ The landmark study that demonstrated a mortality benefit of high-dose CCB (and also anticoagulation) in group 1 PH: Rich S, et al. The effect of high doses of calcium-channel blockers on survival in primary pulmonary hypertension. *N Engl J Med.* 1992;327:76–81. |
| | ■ Investigation definitively demonstrating the utility of vasoreactivity testing for identifying patients most likely to benefit from long-term high-dose CCB therapy: Morales-Blanhir J, et al. Clinical value of vasodilator test with inhaled nitric oxide for predicting long-term response to oral vasodilators in pulmonary hypertension. *Respir Med.* 2004;98(3):225–234. |

## MISTAKE: ANTICOAGULATION FOR ALL PATIENTS WITH PULMONARY ARTERIAL HYPERTENSION

| Case Example | A 67-year-old female with systemic sclerosis complicated by PAH presents to your clinic to establish care. You notice that the patient is not on anticoagulation despite being classified as group 1 PH (PAH). You inform the patient that there is likely a mortality benefit to anticoagulation with warfarin and the patient agrees to start warfarin. Three months later, the patient presents with large-volume hemoptysis. Anticoagulation is stopped. |
| --- | --- |
| Reasoning Error(s) | ■ Reliance on older data and/or guidelines supporting anticoagulation in all PAH patients |
| | ■ Lack of knowledge of the most recent data on anticoagulation in PAH |
| | ■ Lack of patient-tailored decision on anticoagulation |
| How to Avoid the Mistake | ■ Understand that the older data on anticoagulation in PAH have been called into question based on methodologic flaws. Most of the current evidence for anticoagulation in PAH stems from registries (e.g., REVEAL, COMPERA) and suggests a possible mortality benefit in IPAH. Notably, no benefit of anticoagulation (and even decent data showing harm) has been seen in patients with PAH due to connective tissue disease or systemic sclerosis. |
| | ■ Given the moderate evidence for anticoagulation in IPAH, the risks and benefits should be discussed with each patient. Additional reasons favoring anticoagulation (e.g., concomitant atrial fibrillation or DVT) may favor anticoagulation. |

**Antidote**          ■ Not applicable

**Common Scenarios** ■ Not applicable

**Note(s)**           ■ Warfarin is the anticoagulant of choice when treating idiopathic pulmonary arterial hypertension. This is due to the lack of data on the efficacy of DOACs in this population. The target INR varies but ranges from 1.5–2.5 to 2–3.
                      ■ Lifetime anticoagulation remains the backbone therapy for all patients with CTEPH. DOACs are acceptable given indirect data on their efficacy for treating venous thromboembolism.

## MISTAKE: USING PHENYLEPHRINE FOR HYPOTENSION IN PULMONARY HYPERTENSION

**Case Example**      A 50-year-old female with severe PH is admitted to your service for multilobar bacterial pneumonia. The patient is started on broad-spectrum antibiotics but soon becomes hypotensive to 80/55. You initiate phenylephrine and quickly uptitrate to the max dose. Notably her hypoxemia worsens. She is noted to have a PFO, and there appears to be more shunting from right to left. You contact the fellow on call, who recommends correction of acidosis, transition to vasopressin, and a decrease in PEEP on the ventilator settings.

**Reasoning Error(s)** ■ Not treating all types of PVR elevation
                      ■ Not considering the mechanism of different vasopressors and their compatibility with the pathophysiology of PH
                      ■ Lack of familiarity with the ideal pressor in PH

**How to Avoid the Mistake** ■ Remember that phenylephrine is a pure α-agonist that leads to vasoconstriction. This is often helpful for sepsis and other low-SVR syndromes but, in the case of PH, phenylephrine further increases the PVR, worsening the PH and RV afterload. This effectively creates a situation analogous to obstructive shock and may actually worsen the blood pressure.
                      ■ The first approach in a patient with low SVR is to ensure that your therapies do not significantly increase PVR. Acidosis, high PEEP, and pressors such as phenylephrine. Some data suggest vasopressin is an optimal medication to choose due to the relative absence of vasopressin receptors in the pulmonary vasculature. This allows vasopressin to provide vasoconstriction predominantly of the systemic vasculature, thereby increasing blood pressure without increasing PVR. Some centers use epinephrine and norepinephrine, though the data for these medications relative to PVR are unclear.

**Antidote**          ■ Stop phenylephrine
                      ■ Switch to alternative vasopressor (e.g., vasopressin)
                      ■ Correct acidosis
                      ■ Minimize vent settings to prevent increased intrathoracic pressure-mediated RV afterload increase

**Common Scenarios** ■ Not applicable

**Note(s)**
- Inotropes may also be considered, particularly in the setting of PH crisis, which is an acute increase in PVR leading to shock, or in severe right heart failure. Reasonable options include dobutamine and milrinone, both of which are particularly beneficial in PH crisis given they also improve RV function and decrease afterload to the RV via dilation of the pulmonary vasculature. However, careful monitoring of the SVR is needed, especially with milrinone.

## MISTAKE: NONINVASIVE POSITIVE-PRESSURE VENTILATION IN SEVERE PULMONARY HYPERTENSION

**Case Example**

A 66-year-old male with severe PH presents in respiratory distress in the setting of atypical pneumonia. The patient is initially tried on nasal cannula but saturates only at 90% on 15 L and is thus transitioned to BiPAP 18/12 mmHg. The patient's oxygenation increases to 99% but his blood pressure drops precipitously to 79/60. The BiPAP is quickly switched over to high-flow nasal cannula with nonrebreather mask and the patient's blood pressure recovers to 97/60. However, his saturation continues to fall. BiPAP is re-trialed at 15/5 with improvement of saturation to 94%.

**Reasoning Error(s)**
- Not considering the impact of high settings of positive pressure on PH pathophysiology
- Lack of knowing a reasonable alternative to provide adequate oxygen support

**How to Avoid the Mistake**
- Understand that positive-pressure ventilation increases intrathoracic pressure, decreases preload, and increases RV afterload. In severe PH, the acute decrease in preload coupled with an increase in RV afterload may lead to hemodynamic collapse. In particular, patients with pulmonary arterial pressures that are near or exceed the systemic pressures are at very high risk.
- Use alternatives to positive-pressure ventilation if at all possible. Alternative oxygen therapy includes nonrebreather and high-flow nasal cannula (usually acceptable since the positive pressure provided is minimal). Combination of nonrebreather on top of high-flow nasal cannula may also be attempted.

**Antidote**
- Transition to maximum alternate oxygen support

**Common Scenarios**
- Intubation
- BiPAP

**Note(s)**
- High-flow nasal cannula delivers a very small amount (approximately 1 mmHg per 10 L of flow up to 6 mmHg) of positive end-expiratory pressure (PEEP) and thus is not contraindicated in severe PH even though it is technically positive-pressure ventilation.

## MISTAKE: INTUBATION IN SEVERE PULMONARY HYPERTENSION

**Case Example**

A 66-year-old male with severe PH presents in respiratory distress in the setting of atypical pneumonia. The patient is initially tried on nasal canula but saturates at 80% on 15 L. Given the terrible oxygen saturation, the decision is made to intubate. The patient's blood pressure is 97/60. During the induction, he is given a muscle relaxant and his blood pressure drops to 70/40 mmHg. He then has a cardiac arrest.

**Reasoning Error(s)**

- Lack of understanding the complex pathophysiology interplay with intubation and PH
- Nonideal choices of induction agent
- Lack of preparation in terms of goals of care and risk/benefit discussions

**How to Avoid the Mistake**

- Understand that intubation should be delayed for as long as possible (or altogether) in patients with severe PH. This is due to the very high chance for hemodynamic collapse. Intubation not only lowers RV pre-load (which is exacerbated further in the case of RV failure, which is common in severe PH) but also requires induction, which also causes hypotension. A sudden drop in SVR results in a significant imbalance of the SVR:PVR ratio and the LV is unable to fill. Hypotension may also worsen RV oxygen-demand mismatch, further reducing biventricular contractility. Last, during intubation, the transient hypoxia worsens PVR via hypoxic vasoconstriction. All of these mechanisms contribute to a very high chance of hemodynamic collapse and cardiac arrest.
- If an intubation is unavoidable, careful consideration should be given to minimizing hypotension. Prior to intubation, having vasopressin available (or infusing) and additional pressors available. Sedation medications to be avoided include muscle relaxants and only rarely using propofol. Etomidate may be preferential. In rare circumstances, significant topical analgesia and an awake intubation can be considered. Ketamine is also a consideration as it maintains respiratory drive and thus minimizes hypoxic vasoconstriction.
- In all circumstances, there should be a forthright discussion with the patient and family on risks and benefits of intubation. Patients with severe PH should have extended goals of care conversations prior to critical illness.

**Antidote**

- If hemodynamic collapse occurs, vasopressin is the first-line pressor. Other agents such as norepinephrine and epinephrine can be considered. Inotropes can be considered if there is low cardiac output and right heart failure.

**Common Scenarios**

- Not applicable

**Note(s)**

- If intubation is successful, ventilation should be performed with the minimal possible PEEP and tidal volumes to minimize the hemodynamic effects.

## MISTAKE: PERMISSIVE HYPERCAPNIA IN PULMONARY HYPERTENSION

| | |
|---|---|
| **Case Example** | A 66-year-old male with severe PH presents in respiratory distress in the setting of COVID-19 and acute respiratory distress syndrome (ARDS). The patient is initially tried on nasal cannula but saturates at 80% on 15 L. Given the terrible oxygen saturation, the decision is made to intubate. The patient's blood pressure is 97/60. Prophylactic dobutamine and vasopressin are started, and the patient is successfully intubated while awake. Postintubation ABGs demonstrate pH 7.21 and a $pCO_2$ of 78 mmHg. Given pH is >7.15, you tell your intern that the ventilator settings need not be modified in accordance with the principle of permissive hypercapnia to decrease lung injury. Though the dobutamine and vasopressin are attempted to be weaned, their doses actually increase over the next hour as the PVR increases further from the hypercapnia. |
| **Reasoning Error(s)** | ■ Forgetting to consider the effect of permissive hypercapnia on PH pathophysiology<br>■ False sense of assurance postintubation |
| **How to Avoid the Mistake** | ■ Understand that hypercapnia (and hypoxia and acidemia) leads to pulmonary vasoconstriction. In the setting of PH, the concept of permissive hypercapnia does not apply since it will worsen the PVR.<br>■ Pulmonary hypertension patients face a whole set of new challenges once intubation is successfully completed. This includes optimization of gases to ensure adequate oxygenation and ventilation while protecting the alveoli which can often have conflicting priorities. Close attention to every clinical action is required, particularly due to the rare nature of intubated PH patients, which increases the unfamiliarity and thus error rate with even routine clinical actions (e.g., ventilator management). |
| **Antidote** | ■ Increase ventilation (increase tidal volume and/or respiratory rate) |
| **Common Scenarios** | ■ Not applicable |
| **Note(s)** | ■ Even if a patient with PH is in ARDS, the ARDSNET protocol should not be followed as the underlying principles such as permissive hypercapnia are incongruent with the physiology and treatment goals for PH. |

# Pericardial Disease

Bliss J. Chang

## Diagnosis

### MISTAKE: DIAGNOSING ACUTE PERICARDITIS WITHOUT FORMAL CRITERIA

**Case Example**  A 50-year-old female presents with sharp chest pain radiating to her back that began a day ago. She also reports a new dry cough that worsens the chest pain. An ECG reveals subtle ST elevations in a few contiguous leads but does not fit with classic changes seen in pericarditis. Exam is unremarkable (chest pain unchanged with palpation), and troponins are negative. A bedside TTE demonstrates a small pericardial effusion. Confused, you consult your colleague, who astutely diagnoses her with acute pericarditis.

**Reasoning Error(s)**  
- Lack of knowledge regarding the existence and/or specifics of formal criteria for a diagnosis of pericarditis
- Lack of familiarity with atypical presentations of acute pericarditis

**How to Avoid the Mistake**  
- Learn the formal criteria for diagnosing acute pericarditis. Two of four signs/symptoms must be met:
  - Chest pain (most often sharp, pleuritic, acute onset, and improved with leaning forward)
  - Friction rub
  - Diffuse ST elevations
  - New or worsening pericardial effusion
- Refrain from the temptation of skipping formal diagnostic criteria, especially when facing cases with atypical presentations and/or unclear explanations.

**Antidote**  
- Not applicable

| | |
|---|---|
| **Common Scenarios** | ■ Not applicable |
| **Note(s)** | ■ In developed countries, the most common cause of acute pericarditis is idiopathic. However, idiopathic likely represents an undetected viral cause. Viral infections, such as Coxsackievirus or echovirus infection, are among the most common causes. |
| | ■ In developing countries, tuberculosis is the most common cause of acute pericarditis. Tuberculosis is unique in that it has an especially high rate of causing chronic constrictive pericarditis due to calcification of the pericardium. |
| | ■ Incessant pericarditis is when symptoms do not fully resolve for at least 4 to 6 weeks. Patients whose symptoms improve but do not fully resolve still fall under incessant pericarditis. On the other hand, recurrent pericarditis refers to patients who have a minimum 4 to 6 week period of complete symptomatic remission before return of symptoms. |

## MISTAKE: RULING OUT PERICARDITIS IN THE ABSENCE OF DIFFUSE ST ELEVATIONS

| | |
|---|---|
| **Case Example** | A 42-year-old female presents with chest pain radiating to the back that is relieved with sitting up and forward. An ECG is obtained that demonstrates new ST elevations with PR depressions in the inferolateral leads. Though somewhat consistent with typical ECG findings for pericarditis, due to the absence of ST elevations in the anteroseptal leads, you rule out the possibility of pericarditis. The next day, the patient's ECG now also includes ST elevations and PR depressions in the anterior leads. |
| **Reasoning Error(s)** | ■ Reliance on textbook presentations of pericarditis (global inflammation) |
| **How to Avoid the Mistake** | ■ Understand that pericarditis may present focally, in which case ST elevations and PR depressions may be in a limited set of leads. Elevation in more than one coronary distribution decreases the probability of it being ischemic in nature. |
| | ■ Use clinical context (e.g., how pain changes with sitting up or laying down) to help inform your probability of a diagnosis of pericarditis. |
| **Antidote** | ■ Not applicable |
| **Common Scenarios** | ■ Not applicable |
| **Note(s)** | ■ You may not necessarily hear a rub on auscultation in pericarditis. In fact, in the presence of a pericardial effusion (which is not uncommon), you cannot hear a rub, since the pericardial layers are not rubbing against one another. |

## MISTAKE: MISTAKING ACUTE PERICARDITIS FOR ST-ELEVATION MYOCARDIAL INFARCTION

| | |
|---|---|
| **Case Example** | A 35-year-old female presents with acute-onset chest pain and shortness of breath (SOB). ECG demonstrates diffuse ST elevations, and the ST-elevation myocardial infarction (STEMI) pager is activated. An emergent left heart catheterization reveals clean coronaries, and upon reviewing the ECG you realize that the patient likely has acute pericarditis given her age and the diffuse rather than localized ST elevations. |

| | |
|---|---|
| **Reasoning Error(s)** | ■ Equating all ST elevations as diagnostic of acute coronary syndromes (STEMI) |
| | ■ Not thinking about coronary distributions to help with differentiating pericarditis and STEMI |
| | ■ Lack of knowledge on non–ST-segment ECG findings to differentiate pericarditis and STEMI |
| **How to Avoid the Mistake** | ■ Approach all ST elevations as supportive evidence rather than diagnostic findings. Apply a differential diagnosis to any ST elevation that includes more than simply STEMI, though there should be a high threshold to rule out STEMI given the high consequences. |
| | ■ Remember that STEMIs usually involve a single coronary artery, though it may appear to involve more than one coronary territory depending on the anatomic coverage of the culprit coronary vessel. It would be unusual for a patient to present with a STEMI in multiple and/or all coronary territories. Furthermore, if a patient truly experienced a STEMI in all coronary distributions (such as the exceptionally rare case of embolic showering), the patient is likely to be extremely sick and/or dead on presentation. Similarly, patient characteristics such as age and ASCVD risk can be helpful—a young patient is less likely to experience a STEMI. |
| | ■ Remember that pericarditis usually presents with PR depressions (and a PR elevation in aVR) that accompany ST elevations. Though the PR segment can be affected in STEMI (specifically, atrial infarcts, which are very rare), the PR segment is elevated rather than depressed. Furthermore, the morphology of the ST elevations is more convex (tombstone shaped) in acute coronary syndromes compared to concave (smiling) in pericarditis. |
| **Antidote** | ■ Not applicable |
| **Common Scenarios** | ■ Not applicable |
| **Note(s)** | ■ A wrap-around left anterior descending coronary artery is one that covers a significant proportion of the inferior wall (exact definition varies between studies, ranging from the apical inferior wall up to a quarter of the inferior wall) and may present as an infarct in both anterior and inferior coronary territories. |

## MISTAKE: OVERLOOKING CONSTRICTIVE PERICARDITIS IN UNEXPLAINED HEART FAILURE

| | |
|---|---|
| **Case Example** | A 45-year-old female with hypertension and recurrent pericarditis presents with new SOB and lower extremity edema. A transthoracic echocardiogram (TTE) demonstrates normal left ventricular ejection fraction (LVEF), and a coronary computed tomography (CT) angiogram reveals a coronary artery calcium score of 0. Unsure of what could be contributing to her new symptoms, you switch her amlodipine to losartan and refer her to your colleague. |

| | |
|---|---|
| **Reasoning Error(s)** | ■ Not understanding the pathophysiology and long-term complications of acute pericarditis |
| | ■ Lack of knowledge regarding or consideration of a patient's prior medical history |
| | ■ Dismissing constrictive pericarditis from the differential due to incorrect thinking that it is an irreversible condition |
| **How to Avoid the Mistake** | ■ Understand that while chronic constrictive pericarditis is overall a rare complication of a single acute pericarditis event (excluding tuberculosis pericarditis), it is a complication that should always be considered. Transient constriction may occur with acute pericarditis episodes. Unsurprisingly, as a patient experiences recurrent pericarditis, the probability of progressing to constrictive pericarditis increases as there is gradual fibrosis of the pericardium. Constrictive pericarditis seldom results from a single inflammatory episode, though it is possible, particularly from pericarditis caused by systemic inflammatory disorders such as IgG4-related disease. |
| | ■ Always elicit a thorough medical history, particularly when clinically stumped. Patients with prior pericarditis, especially those with recurrent pericarditis or tuberculosis pericarditis, are at risk of developing constrictive pericarditis, which may be difficult to diagnosis and subtle initially in its presentation. |
| | ■ Understand that constrictive pericarditis is potentially reversible if caught early. Specifically, pericardiectomy at experienced surgical centers may be able to fully resolve constrictive pericarditis |
| **Antidote** | ■ Not applicable |
| **Common Scenarios** | ■ Not applicable |
| **Note(s)** | ■ Though constrictive pericarditis may result from various different pathways, the pathophysiology boils down to a reduction in pericardial compliance, such as through fibrosis (scarring) or calcifications. |
| | ■ The right ventricle (RV) is at baseline a very compliant structure, and its compliance is almost wholly dictated by the pericardium and pericardial space surrounding it. For example, in large pulmonary emboli, the RV frequently dilates significantly due to normal compliance. In the case of constrictive pericarditis, the RV compliance decreases dramatically and can have interesting physiologic consequences, such as increasing the degree of interventricular dependence in hemodynamically significant pulmonary embolism (PE). |
| | ■ Pericarditis is often recurrent. It is common for patients to require treatment for long periods; in patients tracked with cardiac MRI to monitor pericardial enhancement, many patients take several years of anti-inflammatory therapy to fully resolve an episode of pericarditis, which may persist subacutely or wax and wane. |

## MISTAKE: CONFUSING CONSTRICTIVE PERICARDITIS WITH RESTRICTIVE CARDIOMYOPATHY

**Case Example**

A 75-year-old female with multiple prior pericarditis episodes presents with new SOB. A TTE demonstrates preserved LVEF and concentric hypertrophy (interventricular septum [IVS] = 1.4 cm). ECG voltages are borderline positive for left ventricular hypertrophy (LVH). Given the LVH, you attribute the new SOB to an infiltrative process such as amyloidosis and embark on an extensive workup, which turns out to be negative.

**Reasoning Error(s)**

- Lack of detailed understanding of the pathophysiology of constrictive pericarditis and restrictive cardiomyopathy, and their differences
- Not knowing the preferred diagnostic modalities for differentiating constrictive pericarditis from restrictive cardiomyopathy

**How to Avoid the Mistake**

- Remember the key pathophysiologic differences between constrictive pericarditis and restrictive cardiomyopathy, which can be thought of as presenting with a syndrome of right-sided heart failure and left-sided heart failure, respectively. First, the pericardial compliance is unaffected in restrictive cardiomyopathy. This means that as the left ventricular function declines and LV dilation occurs, the NTproBNP will become significantly elevated. Contrast this to a normal to mild elevation in NTproBNP in constrictive pericarditis due to the relatively impaired ability of the ventricles to expand against the stiff pericardium. Similarly, the degree of interventricular dependence is not increased in restrictive cardiomyopathy, unlike constrictive pericarditis, in which cardiac MRI and TTE will demonstrate a septal "bounce" each cardiac beat. Hepatic vein flow reversal is also a great differentiator, with reversal in expiration in constrictive pericarditis as opposed to inspiratory reversal in restrictive cardiomyopathy.
- Consider further evaluation with cardiac catheterization (constriction study), which most usually demonstrates a normal to modest pulmonary arterial systolic pressure in constrictive pericarditis as opposed to a significantly elevated PASP in restrictive cardiomyopathy. Similarly, there is equalization of right and left ventricular end-diastolic pressures (RV/LVEDPs) in constrictive pericarditis as opposed to LVEDP > RVEDP in restrictive cardiomyopathy.

**Antidote**

- Not applicable

**Common Scenarios**

- Not applicable

**Note(s)**

- A septal bounce is an abnormal, paradoxical movement of the septum during every cardiac cycle. This is the key difference when differentiating a septal bounce from causes of abnormal septal motion such as septal flattening with inspiration during states of volume overload.
- Signs of constrictive pericarditis leading to right-sided heart failure overlap with exam findings of left-sided heart failure. However, a more unique finding for constriction as opposed to restriction is Kussmaul's sign (a paradoxical rise of the jugular venous distension during inspiration).
- While respirophasic variation across the mitral valve can be a very helpful differentiator between constrictive pericarditis and restrictive cardiomyopathy, atrial fibrillation (a common comorbidity) can make it difficult or impossible to accurately assess for respirophasic variation.

## MISTAKE: CONFUSING CONSTRICTIVE PERICARDITIS WITH TAMPONADE

**Case Example**      A 55-year-old female presents with recurrent pericarditis presents with new SOB. A TTE demonstrates a moderate pericardial effusion without chamber collapse as well as respirophasic variation across the mitral inflow, though there is no pulsus paradoxus on exam. Given the moderate pericardial effusion and the respirophasic variation, you diagnose the patient with tamponade and she is urgently taken for pericardiocentesis. Unfortunately, the patient's SOB does not improve after drainage.

**Reasoning Error(s)**
- Lack of detailed understanding of the pathophysiology of constrictive pericarditis and cardiac tamponade, and their differences
- Not knowing the preferred diagnostic modalities for differentiating constrictive pericarditis from tamponade

**How to Avoid the Mistake**
- Understand that many of the pathophysiologic contributions are similar between constrictive pericarditis and tamponade. For example, both lead to increased ventricular interdependence, diastolic dysfunction, and elevated venous (central and pulmonary) pressures. Both can also lead to elevated jugular venous distention (JVD) and pulsus paradoxus. Between these two conditions, knowing the differences can be more helpful to proper diagnosis!
- Remember that the key pathophysiologic difference between constrictive pericarditis and tamponade is in diastolic ventricular filling. Specifically, the pulmonary arterial diastolic pressure decreases during inspiration for constrictive pericarditis, whereas it remains constant in tamponade. In other words, the Y-descent (which represents early diastole, i.e., early ventricular filling) is particularly sharp and deep in constrictive pericarditis due to the sudden restriction beyond early diastole, whereas the Y-descent is blunted in tamponade, since the diastolic pressures in all chambers essentially equal the pericardial pressure.
- Consider magnetic resonance imaging evaluation to help distinguish between constrictive pericarditis and tamponade. Pericarditis will demonstrate late-gadolinium enhancement, whereas isolated tamponade does not. However, remember that the gold standard for differentiating the two conditions is right heart catheterization that demonstrates a decrease in pulmonary arterial diastolic pressure during inspiration (i.e., a Y-descent).

**Antidote**
- Not applicable

**Common Scenarios**
- Not applicable

**Note(s)**
- Since both constrictive pericarditis and tamponade can lead to increased ventricular interdependence, both may demonstrate respiratory variation of the mitral inflow on TTE as well as pulsus paradoxus (the clinical manifestation of respirophasic variation across the mitral valve).
- Another helpful clue to tamponade over pericarditis is the presence of pulsus alternans on ECG, though this is not a definitive diagnostic means.
- The sharp Y-descent in constrictive pericarditis occasionally leads to auscultation of a high-pitched sound in early diastole, known as a pericardial knock, that represents the sudden restriction and cessation of ventricular filling.

# Treatment

## MISTAKE: HOSPITALIZING FOR ALL CASES OF ACUTE PERICARDITIS

**Case Example**  A 25-year-old male with a recent coldlike syndrome presents to the emergency department (ED) with acute-onset, sharp chest pain radiating to his back. He notes the pain is pleuritic and improved with sitting forward. ECG demonstrates classic diffuse, concave ST elevations with PR depressions. You diagnose the patient with acute pericarditis and admit the patient given the patient has a significant pathology associated with his heart (what a precious organ!).

**Reasoning Error(s)**
- Lack of understanding features of acute pericarditis that suggest higher risk
- Viewing acute pericarditis as a highly dangerous condition that always requires admission due to the relative rarity and/or association with the heart ("an especially important organ")

**How to Avoid the Mistake**
- Recognize high-risk features of pericarditis that support admission for close monitoring:
  - Fever
  - Subacute onset
  - Large pericardial effusion and/or tamponade
  - Refractory pericarditis
  - Myocardial involvement (myopericarditis; positive troponins)
  - Immunosuppression
  - High bleeding risk: oral anticoagulation, dual antiplatelet therapy
  - Recent precordial trauma.
- Understand that most cases of acute (not subacute) pericarditis in healthy and reliable individuals can be managed outpatient with careful contingencies.

**Antidote**
- Not applicable

**Common Scenarios**
- Not applicable

**Note(s)**
- The most common causes of pericarditis in the developed world are idiopathic and viral. Other causes include autoimmune disorders (e.g., lupus), uremia/renal failure, and medications (e.g., hydralazine, procainamide, methyldopa).
- Uremic pericarditis can be associated with significant pericardial effusions in up to one-third of cases. Fortunately, with the advent of dialysis, cases of uremic pericarditis are much rarer.

## MISTAKE: MONOTHERAPY WITH NONSTEROIDAL ANTIINFLAMMATORY DRUGS AND/OR STEROIDS WITHOUT COLCHICINE FOR ACUTE PERICARDITIS

**Case Example**  A 25-year-old male with a recent coldlike syndrome presents to the ED with acute-onset, sharp chest pain radiating to his back. He notes the pain is pleuritic and improved with sitting forward. ECG demonstrates classic diffuse, concave ST elevations with PR depressions. You diagnose the patient with acute pericarditis and send the patient home on high-dose ibuprofen for 2 weeks with outpatient follow-up.

| | |
|---|---|
| **Reasoning Error(s)** | ■ Not understanding the role of colchicine in pericarditis treatment |
| | ■ Thinking that colchicine treatment is only for refractory disease or second-line |
| | ■ Misconception that colchicine is only added to nonsteroidal anti-inflammatory drug (NSAID) therapy |
| **How to Avoid the Mistake** | ■ Understand that the role of colchicine is not to treat the acute episode of pericarditis but rather to reduce the rate of recurrence. This is based on several studies, including the landmark COPE, ICAP, and COPE trials. Specifically, ICAP demonstrated a remarkable reduction in recurrent pericarditis (16.7% versus 37.5%) with the addition of colchicine to either NSAID or steroid therapy. Furthermore, hospitalization rates were lower (5% versus 14.2%), and 1-week treatment success was higher (85% versus 58.3%). |
| | ■ Remember that colchicine should be added to steroid therapy just as it is with NSAID therapy. |
| **Antidote** | ■ Prescribe colchicine to all patients with pericarditis. |
| **Common Scenarios** | ■ Not applicable |
| **Note(s)** | ■ Notably, patients with pericarditis due to bacterial infection or malignancy were included from the ICAP study. |
| | ■ The typical dose of colchicine is 0.6 mg BID. However, if a patient has intolerance (most commonly GI upset), a smaller dose such as 0.6 mg daily may be tried. It is also important to hold baseline laxatives when initiating colchicine, as they may have a compounding effect. |
| | ■ The duration of colchicine for acute pericarditis is often longer (3 months) than the treatment with NSAIDs (usually 2–4 weeks, pending clinical response). |
| | ■ Steroids should be used only in the case of NSAID intolerance or refractory disease given the higher rate of recurrence. |
| **Further Reading** | ■ Excellent review article on the management of pericarditis: Chiabrando JG, et al. Management of acute and recurrent pericarditis. *JACC*. 2020;75(1):76–92. |

## MISTAKE: ROUTINE USE OF STEROIDS FOR ACUTE PERICARDITIS

| | |
|---|---|
| **Case Example** | A 25-year-old male with a recent coldlike syndrome presents to the ED with acute-onset, sharp chest pain radiating to his back. He notes the pain is pleuritic and improved with sitting forward. ECG demonstrates classic diffuse, concave ST elevations with PR depressions. You diagnose the patient with acute pericarditis and send the patient home on prednisone and colchicine for 2 weeks with outpatient follow-up. At the follow-up the patient is elated that his symptoms have resolved. A month later, the patient represents with another episode of acute pericarditis. |
| **Reasoning Error(s)** | ■ Not understanding the downside to steroid treatment of pericarditis |
| | ■ Lack of familiarity with indications for steroid treatment of pericarditis |

| | |
|---|---|
| **How to Avoid the Mistake** | ■ Understand that steroid treatment of pericarditis is associated with a higher recurrence rate. Furthermore, steroids are associated with significantly more general side effects than NSAID therapy and often require a taper. |
| | ■ Use steroids to treat pericarditis that is refractory to NSAIDs or in patients who cannot tolerate NSAIDs (e.g., renal failure, pregnancy). Notably, refractory treatment is defined as having failed more than two (often more than three) attempts of NSAID therapy. Special indications for treatment with steroids rather than NSAIDs include autoimmune pericarditis and that due to immune checkpoint inhibitors. |
| **Antidote** | ■ Not applicable |
| **Common Scenarios** | ■ Not applicable |
| **Note(s)** | ■ The rate of recurrent pericarditis may be as high as 30%. |
| | ■ Alternative immunosuppressant agents such as interleukin-1 antibodies (anakinra), methotrexate, azathioprine, and IVIG may also be considered in severely refractory disease, though this should always be done in consultation with a pericarditis expert. |
| | ■ If steroid therapy is used for pericarditis, tapering should be done gradually as rapid tapering may further increase the risk of recurrence. |

## MISTAKE: PERICARDIOCENTESIS OF ALL MODERATE OR LARGE PERICARDIAL EFFUSIONS

| | |
|---|---|
| **Case Example** | A 78-year-old male with metastatic lung cancer presents with worsening SOB. Though he is diagnosed with community-acquired pneumonia, a TTE is obtained, which demonstrates a moderate pericardial effusion. There is no respirophasic variation of the mitral inflow and no visible chamber collapse in any part of the cardiac cycle. The patient is hemodynamically stable with blood pressures in the 130s/80s. However, the hospitalist team pages the cardiology team emergently requesting a pericardiocentesis for tamponade contributing to the patient's SOB. |
| **Reasoning Error(s)** | ■ Lack of understanding how to diagnose tamponade |
| | ■ Equating fluid around the heart with tamponade without considering the clinical context, volume, and acuity of accumulation |
| | ■ Not understanding the significance of various echocardiographic findings of tamponade |

| | |
|---|---|
| **How to Avoid the Mistake** | ■ Understand that tamponade is a clinical diagnosis, meaning the patient must exhibit evidence of hemodynamic compromise (hypotension, tachycardia, elevated venous pressures—JVD). The mere presence of fluid around the heart does not indicate tamponade or hemodynamic compromise; among the most important factors in whether pericardial effusions affect hemodynamics is the rate of accumulation (a slow accumulating effusion can be large without hemodynamic consequence, whereas a small but fast-growing effusion can cause chamber compromise). Furthermore, echocardiographic signs such as respirophasic variation of the mitral inflow must be contextualized. |
| | ■ Not all echocardiographic signs of tamponade are equally valuable. Respirophasic variation of the mitral inflow is the earliest and most common sign, which can be thought of as an early pulsus paradoxus; this does not equate to a diagnosis of tamponade but rather is an early warning to continue monitoring for clinical signs and symptoms of tamponade. Advanced signs such as RV collapse during systole are highly concerning, even in the absence of clinical signs or symptoms, though this is seldom the case. |
| **Antidote** | ■ Not applicable |
| **Common Scenarios** | ■ Not applicable |
| **Note(s)** | ■ Not all chamber collapse equates to high concern for tamponade. For example, collapse of the right atrium during systole (atrial diastole) occurs early in pericardial pressure buildup, since that is a low-pressure part of the cardiac cycle. |
| | ■ Tamponade physiology (both signs and symptoms) may be masked in the setting of elevated intra-cardiac pressures, such as in significant pulmonary hypertension. |
| | ■ A left-sided pleural effusion can mimic the presence of a posterior (inferolateral) effusion on the parasternal long-axis view. Use the descending thoracic aorta to differentiate between pericardial (anterior to the thoracic aorta) and pleural (posterior) effusions. |

# Vascular Cardiology

Paul Yong Kyu Lee

| Mistake: Forgetting Pregnancy Counseling in Connective Tissue Disorders | Mistake: Overlooking Factors Favoring Early Surgical Intervention of Aortic Aneurysm |
|---|---|

# Peripheral Artery Disease: Diagnosis

## MISTAKE: UNDERDIAGNOSIS OF PERIPHERAL ARTERY DISEASE: SYMPTOM MISATTRIBUTION AND ATYPICAL PRESENTATIONS

**Case Example**

A 67-year-old male with coronary artery disease (CAD), hypertension (HTN), and diabetes mellitus type 2 (T2DM) presents to the clinic to establish care. Knowing that the patient has CAD, you obtain a detailed history about the nature of his CAD, including past myocardial infarction, revascularization, and a thorough assessment of risk factors. The patient then mentions that he recently started having cramping of his calf with walking, but you dismiss it as a combination of normal aging and muscle cramps. The patient continues to have worsening calf pain and is diagnosed with peripheral artery disease (PAD) by a colleague 1 year after later.

**Reasoning Error(s)**

- Thinking that blockages of the legs are not fatal (unlike myocardial infarction or stroke) or would not change clinical outcomes
- Not realizing PAD is a common diagnosis, especially in certain populations
- Minimizing and/or misattribution of symptoms to more common diagnoses such as deep vein thrombosis, lumbar stenosis, aging, or musculoskeletal (e.g., arthritis, muscle strain, or cramp)
- Focusing only on the classic symptoms associated with PAD
- Lack of familiarity with PAD as an entity
- Lack of understanding of PAD and its mechanism

**How to Avoid the Mistake**

- Improve your understanding of PAD. Simply, PAD can be thought of as blockages that occur in the blood vessels that supply the extremities, most commonly the lower extremities but also sometimes the arms. In other words, PAD is CAD of the extremities. The mechanism of PAD is complex and similar to CAD but can be thought of as plaque buildup.
- Understand both classic and atypical presentations of PAD akin to how you think about myocardial ischemia. Classic symptoms include claudication, which may be described as crampy or achy. Stable angina is to stable CAD as intermittent claudication is to PAD. Atypical symptoms may include descriptors of claudication in less familiar ways: fatigue, weakness, and pressure. If PAD is very proximal, it can result in thigh and buttock pain.
- Understand that PAD is actually very common in patients with known CAD—up to 42% of patients with CAD have PAD, and there are an estimated 200 million people worldwide with PAD. With this knowledge, screen for PAD in all patients with known CAD!
- Develop reflexes similar to that when you hear "chest pain." As you would obtain an ECG, troponins, and thorough history to rule out ischemia, you should similarly obtain an arterial-brachial index (ABI) and a thorough history and physical to entertain possible PAD. Think of the ABI as the ECG of PAD (both noninvasive first steps in workup).

| | |
|---|---|
| **Antidote** | ■ Screen for PAD. |
| **Common Scenarios** | ■ Not applicable |
| **Notes** | ■ Generally, PAD occurs after CAD has occurred. However, it is possible as the first manifestation of atherosclerosis (particularly in smokers and diabetes) and should not be ruled out in the absence of CAD. |
| | ■ PAD has a strong predictive value for future myocardial infarction and stroke. |
| | ■ We highly recommend performing a deep dive into PAD, such as through the review article below, given formal education on PAD is traditionally very lacking. This has been shown in numerous studies to result in poor practitioner awareness of PAD as a clinical entity and a markedly low rate of clinical diagnosis and treatment of PAD. |
| **Further Reading** | ■ Excellent practical and contemporary review on PAD: Criqui MH, et al. Lower extremity peripheral artery disease: a contemporary epidemiology, management gaps, and future directions—a scientific statement from the American Heart Association. *Circulation.* 2021;144(9):e171–191. |

## MISTAKE: FORGETTING TO CHECK ARTERIAL-BRACHIAL INDEX IN PATIENTS AT RISK OR SUSPECTED OF PERIPHERAL ARTERY DISEASE

| | |
|---|---|
| **Case Example** | A patient comes in to the clinic complaining of calf pain while walking. Correctly, you suspect PAD, and obtain a detailed walking history and physical exam (obtaining weak lower extremity pulses). However, you do not examine further and tell the patient to return in a year for follow-up. |
| **Reasoning Error(s)** | ■ Lack of access to equipment to obtain ABI in clinic |
| | ■ Not understanding the importance of ABI measurements in PAD management |
| | ■ Thinking there is not enough time to check an ABI |
| **How to Avoid the Mistake** | ■ Understand the importance of obtaining an ABI in patient with suspected PAD. The ABI is the first step in diagnosing PAD and also informs management. A diagnosis of PAD and hence life-changing therapy cannot begin without an ABI. |
| | ■ Determine the best way to obtain ABIs in your practice setting. This may include a nominal investment to obtain ankle blood pressure (BP) cuffs and Doppler ultrasound or referring to a provider or clinic that is able to obtain an ABI. You can also often use a standard BP cuff to measure the ABI in most patients. Your inability to obtain an ABI is not an excuse for inaction. |
| | ■ Understand that PAD is a disease with very high morbidity and mortality. Just as you would feel obligated to check an ECG in a patient with chest pain, you should feel obligated to check an ABI when PAD is suspected. |
| **Antidote** | ■ Not applicable |
| **Common Scenarios** | ■ Not applicable |

Notes

- The American Heart Association/American College of Cardiology (AHA/ACC) recommends a screening ABI in the following asymptomatic patients:
  - Age >65 years
  - Age 50–64 years with at least one risk factor (smoking, diabetes, hypertension, hyperlipidemia, family history of PAD)
  - Age <50 years with diabetes and at least one additional risk factor
  - Known atherosclerotic disease in another vasculature (coronary, carotid, renal, mesenteric, subclavian)

Further Reading

- Great article on working up PAD: Wennberg PW. Approach to the patient with peripheral arterial disease. *Circulation*. 2013;128(20):2241–2250.

## MISTAKE: MEASURING THE BRACHIAL SYSTOLIC PRESSURE IN ONE ARM FOR ARTERIAL-BRACHIAL INDEX CALCULATION

Case Example

A patient endorses a history of calf pain while walking. Correctly, you decide to obtain an ABI. However, you use only the left arm to measure the ABI and find the ABI to be 1.0. Based on this, you rule out the diagnosis of PAD.

Reasoning Error(s)

- Assuming upper extremity BPs are always the same
- Lack of experience or knowledge measuring ABIs
- Rushing due to perceived lack of time

How to Avoid the Mistake

- Understand the proper technique for measuring ABIs. For all BP measurements for determining the ABI, the patient should be supine. The ankle BP is measured based on two arteries (dorsalis pedis and posterior tibial) using a Doppler ultrasound.
- Understand that PAD affects the arteries to all extremities (upper or lower), though lower extremities are much more commonly affected. Furthermore, other types of stenosis such as subclavian artery stenosis may cause unequal BPs in the upper extremities, possibly leading to falsely elevated ABI (since the denominator, i.e., arm BP is decreased). Always use the highest brachial pressure when calculating ABI.
- Remember that a test is only as good as its quality. Rushing may lead to technical errors that invalidate the test (and thus be a complete waste of time let alone lead to improper management of the patient). Take the time to perform (and verify if needed) any maneuvers correctly the first time.
- Since PAD is a common disease, you should have ample practice obtaining ABIs. The more you practice, the better you will become!

Antidote

- Calculate the ABI based on the higher BP in either arm

Common Scenarios

- Not applicable

Notes

- The formula for ABI (to be calculated separately for each leg) is below. Notably, the higher ankle BP refers to the higher of the pressures measured at the dorsalis pedis and posterior tibial arteries.
  - $$ABI = \frac{Higher\ Ankle\ BP}{Higher\ Arm\ BP}$$
- Depending on the source, the normal range for ABI is approximately 0.9–1.4. A value <0.9 is diagnostic of PAD, and a value <0.5 reflects severe PAD.

## MISTAKE: NOT OBTAINING A TOE-BRACHIAL INDEX FOR ABNORMALLY HIGH ARTERIAL-BRACHIAL INDEX (>1.4)

**Case Example**

A 76-year-old male smoker with diabetes, HTN, and hyperlipidemia (HLD) comes to the clinic complaining of calf pain with exertion. Correctly you suspected intermittent claudication secondary to PAD, given his risk factors. You obtain an ABI, making sure to measure the brachial pressure of both arms and using the higher number in your calculation of ABI. However, the ABI is normal at 1.5. Based on this, you rule out PAD in the patient.

**Reasoning Error(s)**

- Assuming that an ABI that is not <0.9 rules out PAD
- Inability to interpret a high ABI and assuming it means something other than PAD
- Lack of understanding the mechanism behind a high ABI

**How to Avoid the Mistake**

- Understand the mechanism and meaning behind an abnormally high ABI. As you have deduced, values >1.4 indicate a markedly higher pressure in the ankle compared to the arms. This occurs when the arteries supplying the lower extremities are difficult to compress (perhaps even totally noncompressible), such as when they become calcified. This leads to an inability to interpret the ABI for diagnosing or ruling out PAD (would lead to false negatives).
- Realize that an alternative to the ABI is to obtain a TBI that is based off a small toe cuff on the great toe, whose vasculature is almost always unaffected by calcification and/or fibrosis. This is an excellent workaround to the ABI that has been validated in many studies to be equally if not better than the ABI.
- Develop a habit of inquiry and clarification when you do not understand a concept rather than assuming or letting the situation slip away.

**Antidote**

- When in doubt, perform a TBI.

**Common Scenarios**

- Not applicable

**Notes**

- High ABI is most often found in diabetic, end-stage renal disease, or very elderly patients.
- Unlike ABI, the exact TBI cutoff for diagnosis of PAD is unclear though <0.7 is generally considered diagnostic. Many centers may have their own cutoffs based on experience with their patient populations.

## MISTAKE: FAILURE TO USE EXERCISE ARTERIAL-BRACHIAL INDEX TESTING IN PATIENTS WITH SUSPECTED PERIPHERAL ARTERY DISEASE BUT NORMAL ARTERIAL-BRACHIAL INDEX

**Case Example**

A 76-year-old male smoker with diabetes, HTN, and HLD comes to the clinic complaining of calf pain with exertion. Correctly you suspected intermittent claudication secondary to PAD, given his risk factors. You obtain an ABI, making sure to measure the brachial pressure of both arms and using the higher number in your calculation of ABI. However, the ABI is normal at 1.2. Based on this, you rule out PAD in the patient.

**Reasoning Error(s)**

- Assuming that the ABI is a perfect diagnostic test and/or lack of knowledge regarding its sensitivity/specificity
- Solely using a test without factoring in clinical context
- Lack of awareness regarding a postexercise ABI

| | |
|---|---|
| **How to Avoid the Mistake** | ■ Understand that while the ABI boasts great sensitivity and specificity, it is not perfect and misses some cases. It is approximately >90% sensitive and >95% specific for detecting at least 50% stenosis of the lower extremities. |
| | ■ In a patient with a normal ABI (measured correctly) but a high pretest probability, you can try an exercise ABI (obtain the ABI before and after walking on a treadmill). A significant decline in ABI (e.g., >20%) is diagnostic of PAD. |
| | ■ When interpreting the results of any test, ask yourself whether it makes sense. If your suspicion for a disease process is strong, determine additional modalities of confirming or refuting your hunches. |
| **Antidote** | ■ Not applicable |
| **Common Scenarios** | ■ Not applicable |
| **Notes** | ■ Similar to an exercise stress test for CAD, an exercise test for PAD provides important long-term prognostic information. |

## MISTAKE: ANGIOGRAPHY FOR ASYMPTOMATIC PERIPHERAL ARTERY DISEASE

| | |
|---|---|
| **Case Example** | A 59-year-old female with a 100-pack-year smoking history, CAD, and diabetes presents for routine follow-up. She has no lower extremity symptoms but given her significant atherosclerotic history and risk factors in conjunction with her age, you perform an ABI. The ABI is 0.7, suggestive of PAD, but the patient requests an angiogram to confirm. You refer the patient for an angiogram, which becomes complicated by an arterial aneurysm. |
| **Reasoning Error(s)** | ■ Thinking that visualization of the vasculature would improve management |
| | ■ Forgetting that an ABI < 0.9 alone is diagnostic of PAD |
| | ■ Favoring invasive and more "definitive" management |
| | ■ Patient insistence despite no medical indication |
| **How to Avoid the Mistake** | ■ Understand that invasive angiography is unnecessary to diagnose PAD in the presence of an ABI <0.9 (specificity >95%) even in the absence of clinical symptoms such as intermittent claudication. Angiography would not change management as revascularization would not be indicated for asymptomatic PAD and hence visualization of the vasculature is not needed. |
| | ■ Counsel patients on the risks of invasive angiography. Though experienced centers perform these commonly and have very low complication rates, there is no need to expose patients to any extra possibility of adverse effects if the results will not inform management. |
| | ■ For all clinical actions, think about the value provided. Does it affect management? |
| **Antidote** | ■ Not applicable |
| **Common Scenarios** | ■ Not applicable |
| **Notes** | ■ The gold standard to diagnosing PAD is angiography. It uses iodinated contrast similar to a coronary angiogram and thus may affect renal function, particularly in patients with preexisting renal dysfunction. Other risks include vascular complications including dissection, aneurysm, and hematomas. |

## MISTAKE: CONFUSING VASCULAR AND NEUROGENIC CLAUDICATION

**Case Example**   A 50-year-old male with CAD comes to the clinic complaining of lower extremity pain with exertion. He also notes chronic back pain and, suspecting lumbar stenosis and resulting neurogenic claudication, you defer obtaining an ABI.

**Reasoning Error(s)**
- Not knowing the key differentiating features between vascular and neurogenic claudication
- Lack of a differential regarding symptoms
- Lack of thorough history-taking

**How to Avoid the Mistake**
- Understand that claudication simply refers to a crampy pain of the lower extremities. It may be caused by both poor perfusion (PAD) and spinal nerve impingement (e.g., lumbar stenosis). The history is especially helpful. Neurogenic claudication often improves with maneuvers that relieve the spinal compression such as bending forward or walking uphill. It is also less exertional than vascular claudication, which should not occur at rest unless the PAD is extremely severe. Vascular claudication typically improves with rest, whereas neurogenic claudication may not improve as reproducibly and is a more positional feature.
- Always think about a differential diagnosis even if your patient population typically presents with a certain diagnosis.
- When in doubt between vascular and neurogenic claudication, perform an exam and obtain an ABI, which should only be affected in PAD

**Antidote**
- Not applicable

**Common Scenarios**
- Not applicable

**Notes**
- Small studies have demonstrated that a very good differentiating maneuver between vascular and neurogenic claudication is to ask the patient to stand. Pain that is triggered with simply standing is rarely vascular in nature.

## MISTAKE: CONFUSING DIABETIC ULCERS WITH ARTERIAL ULCERS

**Case Example**   A 67-year-old female with uncontrolled diabetes presents to your clinic complaining of an ulcer present on the tip of her big toe. You see the ulcer and immediately attribute it to diabetes and refer the patient to podiatry. Her PAD remains undiagnosed until 1 year later, when a different doctor notices the ulcer, finds the pedal pulses to be absent on physical exam, and then finds the ABI to be 0.6.

**Reasoning Error(s)**
- Assuming that foot ulcers in a diabetic patient are due to diabetes
- Jumping to a diagnosis by association rather than after careful workup
- Lack of experience or knowledge on differentiating diabetic and arterial ulcers

| How to Avoid the Mistake | ■ Understand that diabetes is a significant risk factor for PAD. This means that diabetic patients may be high risk for developing not only diabetic ulcers but also ulcers due to their PAD. |
|---|---|
| | ■ Understand the various ulcers that can present and know the difference in presentation between them. PAD is frequently seen in diabetes. Diabetic ulcers are painless ulcers that tend to present on the plantar surface of the foot (that is why you should be regularly checking for these as they can easily go undetected). On the other hand, arterial ulcers in PAD are seen over the distal aspects of the circulation such as the toes and heels of the feet and are usually painful. |
| | ■ Perform a thorough history and physical exam to help differentiate the type of ulcer. Check for the temperature of the foot (cooler foot is suspicious of PAD), arterial pulses (absent pulses favor PAD), sensation (absent sensation and/or reflexes favor a diabetic ulcer), location of ulcer, and presence of pain. |
| **Antidote** | ■ Not applicable |
| **Common Scenarios** | ■ Not applicable |
| **Notes** | ■ Arterial ulcers are often seen in chronic limb-threatening ischemia (CLTI), the most severe form of PAD. Typically presenting symptoms are ischemic rest pain, tissue ulceration, and gangrene. |
| | ■ Venous ulcers can be seen on the malleoli as well however usually in the presence of venous stasis changes such as edema, dry skin, varicose veins, and brown-blue hyperpigmentation/erythema and are frequently painless. |

## MISTAKE: OVERLOOKING CRITICAL LIMB ISCHEMIA

| Case Example | A 75-year-old male with poorly controlled diabetes and known CAD presents with intermittent lower left extremity pain at rest. PAD comes to your mind (and you correctly associate it with intermittent crampy pain), but you dismiss PAD due to his poorly controlled diabetes. You inform the patient that the pain is due to diabetic neuropathy and start gabapentin. |
|---|---|
| **Reasoning Error(s)** | ■ Not knowing that severe PAD can present with ischemic rest pain rather than intermittent claudication on exertion |
| | ■ Lack of knowledge regarding critical limb ischemia (CTLI) and its presentation |
| | ■ Lack of knowing how to diagnose CLTI |
| **How to Avoid the Mistake** | ■ Understand that severe PAD may present with claudication at rest. Specifically, the most severe form of PAD known as critical limb ischemia presents with pain at rest, dry gangrene, and nonhealing wounds. |
| | ■ Suspect critical limb ischemia in any patient with claudication at rest. Obtain an ABI (<0.40 favors CLTI). Other signs on exam include a diminished or absent pedal flow on duplex ultrasound and a toe BP <30–40 mmHg. |
| | ■ Remember that patients with CLTI should be referred urgently to a vascular specialist to salvage the limb through revascularization if possible. |

| | |
|---|---|
| **Antidote** | ■ Immediate referral for revascularization |
| **Common Scenarios** | ■ Not applicable |
| **Notes** | ■ CLTI carries an extremely poor prognosis. About one-third of patients with CLTI will die or require amputation within 1 year. |

# Peripheral Artery Disease: Treatment

## MISTAKE: FORGETTING AGGRESSIVE RISK FACTOR MODIFICATION

| | |
|---|---|
| **Case Example** | A 56-year-old male heavy smoker comes to your office complaining of calf pain with walking. You perform a detailed physical exam, note a cool foot, absent distal pulses, and perform an ABI, which you find to be 0.7. You prescribe the patient aspirin to reduce his risk of cardiovascular events. However, you do nothing to address his other risk factors. |
| **Reasoning Error(s)** | ■ Not understanding how critical it is to address all the risk factors in PAD<br>■ Lack of knowledge regarding the modifiable risk factors for PAD<br>■ Habit of relying on medical and surgical therapies |
| **How to Avoid the Mistake** | ■ Understand the importance of risk factor modification in treating PAD. In particular, cigarette smoking is the most important modifiable risk factor for PAD; patients who stop smoking have dramatic decrease in their mortality even up to 10 years (e.g., one study found that >80% of patients were still alive at 10 years postcessation). Diabetes, hypertension, and dyslipidemia are the key medical conditions to be managed. Therapeutically, exercise (particularly aerobic) is key to improved functional status.<br>■ Always consider lifestyle modifications in addition to medical therapy. Furthermore, pharmacologic adjuncts should be considered for certain modifiable risk factors such as smoking. |
| **Antidote** | ■ Not applicable |
| **Common Scenarios** | ■ Not applicable |
| **Notes** | ■ Though the management of diabetes and hypertension in PAD patients does not differ from usual, the AHA/ACC favors high-intensity statins in patients with PAD.<br>■ Pharmacologic aids for smoking cessation include:<br>　■ Nicotine replacement (patch, gum, nasal spray, inhaler)<br>　■ Varenicline (Chantix): may induce vivid dreams; rarely depression, mania, and psychosis<br>　■ Bupropion (Wellbutrin): avoid in patients with eating disorders and history of seizures |

## MISTAKE: LACK OF ANTIPLATELET THERAPY IN SYMPTOMATIC OR ASYMPTOMATIC PERIPHERAL ARTERY DISEASE

| | |
|---|---|
| **Case Example** | A 56-year-old male smoker and diabetic comes to your office complaining of calf pain with walking. You perform a detailed physical exam, noting a cool foot, absent distal pulses, and perform an ABI, which you find to be 0.6. You address his risk factors and prescribe cilostazol and a supervised exercise regimen. |

| | |
|---|---|
| **Reasoning Error(s)** | ■ Lack of understanding the role of antiplatelet therapy in PAD |
| | ■ Thinking that asymptomatic patients with PAD do not need antiplatelet agents |
| | ■ Considering PAD a unique entity rather than a continuum of atherosclerotic disease and CAD (which would obviously merit antiplatelet therapy) |
| | ■ Misunderstanding that cilostazol is an antiplatelet agent for PAD |
| **How to Avoid the Mistake** | ■ Understand that antiplatelet agents decrease the risk of vascular events in patients with PAD regardless of the presence of symptoms (technically a class IIa recommendation in asymptomatic PAD). The first-line antiplatelet agents are either aspirin or clopidogrel monotherapy. Based on results of the CAPRIE trial, which demonstrated superiority of clopidogrel over aspirin for decreasing vascular events, some clinicians favor clopidogrel monotherapy. |
| | ■ Realize that cilostazol, while it has antiplatelet activity, is primarily a phosphodiesterase inhibitor. It is recommended as a separate agent in addition to antiplatelet therapy in patient experiencing claudication due to evidence for increasing walking distance and decreasing claudication. |
| **Antidote** | ■ Not applicable |
| **Common Scenarios** | ■ Not applicable |
| **Notes** | ■ Dual antiplatelet therapy is unnecessary in patients with concomitant CAD and PAD who are preferred on clopidogrel for the PAD. Clopidogrel is an efficacious substitute for decreasing the incidence of major adverse cardiovascular events in both patients with CAD and PAD. |
| **Further Reading** | ■ Excellent review on antithrombotic therapy in PAD: Hess CN, et al. Antithrombotic therapy for peripheral artery disease in 2018. *JAMA.* 2018;319(22):2239–2330. |
| | ■ Cochrane review on the role of cilostazol for PAD: Brown T, et al. Cilostazol for intermittent claudication. *Cochrane Database Syst Rev.* 2021;6. |

## MISTAKE: NOT PRESCRIBING STATINS IN ISOLATED SYMPTOMATIC OR ASYMPTOMATIC PERIPHERAL ARTERY DISEASE

| | |
|---|---|
| **Case Example** | A 56-year-old male smoker and diabetic comes to your office complaining of calf pain with walking. You perform a detailed physical exam, noting a cool foot, absent distal pulses, and perform an ABI, which you find to be 0.6. You address his risk factors and prescribe clopidogrel, cilostazol, and a supervised exercise regimen. |
| **Reasoning Error(s)** | ■ Not realizing that high-intensity statins are first-line standard of care for PAD |
| | ■ Thinking that statins are only indicated in symptomatic PAD |
| | ■ Considering PAD a unique entity rather than a continuum of atherosclerotic disease and CAD (which would obviously merit statin therapy) |

**How to Avoid the Mistake**
- Understand that statins significantly reduce vascular events in PAD. Notably, this is based upon strong evidence that is not extrapolated from the cardiovascular literature. Statins also reduce the rates of revascularization though a decrease in amputation risk has yet to be shown definitively.
- Realize that statins are indicated in symptomatic as well as asymptomatic PAD, similar to how patients with asymptomatic CAD are treated with statins.

**Antidote**
- Not applicable

**Common Scenarios**
- Not applicable

**Notes**
- Though proprotein convertase subtilisin/kexin type 9 (PCSK9) inhibitors are not included in the latest 2016 AHA/ACC guidelines on the management of PAD, there is strong evidence that PCSK9 inhibitors significantly reduce major vascular events in PAD. In patients who are unable to tolerate statins, consider PCSK9 therapy.

## MISTAKE: PRESCRIBING CILOSTAZOL FOR PERIPHERAL ARTERY DISEASE IN PATIENTS WITH HEART FAILURE WITH REDUCED EJECTION FRACTION

**Case Example**

A 56-year-old male with heart failure with reduced ejection fraction (HFrEF), symptomatic PAD, and type 2 diabetes presents to your office complaining of calf pain with walking. You perform a detailed physical exam, noting a cool foot, absent distal pulses, and perform an ABI, which you find to be <0.8. You correctly prescribe aspirin as you read in a certain book that aspirin decreases risk of cardiovascular adverse effects and offer a trial of cilostazol as you correctly note that it can improve the functional status of PAD patient with intermittent claudication. You smile to yourself, proud that you have done everything in your power to help this patient with PAD. However, you learn later that cilostazol is contraindicated in heart failure, and your smile fades into dread.

**Reasoning Error(s)**
- Lack of awareness that cilostazol is contraindicated in any stage of HFrEF
- Not understanding the reason behind cilostazol's contraindication in HFrEF
- Lack of comfort with a seldom used medication

**How to Avoid the Mistake**
- Understand that cilostazol is contraindicated in HFrEF due to an increase in mortality and risk for serious complications such as ventricular tachycardia. It has also been associated with increased heart failure hospitalizations.
- For any medication that you prescribe, be intimately familiar with the risks and benefits. This is especially true for medications that you do not use as often.

**Antidote**
- Discontinue cilostazol

**Common Scenarios**
- Not applicable

**Notes**
- Common side effects of cilostazol include headaches, dizziness, and diarrhea. Up to one in five patients discontinue cilostazol treatment by 3 months.

## MISTAKE: ANTICOAGULATION FOR REDUCING CARDIOVASCULAR EVENTS IN PERIPHERAL ARTERY DISEASE

| | |
|---|---|
| **Case Example** | A 70-year-old male with symptomatic PAD presents for routine follow-up. His lower extremity claudication has been stable over the past 6 months and he is adherent to clopidogrel, cilostazol, and a supervised exercise therapy program. Today, you introduce the idea of starting rivaroxaban to reduce the rate of major cardiovascular events. |
| **Reasoning Error(s)** | ■ Lack of knowledge of the evidence for and against anticoagulation in PAD |
| | ■ Lack of patient-centered risk/benefit discussion around new evidence |
| **How to Avoid the Mistake** | ■ Understand that the use of anticoagulation in PAD to reduce cardiovascular events is controversial. While the latest 2016 AHA/ACC guidelines on the management of PAD recommend against the use of anticoagulation with a Grade III recommendation (harm), much of that recommendation was based on older studies and involved warfarin (such as the Warfarin Antiplatelet Vascular Evaluation Trial, which demonstrated only an increase in major bleeding) as opposed to direct oral anticoagulantss. Recent evidence such as the VOYAGER-PAD trial have demonstrated that low-dose rivaroxaban (2.5 mg twice daily) in conjunction with aspirin reduces major cardiovascular events without an increase in major bleeding in patients with PAD with prior revascularization. COMPASS-PAD also demonstrated similar reduction in major cardiovascular and limb events although major bleeding was increased (nonfatal, noncritical). |
| | ■ In the appropriate population (PAD with prior revascularization), consider a patient-centered discussion about the addition of low-dose rivaroxaban to reduce cardiovascular events. |
| **Antidote** | ■ Not applicable |
| **Common Scenarios** | ■ Not applicable |
| **Notes** | ■ In August 2021, the US Food and Drug Administration officially approved PAD as a formal indication for low-dose rivaroxaban. |

## MISTAKE: NON–EVIDENCE-BASED THERAPIES: PENTOXIFYLLINE, B VITAMINS, EDTA

| | |
|---|---|
| **Case Example** | A 67-year-old male with hypertension and PAD comes in for follow-up. His lower extremity claudication has worsened significantly despite being on a supervised exercise regimen and clopidogrel. You decide to add cilostazol and pentoxifylline. |
| **Reasoning Error(s)** | ■ Well-intentioned action that is actively refuted by the evidence (confusion between lack of evidence and evidence against a treatment) |
| | ■ Forgetting about polypharmacy and/or unintended medication adverse events |

| How to Avoid the Mistake | ■ Understand the difference between lack of evidence and evidence of lack of efficacy for a treatment. Pentoxifylline and chelation therapy (e.g., ethylenediaminetetraacetic acid [EDTA]) have been studied thoroughly in PAD and have been shown to lack benefit. They are thus a Class III (no benefit) recommendation in the 2016 AHA/ACC guidelines. |
|---|---|
| | ■ Always be mindful of polypharmacy. Patients with PAD often have numerous other comorbidities and are on a myriad of medications. Thus, medications without evidence of benefit should be avoided to minimize medication burnout and maximize adherence and quality of life. Furthermore, remember that all medications, no matter how trivial they may seem, possess adverse effects. |
| Antidote | ■ Not applicable |
| Common Scenarios | ■ Not applicable |
| Notes | ■ While supplementation with high-dose B vitamins is unlikely to reduce major cardiovascular events or claudication symptoms, a daily multivitamin may be considered for overall health and may also ensure that B vitamins are not deficient. |
| Further Reading | ■ A randomized controlled trial from 2000 demonstrated the lack of benefit of pentoxifylline for PAD while showing a benefit with cilostazol: Dawson DL, et al. A comparison of cilostazol and pentoxifylline for treating intermittent claudication. *Am J Med.* 2000;109(7):523–530. |

## MISTAKE: NOT PRESCRIBING A SUPERVISED EXERCISE PROGRAM IN PERIPHERAL ARTERY DISEASE

| Case Example | A 57-year-old female smoker presents to the clinic with intermittent claudication. You make the diagnosis of PAD. You address all the risk factors for PAD and send the patient home with clopidogrel and varenicline (to help stop smoking). |
|---|---|
| Reasoning Error(s) | ■ Overreliance on pharmacologic therapies |
| | ■ Forgetting that a supervised exercise regimen is superior to a home exercise regimen in PAD |
| | ■ Lack of understanding the data on the importance of exercise for PAD |
| | ■ Lack of understanding the mechanism of improvements secondary to exercise in PAD |
| How to Avoid the Mistake | ■ Understand that exercise therapy (in particular, supervised exercise therapy) is one of the best therapies for improving functional status (e.g., walking status) and decreasing claudication in PAD. Multiple mechanisms are thought to play a role, ranging from increased nitric oxide–dependent vasodilation to decreasing whole body inflammation. It is also thought that aerobic exercise may improve the formation of collateral circulation that may significantly reduce the burden of blocked arteries. |
| | ■ Remember that a supervised exercise program has been shown to be superior to home exercise in improving clinical outcomes for PAD. Supervised exercise programs are actually covered by insurance for patients with PAD! |
| | ■ Always consider a holistic approach to patient care that not only uses medications but also lifestyle modifications. |

| | |
|---|---|
| **Antidote** | ■ Not applicable |
| **Common Scenarios** | ■ Not applicable |
| **Notes** | ■ The standard measure of functional capacity in patients with PAD is the 6-minute walk test (6MWT). This takes place on a hard, flat surface where the patient is encouraged to walk as far as they can at their own pace. Interestingly, the 6MWT was originally developed based on patients 60–90 years old. |
| **Further Reading** | ■ Excellent study demonstrating the efficacy of a supervised exercise regimen in PAD patients with and without intermittent claudication: McDermott MM, et al. Treadmill exercise and resistance training in patients with peripheral arterial disease with and without intermittent claudication. *JAMA*. 2009;301(2):165–174. |

## MISTAKE: NOT REFERRING REST PAIN FOR SURGICAL REVASCULARIZATION (OVERLOOKING CHRONIC LIMB-THREATENING ISCHEMIA)

| | |
|---|---|
| **Case Example** | A 56-year-old male with long-standing PAD and intermittent claudication now complains of pain at rest that requires him to dangle his legs at night to achieve relief. He is already on clopidogrel, cilostazol, and max-dose rosuvastatin. He quit smoking a few years ago and has not relapsed. He watches his diet carefully and has been free of diabetes. On exam, you are unable to palpate pedal pulses but there are no wounds or ulcers. Given the lack of ulceration or gangrene, you schedule the patient for a 3-month follow-up and defer referral to a specialist. |
| **Reasoning Error(s)** | ■ Not understanding the criteria for CLTI<br>■ Thinking that rest pain is different from CLTI (i.e., relying on buzz words/terms)<br>■ Tunnel vision on pharmacologic therapy<br>■ Overthinking referral to PAD experts |
| **How to Avoid the Mistake** | ■ Understand that rest pain indicates CLTI and can also be diagnosed in the presence of a severely reduced ABI (≤0.5) and tissue loss (e.g., arterial ulceration). Ulceration and gangrene are not required for a diagnosis of CLTI.<br>■ Avoid learning clinical management based on buzz words or phrases. Know that revascularization is conceptually intended for patients with PAD who are functionally debilitated despite a supervised exercise regimen and optimal medical therapy.<br>■ Feel free to refer a patient whom you think may benefit from revascularization to a vascular specialist. It is better to overrefer than to not refer someone who needs revascularization; in other words, if you do not overrefer, you are likely missing referral of patients who need urgent revascularization. |
| **Antidote** | ■ Not applicable |
| **Common Scenarios** | ■ Not applicable |

**Notes**
- Among patients with PAD who experience claudication, approximately 10% will progress to critical limb ischemia (pain at rest) within 5 years.
- Patients may also be referred for revascularization in the setting of functional limitations despite optimal medical therapy and inadequate response to supervised exercise therapy (i.e., rest pain is not the only criteria).

**Further Reading**
- The 2016 AHA/ACC PAD guidelines are certainly worth reading: Gerhard-Herman MD, et al. 2016 AHA/ACC guideline on the management of patients with lower extremity peripheral artery disease: executive summary: a report of the American College of Cardiology/American Heart Association Task Force on Clinical Practice Guidelines. *Circulation.* 2017;135(12):e686–e725.

## MISTAKE: REVASCULARIZATION FOR SLOWING PROGRESSION OF PERIPHERAL ARTERY DISEASE TO CHRONIC LIMB-THREATENING ISCHEMIA

**Case Example**
A 56-year-old male with PAD presents with intermittent claudication. At prior visits, you have addressed his risk factors (hypertension, diabetes, hyperlipidemia) and convinced the patient to stop smoking. However, the patient is not satisfied and adamantly states that he wants his claudication to be cured and that he is afraid his disease will continue to progress. You discuss revascularization methods, noting that it is possible to decrease the degree of stenosis now and thus worsening of PAD.

**Reasoning Error(s)**
- Well-intentioned and logical thinking that does not bear out empirically
- Lack of understanding why revascularization is not performed on any stenosis

**How to Avoid the Mistake**
- Understand that revascularization is performed on arteries with hemodynamically significant stenoses with knowledge of the risk of complications including distal embolization of plaque. The risk is approximately 1%–3% for revascularization of the lower extremities. Notably, the risk of cardiovascular events and mortality is higher in patients with intermittent claudication than in those without, but revascularization of claudication neither prevents CLTI nor reduces cardiovascular morbidity and mortality. For these reasons, revascularization is usually performed only in either critical limb ischemia or refractory functional limitations despite optimal medical therapy.
- Always try to verify your critical thinking with the available evidence. You may be surprised that empiric results often do not align with theory (usually driven by a lack of human understanding that limits theory). This is also a great way to come up with new ideas to advance the field.

**Antidote**
- Not applicable

**Common Scenarios**
- Not applicable

| Notes | ■ Revascularization may be performed endovascularly or surgically. The correct revascularization for the patient will be dictated by anatomy and patient comorbidity. Ongoing research suggests equipoise between open surgical and endovascular revascularization, and vascular specialists primarily consider patient-related factors to decide between modalities. |
|---|---|
| Further Reading | ■ One of the first epidemiologic studies that investigated the cardiovascular outcomes in PAD patients: Leng GC, et al. Incidence, natural history, and cardiovascular events in symptomatic and asymptomatic peripheral arterial disease in the general population. *Int J Epidemiol.* 1996;25(6):1172–1181. |

## MISTAKE: LACK OF EMPHASIS ON EDUCATING PATIENTS ABOUT PERIPHERAL ARTERY DISEASE

| Case Example | You diagnose a patient with PAD on a busy clinic day. You counsel them on the appropriate pharmacotherapy needed to address her risk factors. You give a brief explanation on PAD and send the patient home with a statin and supervised exercise program. At the next clinic visit, the patient returns and notes noncompliance with her treatment plan, stating that she thought PAD is "just a bit less blood flow to my legs." |
|---|---|
| Reasoning Error(s) | ■ Lack of knowledge regarding the public knowledge gap on PAD<br>■ Focus on prescription without education<br>■ Not considering the role of patient adherence in medical outcomes |
| How to Avoid the Mistake | ■ Understand that there is a huge shortcoming in public knowledge about PAD. In the First National PAD Public Awareness Survey conducted in 2007, public knowledge regarding the increased risk for major cardiovascular events. For example only 14% of the public knew that PAD was associated with amputation and/or death.<br>■ Realize that physicians are ultimately advisors and patient understanding, self-motivation, and adherence are key to health maintenance.<br>■ Educate patients about not only PAD but all of their key medical conditions on an ongoing basis. Given limited time for patient visits, plan out an agenda that includes small bits of education and counseling each visit. |
| Antidote | ■ Not applicable |
| Common Scenarios | ■ Not applicable |
| Notes | ■ PAD is not only a knowledge gap for patients but also for providers! As a topic hardly emphasized in medical school and on clinical rotations, it can often fall through the cracks. Ensure that you understand PAD and its management. |
| Further Reading | ■ Study on public awareness of PAD: Hirsch AT, et al. Gaps in public knowledge of peripheral arterial disease. *Circulation.* 2007;116(18):2086–2094. |

# Aortic Disease: Aortic Dissection

## MISTAKE: RULING OUT ACUTE AORTIC DISSECTION WITH A CHEST RADIOGRAPH

**Case Example**

A 58-year-old male smoker presents with acute-onset chest pain radiating to the back. His vitals are notable for a markedly elevated BP (201/111) and 15-point asymmetry in BP between the arms. You immediately think of aortic dissection; however, the ECG does not show any abnormalities and the chest radiograph shows no mediastinal widening. You become less suspicious of a dissection; you do not order a computed tomography angiography (CTA) and explore other explanations for his pain.

**Reasoning Error(s)**
- Not realizing the sensitivity of a method touted commonly in early training (e.g., medical school) as a good screening test
- Using inappropriate testing for a case with high suspicion
- Lack of understanding what a chest radiograph (CXR) demonstrates for aortic dissection
- Missing a subtle or indeterminate widening of the mediastinum due to not comparing to baseline
- Lack of obtaining CTA due to patient instability or contraindications (e.g., renal function)

**How to Avoid the Mistake**
- Understand that the CXR is only approximately 60%–70% sensitive for aortic dissection. Compare this to a 99% sensitivity with CTA. Any case that presents with high suspicion for aortic dissection should immediately use the best test available (CTA). This is similar to working up a pulmonary embolism—you would not obtain a D-dimer if your probability of a pulmonary embolism was high to begin with!
- Recognize that CXR may provide subtle hints to an aortic dissection. It may not always present with an obviously widened mediastinum. Always compare to a prior image if possible to aid in subtle changes.
- Understand that a transesophageal echocardiogram is an alternate diagnostic modality to CTA with nearly 100% sensitivity and specificity for ascending and descending thoracic dissections. It may be performed quickly at bedside and has few contraindications, most notably esophageal disorders and lack of C-spine clearance (e.g., after a fall or motor vehicle accident). MRI/MRA is another alternative with similar sensitivity and specificity.

**Antidote**
- Not applicable

**Common Scenarios**
- Normal-appearing CXR
- Normal ECG

**Notes**
- In addition to visualization of a dissection flap, imaging findings suggestive of an aortic dissection and/or its complications include new aortic insufficiency, aortic root dilation, new pericardial effusion and/or tamponade, and new wall motion abnormalities.

## MISTAKE: OVERLOOKING AORTIC DISSECTION IN HYPOTENSION

**Case Example**
A 58-year-old male comes in with acute tearing chest pain with hypotension. The likelihood of dissection is lower in your mind given that dissection usually presents with hypertension. CXR is notable for enlarged heart and ECG is unremarkable. You notice that his heart sounds are distant and perform a bedside echo, which diagnoses cardiac tamponade. You bolus the patient with fluids to increase preload and prepare for bedside pericardiocentesis. The drainage turns out to be blood; the patient's BP continues to drop and he eventually dies from cardiac arrest on the way to the operating room for a now-apparent aortic dissection.

**Reasoning Error(s)**
- Associating aortic dissection solely with elevated or normal BPs
- Lack of knowledge regarding complications of aortic dissection
- Not considering complications of aortic dissection that may induce hypotension after initial hypertension
- Only considering the current BP and overlooking the presenting vitals

**How to Avoid the Mistake**
- Understand that while more than two-thirds of patients with an aortic dissection present with hypertension, hypertension does not rule out an aortic dissection. Furthermore, complications such as tamponade or aortic rupture may lead to new hypotension that masks a presenting hypertension. In particular, type A dissections are most likely to present with hypotension.
- Pay attention to changes in hemodynamics after presentation (e.g., hypertension that turned into hypotension) as this may provide early clues as to evolving pathology.
- Remember the structural complications related to aortic dissection: tamponade, aortic insufficiency, coronary dissection, aortic rupture, stroke, renal artery dissection.
- If aortic dissection is high on your differential, obtain a CTA or transesophageal echocardiogram (TEE) to rule it out. Also consider obtaining other collateral information such as checking for tamponade with a quick bedside (nonformal) transthoracic echocardiogram (TTE).

**Antidote**
- Not applicable

**Common Scenarios**
- Tamponade
- Aortic rupture

**Notes**
- Among the coronary arteries, the right coronary artery is the most commonly involved in aortic dissection. This is thought to be the case due to aortic dissections more commonly originating above the right sinus of Valsalva (which is the additional space just distal to the aortic valve and proximal to the coronary ostia that allows for continuous blood flow when the aortic valve opens outward into the aorta).

**Further Reading**
- A contemporary study on the likelihood of classically taught presentations for aortic dissection: Hagan PG, et al. The International Registry of Acute Aortic Dissection (IRAD): new insights into an old disease. *JAMA*. 2000;283(7):897–903.

## MISTAKE: LACK OF CLOSE MONITORING FOR COMPLICATIONS OF AORTIC DISSECTION

**Case Example**

A 54-year-old male smoker comes in with acute-onset chest pain radiating to the back. Acute aortic dissection is diagnosed via bedside TEE. Blood pressure control with β-blockers is initiated promptly, and you await the cardiac and vascular surgery teams to arrive to assess the patient. The patient continues having significant chest pain and complains about a new chest pressure sensation. You reassure him that the situation is under control and that the surgical team is coming soon. Minutes later, the patient becomes hypotensive and a STAT ECG reveals 3-mm ST elevations of leads II, III, and aVF. You immediately activate the cath lab, and during the catherization, it is noted that the cause of the ischemia is a dissection flap obstructing the right coronary artery. Urgent surgical repair is performed.

**Reasoning Error(s)**

- Stopping after diagnosis of acute aortic dissection and not considering the downstream effects of aortic dissection (i.e., comfort after diagnosing)
- Lack of knowledge regarding common complications of aortic dissection

**How to Avoid the Mistake**

- Understand that aortic dissection can and often does progress after diagnosis. Close serial monitoring for complications is vital to minimizing the morbidity and mortality associated with aortic dissection. Diagnosis and treatment of BP are not enough!
- Learn the most common serious complications of acute aortic dissection (see below in common scenarios) and how to monitor for them.
  - Aortic insufficiency: serial auscultation and/or bedside color Doppler to assess for AI, watch for acute pulmonary edema
  - Acute coronary syndrome: watch for evolution of chest pain character and/or new chest pressure, consider trending troponins and ECG
  - Tamponade: watch for hypotension and worsening tachycardia
  - Stroke: serial neurologic exams, watch for syncope
  - Mesenteric/renal/peripheral ischemia: reassess symptoms and exam serially

**Antidote**

- Not applicable

**Common Scenarios**

- Aortic insufficiency
- Acute coronary syndrome
- Tamponade
- Aortic root dilation
- Aortic rupture
- Stroke
- Mesenteric/renal/peripheral ischemia

**Notes**

- Do not administer heparin for acute coronary syndrome in the setting of aortic dissection. This is for three reasons: 1) the ACS is not caused by plaque rupture; thus, the heparin will not have a role in plaque stabilization; 2) there is mostly neutral evidence on the benefit of heparin in ACS despite its inclusion in the ACS guidelines; and 3) anticoagulation may increase the bleeding in the event of aortic rupture.

## MISTAKE: INADEQUATE BLOOD PRESSURE CONTROL IN AORTIC DISSECTION

**Case Example**

A 58-year-old male presents with agonizing chest pain radiating to his back. An emergent CTA demonstrates an extensive Stanford type B aortic dissection. You carefully analyze the CTA and note that there is no involvement of celiac/mesenteric/renal/limb branches of the aorta and confirm this with the radiologist on call. You let vascular surgery be aware of the patient and ask that they evaluate the patient. You note that in hypertensive emergencies, the BP should be lowered 20%–25% within an hour, gradually to 160/100 within the next few hours, and carefully brought to normal in the next 24–48 hours. You start the patient on IV nicardipine and cautiously titrate to prevent sudden drops on BP. In several hours, the patient suddenly becomes hemodynamically unstable and immediately brought to the OR. The dissection was found to have propagated and ruptured.

**Reasoning Error(s)**
- Lack of knowledge regarding ideal BP goals for aortic dissection
- Confusing BP goals in dissection with hypertensive emergency or outpatient BP goals
- Not understanding the rationale for BP lowering in aortic dissection
- Not considering relative hypertension (soft baseline BPs)
- Thinking that BP control is only for type B aortic dissection

**How to Avoid the Mistake**
- Understand that the systolic BP goal for aortic dissection is generally <120 mmHg within the first hour with associated lower heart rates approaching 60 bpm. Theoretically, the goal is to reduce the BP to the minimal amount necessary for adequate organ perfusion. Thus in patients with baseline soft pressures, a much lower BP may not only be possible but, in fact, necessary (if a normal BP is relative hypertension for them). Last, aortic dissection does not fall under the purview of hypertensive emergency and BP should be lowered much more rapidly.
- Check prior records for a sense of the patient's baseline BP. If the baseline pressures are soft, we strongly recommend considering a lower BP goal. Monitor carefully for signs of end-organ hypoperfusion.
- Understand that though surgical management is indicated for type A dissections, BP management should occur while awaiting surgery to minimize propagation of the dissection.

**Antidote**
- Not applicable

**Common Scenarios**
- Not applicable

**Notes**
- Aortic dissection is a very painful condition! Ensure that you control the patient's pain—this can be a significant contributor to high and labile BPs.
- Minimize patient movements as it may lead to labile BPs that increase aortic shear stress.
- Resistant hypertension in the setting of descending aortic dissection should concern you for involvement of the renal arteries.

## MISTAKE: NOT USING A β-BLOCKER FIRST-LINE FOR BLOOD PRESSURE LOWERING

**Case Example**   A 58-year-old male presents with agonizing chest pain radiating to his back. An emergent CT scan demonstrates an extensive Stanford type B aortic dissection. You measure the patient's BP to be 129/78 and heart rate to be 78 bpm. You immediately begin BP control with IV captopril and are happy to see the systolic BP settle in the 110s.

**Reasoning Error(s)**
- Lack of understanding regarding the rationale for using β-blockers first
- Not knowing the evidence behind various antihypertensive medications in acute aortic dissection
- Confusing first-line outpatient antihypertensive agents with that for aortic dissection
- Using β-blockers that are not fast onset

**How to Avoid the Mistake**
- Understand that IV β-blockers (esmolol, labetalol, metoprolol, propranolol) are first-line for BP lowering in acute aortic dissection due to their ability to not only lower BP but also reduce heart rate and force of systole, which reduces aortic wall stress (primarily driven by the force that the aorta receives from the heart).
- Remember that starting BP control in aortic dissection with a vasodilator can cause reflex tachycardia, which will worsen the force imparted on the aortic wall and hence the dissection. This reflex tachycardia is due to the baroreceptors compensating for what they interpret as a decrease in BP due to the vasodilation and causing a compensatory tachycardia. Vasodilators do have their role in aortic dissection AFTER β-blockade is established (ideally once HR <60), which will prevent reflex tachycardia.
- Understand that β-blockers are the only medications with evidence for reducing acute aortic dissection-related complications.
- Remember to use IV β-blockers to ensure fast onset and easy titration

**Antidote**
- Switch to IV β-blocker

**Common Scenarios**
- Not applicable

**Notes**
- If the heart rate falls under 60 with β-blocker therapy, other IV antihypertensives should be used to achieve the desired BP goal (usually 100–120 mmHg). Vasodilators such as ACE inhibitors (captopril), dihydropyridine (DHP) calcium channel blockers (CCBs) (e.g., nicardipine), and nitroprusside/nitroglycerin are preferred.
- If the heart rate is elevated despite achieving BP control, use non-DHP CCBs (e.g., diltiazem) for additional rate control as well as BP control.

## MISTAKE: NOT USING NONDIHYDROPYRIDINE CALCIUM CHANNEL BLOCKERS IN PATIENTS INTOLERANT OF β-BLOCKERS

**Case Example**   A 58-year-old male presents with agonizing chest pain radiating to his back. An emergent CT scan demonstrates an extensive Stanford type B aortic dissection. You measure the patient's BP to be 160/78 and heart rate to be 78 bpm. You immediately begin BP control with IV esmolol but notice urticaria developing and immediately stop the medication. The patient is instead started on IV captopril for BP control.

**Reasoning Error(s)**
- Lack of understanding why non-dihydropyridine calcium channel blockers (non-DHP CCB) are the preferred alternatives to β-blockers in aortic dissection

| How to Avoid the Mistake | ■ Understand that non-DHP CCBs are physiologically very similar to β-blockers and serve as the alternative antihypertensive of choice in acute aortic dissection. In particular, control of the heart rate is essential to minimizing aortic wall stress and thus a BP agent with negative chronotropic effects (β-blocker, non-DHP CCB) is preferred. |
| --- | --- |
| Antidote | ■ Use verapamil or diltiazem |
| Common Scenarios | ■ Not applicable |
| Notes | ■ Unlike β-blockers, which were associated with decreased mortality in all types of aortic dissection in the International Registry of Acute Aortic Dissection, non-DHP CCBs were associated with improved survival in only type B dissections. Other antihypertensives were not shown to have any mortality benefit. |

## MISTAKE: USING β-BLOCKER/NONDIHYDROPYRIDINE CALCIUM CHANNEL BLOCKER IN AORTIC DISSECTION COMPLICATED BY ACUTE AORTIC INSUFFICIENCY

| Case Example | A 58-year-old male presents with agonizing chest pain radiating to his back. An emergent CT scan demonstrates an extensive Stanford type A aortic dissection with aortic root involvement resulting in significant aortic insufficiency. You measure the patient's BP to be 129/78 and heart rate to be 78 bpm. You immediately begin BP control with IV esmolol, and soon the patient's oxygen saturation drops precipitously. CXR confirms flash pulmonary edema. |
| --- | --- |
| Reasoning Error(s) | ■ Lack of understanding contraindications to management of aortic insufficiency<br>■ Lack of a contingency plan for managing hypertension in acute aortic dissection complicated by aortic insufficiency<br>■ Mixing up non-DHP and dihydropyridine (DHP) CCBs<br>■ Not recognizing the signs of aortic insufficiency |
| How to Avoid the Mistake | ■ Understand that while not absolutely contraindicated, β-blockers and non-DHP CCBs may worsen regurgitation (by prolonging diastole), blunt the reflex tachycardia in aortic insufficiency, and even precipitate cardiogenic shock. In fact, tachycardia can be a compensatory mechanism to maintain cardiac output.<br>■ If BP control is needed for aortic dissection in the setting of aortic regurgitation, use vasodilators such as IV nitroglycerin/nitroprusside, captopril, or nicardipine. Remember, DHP CCBs are not contraindicated!<br>■ Recognize the need to balance controlling heart rate with preventing further hemodynamic deterioration. Higher heart rates are usually acceptable in the presence of acute aortic insufficiency because patients are taken urgently to surgery and thus significant extension of the dissection due solely to the heart rate would be unusual. Vasodilators are more appropriate given that they will not suppress compensatory tachycardia.<br>■ Remember that non-DHP CCBs (verapamil and diltiazem) affect the heart via negative inotropy and chronotropy.<br>■ Learn how to suspect aortic insufficiency on exam: wide pulse pressures, diastolic decrescendo murmur, and/or symptoms of cardiogenic shock (hypotension and symptoms/findings of pulmonary edema). |

**Antidote**
- Consider switching to alternative vasodilator antihypertensive (IV nitroprusside/nitroglycerin, captopril, nicardipine).

**Common Scenarios**
- Not applicable

**Notes**
- A low diastolic BP (and hence a wider pulse pressure) is a marker of more severe aortic insufficiency.

## MISTAKE: USING INOTROPES IN AORTIC DISSECTION

**Case Example**

A 64-year-old female presents to the emergency department with sudden-onset chest pain. Vitals are notable for heart rate of 120 and BP of 91/52. CTA reveals an ascending dissection extending to the aortic root, and cardiothoracic surgery is notified right away for emergent repair. You notice crackles on exam and an elevated JVP, along with a diastolic murmur. You are concerned for cardiogenic shock secondary to acute aortic regurgitation and start dobutamine to increase cardiac output. The BP of the patient increases; however the patient is found to have new neurologic deficits. During emergent repair, the dissection is seen to have propagated to the level of the left common carotid artery causing blockage of its ostium.

**Reasoning Error(s)**
- Lack of understanding of the impact of inotropes on aortic dissection
- Misunderstanding the goal of medical temporization prior to surgery
- Not recognizing that hypotensive aortic dissection usually requires definitive surgical management as soon as possible
- Not considering the etiology of hypotension in aortic dissection

**How to Avoid the Mistake**
- Understand that inotropes increase the force and rate of aortic wall stress that the heart imparts which can worsen the dissection. If hypotensive, first consider the etiology of hypotension (often in dissection this is either tamponade, aortic rupture, or aortic insufficiency). Though surgery should be performed urgently, complications of dissection causing hypotension should always be communicated to the surgical team (which may further expedite surgery).
- Understand that most hypotensive aortic dissections are type A and thus urgent surgery is the treatment. Your goal is not to resuscitate the patient to a normal BP; rather, ensure that the most vital organs (in particular, the brain) maintain the minimal perfusion necessary until definitive management with surgery. This may be accomplished with judicious use of intravenous fluids.

**Antidote**
- Judicious use of IV fluids
- Emergent surgical management

**Common Scenarios**
- Not applicable

**Notes**
- Though afterload reduction (i.e., with vasodilators) may improve forward flow and thus hypotension in aortic insufficiency, this should not be attempted in concomitant aortic dissection unless as a last resort.

## MISTAKE: AGGRESSIVE FLUID RESUSCITATION FOR HYPOTENSION IN AORTIC DISSECTION

| | |
|---|---|
| Case Example | A 58-year-old male presents with agonizing chest pain radiating to his back. An emergent CT scan demonstrates an extensive Stanford type A aortic dissection with aortic root involvement resulting in significant aortic insufficiency. You measure the patient's BP to be 90/58 and order 2 L of lactated Ringer's to be run as fast as possible. The patient's hypotension initially resolves but repeat labs demonstrate a new acute kidney injury. Urgent repeat CT scan demonstrates significant extension of the dissection, now including the right renal artery. |
| Reasoning Error(s) | ■ Not considering the consequences of a common clinical action in a less familiar disease process (i.e., mindless clinical habits)<br>■ Lack of understanding why fluids may worsen aortic dissection if not used judiciously<br>■ Temporizing rather than finding the etiology of hypotension |
| How to Avoid the Mistake | ■ Understand that the majority (~70%) of aortic dissections, particularly Stanford Type B, present with hypertension. Thus aortic dissection with concomitant hypotension should immediately raise concern for complications such as aortic rupture or cardiac tamponade.<br>■ When dealing with less familiar disease states, consider the risks and benefits to every clinical action thoroughly to minimize unintended harm. For example, excess fluids in aortic dissection may cause further distention of the aorta, which can lead to increased aortic wall stress and further propagation of the dissection.<br>■ If using significant intravenous fluids, perform careful serial exams and/or imaging to check for stability of the dissection. |
| Antidote | ■ Not applicable |
| Common Scenarios | ■ Not applicable |
| Notes | ■ There are no data investigating the impact of rate of fluid resuscitation on outcomes in aortic dissection. However, hemodynamics permitting, it is reasonable to run fluids over a brisk (e.g., 1 L over 1 hour) but not overly brisk rate (e.g., 1 L as fast as possible within 20 minutes) to minimize the theoretical risk of an abrupt increase in aortic wall stress. |

## MISTAKE: NOT ONBOARDING THE SURGICAL TEAM IMMEDIATELY UPON DIAGNOSIS OF AORTIC DISSECTION

| | |
|---|---|
| Case Example | A 55-year-old male with long-standing hypertension and 70-pack-year smoking history presents with acute onset abdominal pain radiating to the back. CT angiography demonstrates a Stanford Type B aortic dissection. You remember from medical school that Type A dissection requires emergent surgery but that Type B can be managed medically. As such, you start β-blockers for mild hypertension and do not alert vascular surgery of the patient. As you medically manage this patient, the patient suddenly becomes hemodynamically unstable. Suspecting aortic rupture, you immediately let vascular surgery know. Before the patient can go to the operating room, the vascular team sends their intern to eyeball the patient, but he undergoes cardiac arrest despite aggressive fluid resuscitation. |

| | |
|---|---|
| **Reasoning Error(s)** | ▪ Not knowing the importance of having the surgical team onboard for all dissections<br>▪ Lack of a team-centered approach to managing a highly morbid condition<br>▪ Believing that descending aortic dissection (Stanford Type B) does not require surgical evaluation or intervention<br>▪ Lack of awareness of reasons for surgical intervention in Type B dissections |
| **How to Avoid the Mistake** | ▪ Understand that after the first few hours, the mortality in acute aortic dissection increases by approximately 1% every hour. The morbidity and mortality add up quickly given the relative rarity of aortic dissection that leads to it being overlooked initially unless a high index of suspicion is present.<br>▪ In any aortic dissection case, always alert surgery immediately. This includes Type B dissections, which are theoretically and traditionally taught as less urgent and morbid, and able to be often managed medically. Many complications can occur and having surgery aware is always beneficial.<br>▪ Remember specific indications for surgical intervention of Type B dissections:<br>  ▪ Aortic rupture<br>  ▪ Rapid expansion of the dissection<br>  ▪ End-organ dysfunction due to hypoperfusion (e.g., extension of the dissection flap to the renal artery)<br>  ▪ Refractory hypertension<br>  ▪ Refractory chest or back pain |
| **Antidote** | ▪ Alert the surgical team as soon as possible. |
| **Common Scenarios** | ▪ Not applicable |
| **Notes** | ▪ In the largest registry of aortic dissection to date (IRAD), type A dissection carried a 26% mortality even with surgery, whereas medical management alone carried a 58% mortality.<br>▪ Refractory hypertension in acute aortic dissection may be caused by renovascular hypertension in the setting of a dissection flap that extends to the renal artery. |

## MISTAKE: FORGETTING TO TREAT PAIN IN AORTIC DISSECTION

| | |
|---|---|
| **Case Example** | A 58-year-old male presents with agonizing chest pain radiating to his back. An emergent CTA demonstrates an extensive Stanford type A aortic dissection. You immediately consult surgery and optimize BP, but the patient begins crying due to his pain. His heart rate and blood pressure increase as a result. |
| **Reasoning Error(s)** | ▪ Focusing too much on the pathophysiologic aspect of patient care<br>▪ Lack of empathy when treating patients<br>▪ Not realizing the medical benefit of serial pain assessments in aortic dissection<br>▪ Lack of knowledge regarding the severity of pain in aortic dissection leading to inadequate therapy (e.g., starting with Tylenol [acetaminophen]) |

| | |
|---|---|
| **How to Avoid the Mistake** | ■ Understand that aortic dissection is an extremely painful condition! The first-line pain medications for most patients are opioids. Treating pain also prevents worsening dissection by decreasing heart rate and BPs. |
| | ■ Understand that serial assessment of pain is not only essential for patient comfort but also preserves a therapeutic alliance and provides valuable information on whether the dissection may be evolving or in need of alternate management (e.g., surgery for refractory pain in type B dissection). |
| | ■ Practice holistic patient care that emphasizes not only providing scientific care but also empathetic and humanistic care. Take a step back and think about what additional actions you should take in addition to managing the acute medical condition. |
| **Antidote** | ■ Adequate pain control (often with opioids) |
| **Common Scenarios** | ■ Not applicable |
| **Notes** | ■ Remember, the same precautions apply to administering pain medications to patients with aortic dissection as any other patient. For example, if the dissection involves the right coronary artery and the patient suffers an inferior infarct, be judicious about using opioids as they may decrease preload and cause hypotension. |

## Aortic Disease: Aortic Aneurysm

### MISTAKE: OVERLOOKING THORACIC AORTIC ANEURYSM SCREENING IN PATIENTS WITH CONNECTIVE TISSUE DISORDERS

| | |
|---|---|
| **Case Example** | A 19-year-old male with Marfan syndrome presents to your clinic to establish care over a previously discovered bicuspid aortic valve. He has no complaints at all and does not recall any cardiac family history or that of sudden death. You perform a physical exam and do not note any murmurs besides a clicking of the aortic valve. Seeing that he has no problems and is up to date on his vaccinations, you schedule a follow-up appointment in 1 year. Six months later, however, the patient undergoes emergent surgery in the setting of a ruptured thoracic aortic aneurysm. |
| **Reasoning Error(s)** | ■ Not considering screening for aortic aneurysms in patients with connective tissue disorders |
| | ■ Lack of knowledge of the various connective tissue disorders that predispose to aortic aneurysms |
| **How to Avoid the Mistake** | ■ Understand that while risk factors include hypertension, smoking, and older age, connective tissue disorders pose significant increased risk of aortic aneurysm. |
| | ■ Learn common connective tissue disorders that predispose to development of aortic aneurysm: Marfan, Ehlers-Danlos, Loeys-Dietz, Shprintzen-Goldberg, Turner, and osteogenesis imperfecta syndromes. Other conditions include an isolated bicuspid aortic valve (approximately 50% of patients with a bicuspid aortic valve develop a thoracic aortic aneurysm throughout their lifetime). |

**Antidote**        ■ Not applicable

**Common Scenarios** ■ Bicuspid aortic valve
                     ■ Marfan syndrome
                     ■ Ehlers-Danlos syndrome
                     ■ Turner syndrome
                     ■ Family history of aortic disease

**Notes**           ■ Consider offering genetic testing to patients who present with an aor-
                     tic aneurysm prior to the age of 50 without a clear history of familial
                     aortic disease. Also consider screening for aortopathy in first-degree
                     relatives.
                    ■ Bicuspid aortic valve is the most common congenital heart defect,
                     occurring in 1%–2% of the general population. Given how common
                     this disorder is, you are bound to come across many patients with
                     bicuspid aortic valves throughout your career. Be sure to screen them
                     for thoracic aortic aneurysms annually with a TTE!
                    ■ Interestingly, aortic aneurysms are usually proximal (thoracic) in
                     patients with connective tissue disorders.

**Further Reading** ■ A great summary of genetic causes of thoracic aortic aneurysm:
                     Fletcher AJ, et al. Inherited thoracic aortic disease. *Circulation*.
                     2020;141(19):1570–1587.

## MISTAKE: FORGETTING MEDICAL MANAGEMENT OF AORTIC ANEURYSM

**Case Example**    A 67-year-old male with long-standing hypertension presents to your
                    clinic to establish care. Notable in his history is an incidentally found
                    thoracic aortic aneurysm on TTE measuring 4.7 cm about 6 months
                    ago. His BPs are elevated in the clinic today (139/95), and he cor-
                    roborates with a home BP log. You inform the patient that his BP is a
                    little elevated; however, he prefers not to start a new BP medication.
                    You decide it is reasonable to monitor his BPs more given that his BP
                    is not markedly elevated and given his age. You schedule a follow up
                    TTE in a week, which is about 6 months after the aneurysm was first
                    found.

**Reasoning Error(s)** ■ Thinking that management of asymptomatic aortic aneurysm only
                        involves surveillance
                       ■ Lack of knowledge of medical management of aortic aneurysm
                       ■ Lack of understanding the reason hypertension management is impor-
                        tant in aortic aneurysm

**How to Avoid the Mistake**
- Understand that hypertension management is especially important in aortic aneurysm to decrease the rate of aortic aneurysm dilation. In particular, β-blocker therapy is paramount due to not only controlling the BP but also the heart rate (for goal 60 bpm) and reducing peak systolic force. ACE inhibitor or ARB therapy should also be initiated given data that it may reduce risk of rupture. The goal BP in thoracic aortic aneurysm is <130/80 mmHg, and consideration should be given to reducing the BP further to the lowest tolerated levels without hypoperfusion.
- Understand the modifiable risk factors for aneurysm expansion and rupture beyond hypertension: smoking and atherosclerosis. Therefore, it is of utmost important to emphasize smoking cessation, provide pharmacologic therapy for to aid smoking cessation as desired, and consider starting a statin (certainly for abdominal aortic aneurysms; lack of evidence on thoracic aortic aneurysms).
- Develop a habit of thinking about prevention in all diseases. In aortic aneurysm, surveillance is important but so are any measures that can decrease the rate of aneurysm dilation or rupture.

**Antidote**
- Blood pressure control to <130/80

**Common Scenarios**
- Not applicable

**Notes**
- Remember to avoid β-blockers if thoracic aortic aneurysm is accompanied by significant aortic insufficiency as it will block compensatory tachycardia and decrease diastolic time (during which regurgitation occurs).
- There is some evidence derived from studies in mice models that CCBs may increase the risk of aortic dissection and rupture in Marfan syndrome.

## MISTAKE: FORGETTING PREGNANCY COUNSELING IN CONNECTIVE TISSUE DISORDERS

**Case Example**
A 31-year-old female presents to your clinic for an annual follow-up visit. She was diagnosed with bicuspid aortic valve in childhood. The most recent annual screening found a thoracic aortic aneurysm that was 43 mm in diameter. The patient mentions that she and her husband are trying to conceive. You congratulate her and make sure she is taking her prenatal vitamins. You schedule a follow-up appointment in 1 year.

**Reasoning Error(s)**
- Lack of familiarity with the physiologic changes that occur in pregnancy and their impact on aortic aneurysms (abdominal or thoracic)
- Lack of knowledge on what determines risk for worsening aortic disease in pregnancy

**How to Avoid the Mistake**

- Understand that pregnancy leads to a physiologic increase in cardiac output, heart rate, and total circulating volume that increases aortic wall stress. Pregnancy can also be associated with preeclampsia or eclampsia, which can further worsen the stress on the aortic wall. Therefore, patients who wish to conceive in the presence of an aortic aneurysm should be counseled carefully on the risks of pregnancy.
- Ask for help from colleagues or refer to a specialist (the emerging field of cardio-obstetrics) when in doubt regarding how to best counsel patients with connective tissue disorders looking to become pregnant. In general, the size of aneurysmal dilation and recent rate of expansion will determine the risk during pregnancy.

**Antidote**

- Careful counseling on the risks of pregnancy

**Common Scenarios**

- Not applicable

**Notes**

- Even without a known aortic aneurysm, a discussion is worthwhile with patients who wish to become pregnant as they are still at increased risk by virtue of their connective tissue disorder.

## MISTAKE: OVERLOOKING FACTORS FAVORING EARLY SURGICAL INTERVENTION OF AORTIC ANEURYSM

**Case Example**

A 61-year-old male presents to your clinic for an annual checkup. A recent coronary angiogram was significant for triple-vessel disease. He mentions that he has an abdominal aortic aneurysm that is 4.6 cm in diameter in a recent surveillance echocardiogram from an outside hospital. You discuss the risks and benefits of a coronary artery bypass graft surgery (CABG) for his triple-vessel disease but do not discuss the aneurysm, as you note to yourself that elective surgery is advised for patients with an aneurysm of ≥5.5 cm in the ascending aorta.

**Reasoning Error(s)**

- Lack of awareness of reasons for earlier surgical intervention of aortic aneurysms
- Not verifying atypical cases with guidelines and/or experts

**How to Avoid the Mistake**

- Understand the exceptions (<5.5 cm) to thresholds for surgical repair of aortic aneurysms:
  - Rapid growth: >0.5 cm/year
  - Significant symptoms
  - Concomitant open heart surgery (CABG, valve surgery): ≥4.5 cm
  - Connective tissue disorders: ≥4.0 cm (variable)
- For patients with atypical causes of thoracic aortic aneurysm, consult with colleagues and the guidelines to ensure you do not overlook management.

**Antidote**

- Not applicable

**Common Scenarios**

- Rapid growth
- Symptomatic aneurysm
- Concomitant open heart surgery (e.g., CABG, valvular intervention)
- Connective tissue disorders

**Notes**

- While the management of abdominal versus thoracic aortic aneurysms differ, rapid growth and significant symptoms are indications for earlier surgery in both conditions.
- Abdominal aortic aneurysms occur predominantly in men but possess a severalfold increased risk of rupture. Interestingly, data from the UK Small Aneurysm Trial suggest that rupture occurs at smaller diameters in women compared to men (5 versus 6 cm, respectively).

## CHAPTER 14

# Venous Thromboembolism

Ashkon Alexander Rahbari

# Anticoagulation

## MISTAKE: FORGETTING TO EDUCATE PATIENTS ON DIETARY RESTRICTIONS ON WARFARIN

**Case Example**  A 28-year-old female with two spontaneous abortions and a recent hospital admission for unprovoked pulmonary embolism (PE) is scheduled for a new patient visit with you to establish care. Her discharge summary summarizes her hospital course, and the postdischarge visit with the hematologist indicates a suspicion for antiphospholipid antibody syndrome. She remains on anticoagulation with warfarin while awaiting final testing results. Her most recent INR is therapeutic (2–3), and she endorses no new physical complaints at the time of your visit. Unbeknownst to you, after the appointment she decides to make healthy changes to her diet by eating spinach-containing smoothies twice a day and salad bowls containing substantial portions of Brussels sprouts and kale. Several weeks later, she presents to the emergency department with shortness of breath and pleuritic chest pain. CT angiogram reveals a new subsegmental PE, and a lower extremity venous ultrasound is positive for an occlusive femoral vein thrombus in the left leg.

**Reasoning Error(s)**
- Not understanding the mechanism of warfarin
- Lack of knowledge on dietary effects on warfarin anticoagulation
- Not prioritizing patient education as part of effective medical management

**How to Avoid the Mistake**
- Understand that warfarin acts by inhibiting vitamin K epoxide reductase, which is the enzyme responsible for indirectly activating vitamin K–dependent coagulation factors. Thus, an excess of vitamin K is antagonistic to the efforts of warfarin.
- Learn the common foods with high levels of vitamin K that may interfere with warfarin effectiveness: kale, broccoli, spinach, Brussels sprouts, cabbage. Counsel patients on warfarin regarding the impact of these foods on the efficacy of anticoagulation.
- Realize that patient education significantly improves adherence and decreases inadvertent negative outcomes. Prioritize patient education and seek help for patient education through colleagues such as pharmacists if you are limited by time.

**Antidote**
- Not applicable

**Common Scenarios**
- Not applicable

**Note(s)**
- Medications and over-the-counter supplements are also common culprits that can interfere with the effectiveness of warfarin therapy. These agents may be inducers or inhibitors of warfarin metabolism. Always check for potential interactions for any new ingestions.
- Similar to administering vitamin K, eating a diet high in vitamin K does not have an immediate effect on the INR but rather a slow effect over the following few days. This is because it takes time for the body to synthesize new clotting factors.

## MISTAKE: OVERLOOKING COMMON WARFARIN INTERACTIONS

**Case Example**

A 57-year-old female from Bangladesh is discovered to have rheumatic mitral stenosis and atrial fibrillation. As her new cardiologist, you astutely start her on warfarin and plug her in with the warfarin clinic. The patient's INR is stably between 2.0 and 3.0 until 3 weeks later when it is found to be 1.5 despite medication adherence and dietary considerations. You discover that her PCP recently started treatment for tuberculosis with a regimen including rifampin in light of a positive Quantiferon Gold test.

**Reasoning Error(s)**

- Lack of familiarity with drugs that interact in clinically significant ways with warfarin
- Forgetting the metabolic pathway of warfarin that heavily interacts with other medications
- Relying too heavily on software (e.g., electronic medical record medication interaction checker) without independent efforts to verify
- Lack of time to check for drug–drug interactions despite uncertainty ("it will be okay")

**How to Avoid the Mistake**

- Warfarin is metabolized through the CYP P450 pathway by enzymes 2C9, 1A2, and 3A4. Substances that inhibit or induce these enzymes alter the levels (and thus potency) of warfarin. However, it is paramount to differentiate the substances that lead to clinically significant alterations in warfarin level as opposed to theoretical interactions.
- Learn the common medications that significantly alter warfarin levels as shown under the Common Scenarios below.
- Trust but verify the medication interaction warnings (or lack thereof) by software.
- When unsure about a medication's potential interaction with warfarin, always check. Clinical decisions on these interactions should be based upon data.

**Antidote**

- Check INR and seek expert opinion on tailoring warfarin dosing

**Common Scenarios**

- Inducers (decrease anticoagulation effects):
  - Rifampin
  - Antiepileptics: phenytoin, carbamazepine
  - St. John's wort
- Inhibitors (increase anticoagulation effects):
  - Antifungals: fluconazole, voriconazole
  - Metronidazole
  - Amiodarone
  - Tylenol (especially at doses >1.3–2.0 g/day)

**Note(s)**

- Be mindful when adjusting warfarin and/or interacting medication dosages. The half-life of warfarin is approximately 36 hours and anticoagulant effects will continue after discontinuation of the medication.

# MISTAKE: MAINTAINING PATIENTS ON WARFARIN OVER DIRECT ORAL ANTICOAGULANTS

**Case Example**  A 61-year-old female with nonvalvular atrial fibrillation on warfarin presents to your clinic to establish care after moving from out of state. The patient has been well on 6 years of warfarin therapy with weekly INR monitoring. You tell the patient that she is doing great and schedule a follow-up for next year. A month after the appointment, she presents to the hospital with acute anemia and is found to have a major gastrointestinal (GI) bleed.

**Reasoning Error(s)**
- Lack of constant review of ongoing therapies and their appropriateness
- Overlooking the practical and medical benefits of DOACs as opposed to warfarin
- Lack of patient-centered decision-making

**How to Avoid the Mistake**
- Always review the appropriateness of chronic therapies. Indications for change and preferable alternatives may become available over time. DOACs are a great example where they are preferred over warfarin therapy in most venous thromboembolism and nonvalvular atrial fibrillation due to their convenience (no monitoring with constant blood draws), improved safety profile (specifically, approximately half the risk of intracranial hemorrhage as warfarin and reduced GI bleeding in the case of apixaban), and in some cases, superior outcomes for preventing stroke (e.g., apixaban). These benefits generally outweigh the risks of more difficult reversibility in the case of bleeding.
- Reserve warfarin for situations in which it is preferred over DOAC therapy (e.g., prosthetic valves, valvular atrial fibrillation, antiphospholipid antibody syndrome, or patient preference).
- Always discuss new available treatment options with patients. Patients are usually unaware of alternatives and it is the provider's responsibility to keep patients up to date. Similarly, a lack of complaints regarding the current therapy is not appropriate justification for continuing a therapy.

**Antidote**
- Transition to DOAC

**Common Scenarios**
- Long-standing therapy with warfarin
- Transition of care from another provider
- Patients doing well with little changes to their medication regimen

**Note(s)**
- Transitioning to DOAC therapy from warfarin should be done by stopping warfarin and monitoring closely until the INR is <2.0 at which time the DOAC can be initiated.
- While DOAC use in mechanical heart valves is contraindicated, it is considered acceptable for patients with bioprosthetic heart valves which are less thrombogenic.
- The FRAIL-AF study demonstrated in frail, elderly patients switching from vitamin K antagonist (VKA) therapy to DOAC led to a greater risk of beeding events without benefit in reduction of thromboembolic events, reinforcing that the choice to switch patients from VKA to DOAC is an individualized decision.

**Further Reading**
- An excellent review of the clinical nuances encountered when using DOACs: Chen A, et al. Direct oral anticoagulant use: a practical guide to common clinical challenges. *J Am Heart Assoc.* 2020;9(13):e017559.
- A study on the safety of switching from VKA to DOAC in frail, elderly patients (FRAIL-AF): https://doi.org/10.1161/CIRCULATIONAHA.123.066485.

## MISTAKE: NOT BRIDGING WARFARIN WITH HEPARIN FOR HIGH-RISK INDICATIONS

**Case Example**     A 65-year-old male with rheumatic heart disease status-post mechanical mitral valve replacement presents to the emergency department with nausea, lethargy, and unintended weight loss. A CT scan of the abdomen reveals numerous hypodense lesions present in the liver concerning for metastatic malignancy. Interventional radiology is consulted for biopsy, and the patient's warfarin is held for 5 days prior to the procedure with a plan to resume anticoagulation 48 hours afterward. The biopsy is performed without complication. Three days after the biopsy, the patient develops altered mental status, is found to be hypotensive to 82/45, and develops an oxygen requirement of 4 L NC after previously breathing well on room air. A holosystolic murmur is auscultated most loudly over the apex, and bilateral rales are heard on auscultation of the lungs. A plain film of the chest is remarkable for diffuse pulmonary vascular congestion. The valve team is urgently consulted, and a transesophageal echocardiogram reveals a severe mechanical mitral valve thrombosis.

**Reasoning Error(s)**
- Not considering the individual risk for thromboembolism with interruption of warfarin therapy
- Well-intentioned but incorrect thinking that a procedure with a high risk for bleeding eliminates the necessity for periprocedural anticoagulation in a high-risk patient
- Failing to account for the fact that the patient may initially enter a hypercoagulable state when warfarin therapy is restarted if not bridged appropriately.

**How to Avoid the Mistake**     Consider the patient's indication for warfarin therapy and the need for bridging anticoagulation. Is the patient at high risk for thrombosis with interruption of warfarin (e.g., a mechanical valve)? What is the risk for adverse events if anticoagulation is held for approximately 5–10 days? Develop a plan for bridging anticoagulation in the periprocedural period for high-risk patients. Common approaches include bridging with some form of heparin.

**Antidote**
- Bridge with heparin

**Common Scenarios**
- Mechanical heart valves
- Valvular atrial fibrillation
- Recent cardioembolic stroke
- Proximal and extensive venous thromboembolism

**Note(s)**
- While some patients are at high risk for developing thrombosis with interruption of warfarin, not every patient will benefit from bridging anticoagulation, and may be harmed due to the increased risk of bleeding, particularly after the procedure. In patients who are receiving warfarin for stroke prevention in nonvalvular atrial fibrillation and patients with significant risk for bleeding, it may be preferable to not use bridging anticoagulation.

## MISTAKE: FAILURE TO TAILOR INR TO INDICATION

| | |
|---|---|
| **Case Example** | A 44-year-old male with rheumatic mitral valve disease presents to your anticoagulation clinic after receiving a mechanical mitral valve replacement. The current INR is 3.1 and you inform the patient that he is near goal but that his goal is 2.0–3.0. The warfarin dosing is reduced slightly, and the patient subsequently has INR readings between 2.0 and 3.0. A few months later, the patient presents with valve thrombosis. |
| **Reasoning Error(s)** | ■ Not recognizing indications for nonstandard INR goals<br>■ Thinking that all patients on warfarin should be targeted for INR 2.0–3.0<br>■ Lack of knowledge regarding the patient, such as alternate medications or bleeding history |
| **How to Avoid the Mistake** | Always review the indication for warfarin anticoagulation and tailor the INR goal to the indication and the patient. Common indications for a nonstandard INR goal include mechanical valves in the mitral position as well as high-risk antiphospholipid syndrome (arterial thromboses or presence of multiple antibodies, based on expert opinion which varies). While you may not know off the top of your head the evidence for optimal INR goals in these conditions, you will be fine if you develop a habit of tailoring the INR goal to each patient. Other indications to alter INR goals include concomitant medications such as antiplatelet therapy.<br>■ Obtain a thorough history to ensure you can make optimal decisions for INR goals. Considerations include a thorough medication reconciliation for antiplatelet agents, inducers or inhibitors, and bleeding risk or history. |
| **Antidote** | ■ Not applicable |
| **Common Scenarios** | ■ Mechanical mitral valves<br>■ Antiphospholipid syndrome with 2+ antibodies<br>■ Antiplatelet agents |
| **Note(s)** | ■ In patients with low risk of bleeding, all patients with mechanical mitral valves should also receive antiplatelet therapy with aspirin. The evidence for anticoagulation in patients with bioprosthetic valves is less clear, but guidelines recommend that following bioprosthetic mitral valve replacement, patients should be anticoagulated with warfarin to a target INR of 2.5 (range 2.0–3.0). Following bioprosthetic aortic valve replacement and no other indications for anticoagulation, patients may receive aspirin alone. |
| **Further Reading** | ■ Carnicelli A. *Anticoagulation for Valvular Heart Disease*. American College of Cardiology, 2015; online expert analysis. |

## MISTAKE: USING DIRECT ORAL ANTICOAGULANTS IN SPECIAL HYPERCOAGULABLE STATES

**Case Example**

A 70-year-old female smoker with hypertension and hyperlipidemia presents with worsening exertional dyspnea, orthopnea, and bilateral leg swelling. She has been historically nonadherent with medications and has been out of care often. TTE reveals new moderately reduced systolic function as well as a mass in the left ventricle (LV) apex. A contrast TTE confirms the presence of an apical LV thrombus. You start the patient on apixaban. On hospital day 5, a stroke code is called due to dysarthria and weakness in her right arm and leg.

**Reasoning Error(s)**

- Assuming that DOACs are appropriate for all the same indications as warfarin
- Lack of patient-centered discussion

**How to Avoid the Mistake**

- Review the indications for anticoagulation in which DOACs are inferior to warfarin therapy. These indications include LV thrombus, valvular atrial fibrillation, mechanical valves, and antiphospholipid antibody syndrome. Always double-check when treating conditions with which you are less familiar.
- Given emerging evidence for use of DOAC in indications previously limited to warfarin therapy, a patient-centered discussion may be had if there is a strong preference to avoid frequent INR monitoring or a contraindication to warfarin therapy.

**Antidote**

- Not applicable

**Common Scenarios**

- Valvular atrial fibrillation
- Mechanical valves
- LV thrombus
- Antiphospholipid syndrome

**Note(s)**

- One indication previously reserved for warfarin therapy that now has encouraging evidence for DOAC use is atrial fibrillation in the setting of hypertrophic cardiomyopathy. Another indication with emerging positive evidence is in individuals with very high body mass, since DOACs are prescribed as one dose.
- Although the ability to prescribe DOAC therapy without the need for monitoring is convenient for many patients, in patients with adherence challenges to therapy, the lack of routine laboratory monitoring limits clinical oversight to confirm adherence to DOAC therapy. However, if desired, factor Xa levels may be checked to verify adherence.

**Further Reading**

- Excellent review of emerging evidence for DOAC use in conditions once reserved for warfarin therapy: Wadsworth, D et al. A review of indications and comorbidities in which warfarin may be the preferred oral anticoagulant. *J Clin Pharm Ther.* 2021;46:560–570.
- Cohort study on use of DOACs for treatment of LV thrombus: Robinson AA, et al. Off-label use of direct oral anticoagulants compared with warfarin for left ventricular thrombi. *JAMA Cardiol.* 2020;5(6):685–692.

## MISTAKE: NOT FAVORING APIXABAN IN PATIENTS WITH INCREASED GASTROINTESTINAL BLEEDING RISK

**Case Example**
A 73-year-old male with stable coronary artery disease on aspirin, hypertension, and gastroesophageal reflux presents to the emergency department with shortness of breath, pleuritic chest pain with workup revealing a PE. His creatinine clearance is 64 mL/min. After initially receiving heparin infusion, the patient is transitioned to oral anticoagulation with rivaroxaban. Three weeks following his discharge, the patient is brought in to the emergency department with coffee-ground emesis and symptomatic anemia and is found to have an upper GI bleed.

**Reasoning Error(s)**
- Thinking that all forms of anticoagulation (or all DOACs) possess the same bleeding risk
- Lack of knowledge regarding the safety data for anticoagulants
- Not considering the patient's individual bleeding risk

**How to Avoid the Mistake**
- Understand that each anticoagulant has its own specific safety profile. In general, DOACs possess approximately half the intracranial hemorrhage risk as compared to warfarin while possessing a slightly higher GI bleeding risk. Apixaban is an exception with a significantly lower bleeding risk compared to warfarin. In fact, recent propensity score–matched analyses (Ingason AB, et al, *Ann Intern Med,* 2021) reinforce this, showing apixaban to have the lowest GI bleeding risk among the DOACs and rivaroxaban the highest.
- Assess each patient's individual bleeding risk prior to choosing an anticoagulant. Helpful information includes prior history of bleeding or comorbidities that put a patient at an especially high risk of bleeding. The HAS-BLED score is one helpful tool for estimating the risk of major bleeding in patients with atrial fibrillation but is often helpful tool in patients treated for other indications such as venous thromboembolism.
- Strongly consider the use of apixaban in patients with increased bleeding risk unless not covered by insurance or other specific barriers such as adherence issues.

**Antidote**
- Not applicable

**Common Scenarios**
- Not applicable

**Note(s)**
- The ARISTOPHANES study is the largest retrospective observational study comparing the use of apixaban, dabigatran, rivaroxaban, or warfarin for stroke prevention in nonvalvular atrial fibrillation. Apixaban was associated with a significantly lower risk of GI bleeding in patients at high risk of GI bleeding (HAS-BLED score ≥3).
- Andexanet alfa is the reversal agent for apixaban and rivaroxaban. Idaricizumab is the reversal agent for dabigatran.
- Rivaroxaban is the DOAC of choice in patients who are less adherent as it is only a daily medication as opposed to twice a day for apixaban.

## MISTAKE: DIRECT ORAL ANTICOAGULANTS IN RENAL FAILURE/ END-STAGE RENAL DISEASE

**Case Example**

A 45-year-old female with permanent atrial fibrillation and ESRD on hemodialysis presents to your clinic for follow-up. She has been on warfarin for the past year and notes that the frequent blood draws are annoying. You empathize with her and note that a newer class of medications called DOACs are an excellent and now preferred alternative to warfarin for management of nonvalvular atrial fibrillation. The patient is excited about this new option and you start her on rivaroxaban given she prefers once-a-day dosing. A few months later, the patient is admitted to the hospital with a major GI bleed.

**Reasoning Error(s)**

- Forgetting to consider renal function prior to prescribing
- Lack of knowledge regarding metabolism and clearance of DOACs
- Assuming all DOACs carry the same usability in significant renal dysfunction

**How to Avoid the Mistake**

- Always check the renal (and hepatic) function for patients prior to prescribing DOACs (or any other medication). These are the two most common routes of drug metabolism and may significantly influence the safety and efficacy of medication use.
- Understand the route of metabolism for DOACs. Apixaban is the least renally cleared among the common DOACs, followed by rivaroxaban, edoxaban, and dabigatran in that order. While apixaban is about 25% renally cleared, dabigatran is 80% renally cleared.
- If using a DOAC in severe renal dysfunction, apixaban is the drug of choice. Understand that there is no consensus on the safety of apixaban in severe renal dysfunction though many experts believe it is safe based on retrospective studies demonstrating similar efficacy without increased bleeding risk. Apixaban dosing in renal failure is based largely upon expert opinion and small studies but does not seem to require dose reduction though some experts suggest using the low dose (2.5 mg twice daily). However, some experts recommend against the use of DOACs in ESRD at this time.

**Antidote**

- Switch to apixaban or warfarin.

**Common Scenarios**

- Not applicable

**Note(s)**

- Notably, betrixaban is a newer DOAC that has very little renal elimination (approximately 5%). However, betrixaban is no longer sold in the United States due to poor usage patterns.
- Recent evidence indicates that systemic fluconazole therapy increases the risk of bleeding during Apixaban use by approximately 3.5-fold. This should be considered, particularly in the setting of significant renal dysfunction.

## MISTAKE: DIRECT ORAL ANTICOAGULANTS IN LIVER FAILURE

**Case Example**

A 62-year-old female with hepatitis B cirrhosis and PE 3 months ago is admitted with decompensated cirrhosis. The patient's INR on admission is 2.0 and her albumin is 2.8 g/dL, and her Child-Pugh Class is a C. During her hospitalization, the patient is continued on apixaban since you astutely remember that an elevated INR in liver failure does not indicate the same level of anticoagulation as an equivalent INR on warfarin. On hospital day 6, the patient suffers a variceal hemorrhage.

**Reasoning Error(s)**

- Lack of knowledge regarding the evidence for safety and efficacy of DOACs in liver disease
- Not accounting for the severity of the patient's liver disease when choosing therapy for anticoagulation
- Lack of patient-centered discussion

**How to Avoid the Mistake**

- Understand that evidence regarding the safety and efficacy of DOACs in liver disease is lacking. The major DOAC trials have excluded patients with active liver disease and transaminitis; hence, the guideline contraindication of DOAC use in moderate to severe liver disease. Small recent studies do suggest at least comparable efficacy and safety of DOACs versus warfarin in compensated cirrhosis. Notably, a large Korean study in 2019 (Lee SR, et al, *JACC*) demonstrated a superior safety and efficacy of DOACs in patients with active liver disease.
- Determine the severity of hepatic impairment using the Child-Pugh Score. In patients with a score between 10 to 15, novel oral anticoagulants are certainly not recommended. In this setting, the use of warfarin with an INR goal between 2 and 3 is the desired therapy.
- Recognize that given the limited evidence, DOAC use is mainly based on expert opinion and patient understanding of risks and benefits. Always involve your patient!

**Antidote**

- Not applicable

**Common Scenarios**

- Not applicable

**Note(s)**

- While the use of novel oral anticoagulants in patients with severe hepatic impairment is not recommended, for patients with mild hepatic impairment (Child-Pugh Score 5–6, Class A), evidence suggests novel oral anticoagulants are safe, and for patients with moderate hepatic impairment (Child Pugh Score 7–9, Class B), novel oral anticoagulants should be used with caution, which should involve serial monitoring of liver function tests and multidisciplinary follow-up.

**Further Reading**

- Excellent review on oral anticoagulation in liver disease:
  - Qamar A, et al. Oral anticoagulation in patients with liver disease. *JACC*. 2018;71(19):2162–2175.

## MISTAKE: DIRECT ORAL ANTICOAGULANTS IN PREGNANCY

**Case Example**

A 25-year-old female with hypertension and diabetes in the second trimester of her first pregnancy is admitted to the hospital for severe palpitations. On telemetry, she is discovered to have paroxysmal atrial fibrillation. The inpatient team discharges her for follow-up in your outpatient primary care clinic for an extended discussion regarding anticoagulation. After calculating her CHADSVASC score to be 3 and astutely noting that the gender in the score is thought to play less of an effect on annual stroke risk than previously thought, you offer her apixaban versus rivaroxaban. You note that warfarin is teratogenic and that the patient would be much happier on a newer medication with great (even superior) efficacy for preventing strokes in atrial fibrillation. Several weeks later, the patient informs you that her baby was determined during routine prenatal follow-up to have several congenital defects and intrauterine growth restriction.

**Reasoning Error(s)**

- Forgetting to consider major contraindications to a therapy
- Familiarity with treating mostly older patients who are not pregnant that led to overcomfort
- Lack of knowledge regarding safety and efficacy of DOACs in pregnancy

**How to Avoid the Mistake**

- Remember that DOACs are contraindicated both during pregnancy and during breastfeeding. Though data are scare, they have been associated with various congenital abnormalities and growth restriction. While it is not possible to attribute causality between DOAC use and the birth defects in the case example, it is a fair warning that patients who take DOACs during pregnancy must be aware of the possibility of unknown teratogenic effects.
- For new and unfamiliar medications, always search for contraindications prior to prescribing them. This not only helps with learning about the medication but also prevents medical errors.
- For biologically female patients of child-bearing age on DOACs, strongly consider recommending highly effective contraceptive methods for the duration of DOAC therapy.

**Antidote**

- Contraception
- Stop DOAC and initiate low-molecular-weight heparin (LMWH).

**Common Scenarios**

- Pregnancy
- Breastfeeding

**Note(s)**

- Notably, LMWH does not cross the placenta, enter human-produced breastmilk, or cause teratogenic effects. Thus, LMWH is the anticoagulant of choice for pregnant patients or those seeking to be pregnant in the near future. Consultation should be sought with experts in anticoagulation management in pregnancy as there are several factors that are not well-defined, such as dosing (prepregnancy versus actual weight).
- While unfractionated heparin may be used, it requires PTT monitoring and thus is much more difficult to achieve adequate and practical anticoagulation out of the hospital.

## MISTAKE: NOT INCREASING HEPARIN GTT IN THE CASE OF HEPARIN RESISTANCE

**Case Example**  A 60-year-old female presents with crushing substernal pressure. An ECG reveals prominent ST depressions in the inferior leads associated with a high-sensitivity troponin of 280. You astutely diagnose the patient with type 1 NSTEMI and prescribe full-dose aspirin, atorvastatin 80 mg, and a heparin bolus with drip. You avoid β-blockers in the setting of soft blood pressures and preload dependence with inferior involvement. Six hours later, the PTT returns normal and you uptitrate the heparin drip as per protocol. However, the next PTT still returns normal. You become hesitant to increase the heparin further given the current high doses of heparin.

**Reasoning Error(s)**
- Fear of increasing bleeding risk by increasing the heparin dosing
- Not understanding the mechanism and/or definition of heparin resistance
- Not recognizing potential patient comorbidities that contribute to heparin resistance
- Lack of knowledge regarding treatment of heparin resistance

**How to Avoid the Mistake**
- Understand the that heparin resistance occurs due to various mechanisms such as decreased antithrombin levels, the critical cofactor that heparin's mechanism depends upon. The presence of antithrombin deficiency may contribute to a degree of heparin resistance; conditions include hereditary deficiencies, COVID-19 infection, severe liver disease, and the use of extracorporeal circuits such as ECMO.
- Heparin resistance does not have a universally established definition. Clinically, heparin resistance is a spectrum, and PTT levels that do not increase in response to appropriate dose increases of heparin should raise concern for at least partial heparin resistance.
- The treatment to heparin resistance is to increase heparin levels, often to unfamiliarly high levels. Argatroban may be considered in truly heparin-resistant cases since its mechanism of action does not depend on any cofactors.
- Realize that increasing heparin dosing to high levels does not confer higher bleeding risk since the bleeding risk is determined by the PTT level (or other means of monitoring the degree of anticoagulation). If there is concern for PTT levels inaccurately reflecting anticoagulation, a heparin level (also known as an anti–factor Xa level) may be obtained.

**Antidote**
- If PTT becomes significantly supratherapeutic, turn off the heparin. The half-life is short, and effects should wear off quickly (30–60 minutes). In the case of severe active bleeding, protamine sulfate should be administered.
- In true heparin resistance, consider argatroban in discussion with hematology.

**Common Scenarios**
- Not applicable

**Note(s)**
- Though heparin is a part of the standard ACS protocol, overall evidence (eight large randomized controlled trials thus far) for its benefit is neutral at best in the setting of NSTEMI. Thus, do not be overly alarmed at inadequate ACS treatment in the setting of heparin resistance.
- Heparin resistance refers to unfractionated heparin in a drip form rather than low-molecular-weight heparin for which adequate anticoagulation is typically not monitored.

**Further Reading**
- Excellent review article on heparin resistance: Levy JH, et al. Heparin resistance: clinical perspectives and management strategies. *N Engl J Med*. 2021;385(9):826–832.

## MISTAKE: MISATTRIBUTING THROMBOCYTOPENIA TO HEPARIN-INDUCED THROMBOCYTOPENIA

**Case Example**

A 45-year-old female presents with COVID-19 pneumonia. An occlusive DVT is diagnosed in the left common femoral vein and heparin drip is initiated. Over the next 2 days, the patient's platelet count drops from 150,000–100,000 and the patient's heparin is held for concern of heparin-induced thrombocytopenia. All forms of anticoagulation are held while working up potential HIT. A few days afterwards, the patient experiences worsening hypoxia and is subsequently diagnosed with bilateral PE.

**Reasoning Error(s)**
- Equating any decrease in platelets as related to HIT
- Not knowing the types of HIT and their clinical relevance
- Lack of familiarity with the timeline of HIT
- Lack of understanding the mechanism of HIT
- Not initiating an alternate form of anticoagulation while working up potential HIT

**How to Avoid the Mistake**
- Understand that the clinically relevant (type 2) heparin-induced thrombocytopenia occurs in the setting of an antibody directed against platelet-factor 4 (PF4). The antibody leads to platelet activation, which not only causes thrombocytopenia but also leads to thromboses (both arterial and venous).
- Remember that only type 2 heparin-induced thrombocytopenia is clinically relevant.
  - Type 1 is a transient mild thrombocytopenia (average platelet count of 100,000) that occurs within days of heparin exposure. The thrombocytopenia soon self-resolves and there is no increased risk of thrombosis.
  - Type 2 almost always occurs after a minimum of 5 days (usually 5–10 days) after exposure to heparin. This is because the body requires time to develop sufficient levels of antibody against PF4. The average platelet count in type 2 HIT is around 60,000–80,000 and rarely severe (e.g., <20,000). This is the type that is clinically relevant and associated with thromboses.
- While the gold standard diagnostic assay for HIT is the serotonin release assay (SRA), the heparin antibody test is completed much faster and holds a respectable sensitivity (>90%). In most cases, quick turnaround enables clinicians to continue treating with heparin when clinically indicated.
- All forms of heparin should be discontinued when suspecting type 2 HIT. An alternate anticoagulant should be used if clinically indicated.

**Antidote**
- Work up alternate causes of thrombocytopenia.

**Common Scenarios**
- Not applicable

**Note(s)**
- Rarely, type 2 HIT may occur after heparin is no longer active. Thus, HIT should be diagnosed not based on the current use of heparin but rather the exposure timeline to heparin.

## MISTAKE: NOT USING LOW-MOLECULAR-WEIGHT HEPARIN IN MALIGNANCY

**Case Example**     A 70-year-old female with localized breast cancer presents with acute right calf pain and is diagnosed with an occlusive DVT of the right popliteal vein. You initiate her on apixaban for VTE treatment on discharge. The patient re-presents 4 months later with another DVT in her left leg.

**Reasoning Error(s)**
- Assuming DOACs are the standard means of anticoagulation in all patients
- Lack of knowledge regarding treatment of VTE in malignancy
- Not considering whether the increased hypercoagulability in active malignancy alters the ideal choice of anticoagulant

**How to Avoid the Mistake**
- Understand the CLOT Trial. This was a landmark study in 2003 that compared dalteparin (an LMWH) versus warfarin in patients with active malignancy and acute symptomatic venous thromboembolism. Notably, there was no difference in risk of bleeding but a marked decrease in the rate of VTE at 6 months (8.0% versus 15.8%), primarily driven by a decrease in DVT as opposed to PE.
- Realize that while DOACs are standard for treatment of VTE, exceptions exist such as active malignancy and other specific hypercoagulable disorders such as antiphospholipid syndrome. Always check the latest evidence for the best VTE treatment option in unfamiliar cases.
- From a critical thinking perspective, practice thinking about the pathophysiology of each disease you treat and whether significant differences in pathophysiology may alter optimal clinical management.

**Antidote**
- LMWH

**Common Scenarios**
- Not applicable

**Note(s)**
- Recent data such as those from the Select-D and Hokusai VTE Cancer Trials suggest that DOACs (specifically rivaroxaban and edoxaban thus far) may be as effective at treatment of VTE in active malignancy as LMWH though there may be increased bleeding. However, data is currently lacking and DOAC use is yet to be supported by current guidelines.
- DOACs should be avoided particularly in luminal GI malignancies or genitourinary malignancies due to their increased bleeding risk in several trials.

**Further Reading**
- The landmark CLOT trial is worth a read: Lee AY, et al. Low-molecular-weight heparin versus a coumarin for the prevention of recurrent venous thromboembolism in patients with cancer. *N Engl J Med.* 2003;349:146–153.

# Pulmonary Embolism

## MISTAKE: NOT USING AGE-ADJUSTED D-DIMER CUTOFFS

**Case Example**     A 78-year-old female with stage III CKD presents with pleuritic chest pain. She remains on room air and does not demonstrate respiratory difficulties. A D-dimer of 680 µg/dL is obtained. The patient undergoes a CTA-PE study, which is negative. A few days later, her urine output decreases, and she is soon diagnosed with contrast-induced nephropathy.

| | |
|---|---|
| **Reasoning Error(s)** | ■ Assuming that traditional D-dimer cutoffs apply equally well to all patients<br>■ Inadequate understanding of what factors influence D-dimer levels<br>■ Not knowing how to calculate age-adjusted D-dimer cutoffs |
| **How to Avoid the Mistake** | ■ D-dimer is a small protein that is created in the presence of blood clots. While it is elevated in the presence of DVT or PE, there are many factors that also increase D-dimer levels. These factors can be simply thought of as factors that increase inflammation: sepsis, active malignancy, age, and other highly inflammatory states. Thus, D-dimer levels should be ordered judiciously and interpreted in context.<br>■ Understand the evidence behind age-adjusted D-dimer testing. A meta-analysis (Schouten et al, *BMJ* 2013) demonstrated superior specificity but equal sensitivity of age-adjusted D-dimer testing compared to traditional D-dimer cutoffs (500 µg/L). This means that age-adjusted D-dimer testing decreases the rate of false positives and hence decreases inappropriate CTA imaging.<br>■ Age-adjusted D-dimer cutoffs are calculated by multiplying a patient's age in years by 10. For example, a 70-year-old woman would have an age-adjusted cutoff of 700 µg/dL. |
| **Antidote** | ■ Not applicable |
| **Common Scenarios** | ■ Not applicable |
| **Note(s)** | ■ The age-adjusted D-dimer cutoffs should be used only in patients at least 50 years old. |

## MISTAKE: VIEWING S1Q3T3 AS PATHOGNOMONIC FOR PULMONARY EMBOLISM

| | |
|---|---|
| **Case Example** | A 24-year-old male with severe pulmonary hypertension due to uncorrected tetralogy of Fallot presents with worsening shortness of breath. An ECG demonstrates normal sinus rhythm with an S1Q3T3 and no other notable findings. You order a CTA-PE which returns negative for PE. |
| **Reasoning Error(s)** | ■ Inadequate understanding of what S1Q3T3 means<br>■ Taking commonly taught associations in medical school at face value<br>■ Not knowing the incidence of S1Q3T3 in PE |
| **How to Avoid the Mistake** | ■ Understand that S1Q3T3 is actually a marker of right-heart strain. Therefore, it is quite nonspecific for a particular etiology that may range from pulmonary hypertension to pneumothorax and PE. Another common cause is simply left-sided heart failure.<br>■ S1Q3T3 is only present in 10%–50% (based on small studies) of PE cases. Furthermore, the sensitivity is a mere 30%–50%. While the presence of S1Q3T3 should certainly draw your attention to investigating for a cause of right-sided heart strain, its absence should not prohibit the investigation of PE. |
| **Antidote** | ■ Not applicable |
| **Common Scenarios** | ■ Not applicable |

| | |
|---|---|
| **Note(s)** | ■ S1Q3T3 is also termed the McGinn-White sign. |
| | ■ Laboratory markers of right-heart strain include a troponin leak and elevated NT-proBNP. |
| | ■ Imaging markers include an increased right ventricle (RV)/LV ratio, increased PASP (derived from the TR jet on TTE), and septal flattening (particularly during systole). The McConnel sign, which is hypokinesis of the RV free wall with sparing of the apex, is highly specific (>97%) for PE. |

## MISTAKE: FORGETTING TO SCREEN FOR HYPERCOAGULABILITY RISK FACTORS

| | |
|---|---|
| **Case Example** | A 38-year-old female with no significant past medical history presents with acute-onset shortness of breath and is found with a massive PE. Ultrasound of her lower extremities demonstrate extensive occlusive thrombosis of her left common femoral, femoral, and popliteal veins. She undergoes local catheter-directed thrombolysis and improves rapidly. She is sent home on apixaban 5 mg twice daily for a minimum of 3 months. Two months later, she presents with an acute on chronic PE despite perfect adherence to her apixaban. She is discovered to have a rapidly growing neuroendocrine tumor in her small intestine as well as two of three antiphospholipid syndrome antibodies. |
| **Reasoning Error(s)** | ■ Lack of knowledge regarding hypercoagulability factors |
| | ■ Not knowing when to screen for hypercoagulability factors |
| | ■ Forgetting to think about secondary prevention |
| **How to Avoid the Mistake** | ■ Understand common risk factors for hypercoagulability: recent surgery or immobilization, pregnancy, medications (e.g., hormone replacement), obesity, chronic inflammatory states (e.g., inflammatory bowel disease), malignancy, and genetic causes. |
| | ■ Always screen for common hypercoagulability factors such as prior venous thromboembolism, medications (e.g., estrogen-containing contraceptives, NSAIDs, COX-2 inhibitors, erythropoietin agents and mobility issues. |
| | ■ When in doubt, consult a hematologist on appropriate thrombophilia testing. |
| | ■ Always think about not only managing the immediate scenario but also preventing recurrence. For venous thromboembolism, this includes ensuring appropriate anticoagulation, investigating and minimizing modifiable hypercoagulable risk factors, and considering low-dose prophylactic anticoagulation. |
| **Antidote** | ■ Not applicable |
| **Common Scenarios** | ■ Not applicable |
| **Note(s)** | ■ Fetal loss, particularly in the second or third trimester, may suggest a thrombophilia. |
| | ■ Immobilization in terms of flying on an airplane is specifically defined as lasting a minimum of 6 hours. The risk of VTE increases further, roughly doubling for every additional 2 hours of flight time. |

## MISTAKE: V/Q SCANNING IN SIGNIFICANT PULMONARY DISEASE

**Case Example**
A 37-year-old female with $\alpha_1$-trypase deficiency complicated by COPD and CKD IV secondary to focal sclerosing glomerulonephritis presents with acute shortness of breath and tachycardia. PE is highest on the differential given her recent prolonged hospitalization and oral contraceptives. Given patient's severe CKD, a V/Q scan is pursued. Unfortunately, the test returns as indeterminate.

**Reasoning Error(s)**
- Lack of understanding the principles behind V/Q scans
- Not thinking about comorbidities that may confound results
- Incomplete information on patient comorbidities that would preclude V/Q scanning

**How to Avoid the Mistake**
- Understand that V/Q scans depend on the integrity of the alveoli (and to some degree the interstitium) since the test relies on adequate ventilation (airflow). Pulmonary infiltrates prevent adequate ventilation to those regions and increase the likelihood of an indeterminate study, which usually reflect a 25–30% probability for PE.
- Obtain a chest radiograph prior to V/Q scanning to rule out severe pulmonary disease. Some conditions such as asthma may appear normal on CXR, but these are the minority of patients and you will hopefully have adequate history to rule out such conditions.

**Antidote**
- Not applicable

**Common Scenarios**
- COPD
- Decompensated heart failure
- Pneumonia
- Obesity
- Rarer pulmonary conditions (e.g., interstitial lung disease)

**Note(s)**
- A common misconception is that V/Q scans do not involve radiation. The test involves using radioisotopes, so a pregnancy test is warranted if pregnancy is a possibility. The dose of radioisotope should be lowered to protect the fetus, but the test is not an absolute contraindication.
- Iodinated contrast for CTA-PE may be used in the setting of true ESRD since there is no renal function left to preserve. However, double check that the patient is truly anuric as some patients (especially those on peritoneal dialysis) do make small urine.
- Indications for V/Q scanning beyond detecting PE include ruling out chronic thromboembolic pulmonary hypertension and quantifying right-to-left shunts.
- Empiric anticoagulation may be considered for high-probability PE in patients with low bleeding risk who cannot be diagnosed easily in the setting of prohibitive renal and pulmonary disease.

## MISTAKE: ADMINISTERING EXCESS FLUIDS IN MASSIVE PULMONARY EMBOLISM

**Case Example**
A 45-year-old male is discovered with a saddle pulmonary embolus with clear evidence of right-heart strain on CT imaging (RV/LV ratio of 1.8). The patient receives 2 L of lactated Ringer's but is persistently hypotensive. You continue providing more fluids while administering unfractionated heparin, but the patient's hypotension persists and then begins to worsen.

| | |
|---|---|
| **Reasoning Error(s)** | ■ Not considering a common agent as harmful |
| | ■ Lack of understanding the pathophysiology of PE |
| | ■ Not knowing the standard management for hypotension in PE |
| **How to Avoid the Mistake** | ■ Understand that hemodynamically significant PE is on the spectrum of obstructive shock. As the preload to the right side of the heart increases, the increases pulmonary artery pressures from the pulmonary emboli lead to increased pressures in the RV. The RV is very compliant and will expand to accommodate the increased pressure and volume, bowing into the LV. This diminishes the ability of the LV to fill with blood and paradoxically decreases cardiac output in a phenomenon known as ventricular interdependence. |
| | ■ Though hypotension in PE may initially be managed with IV fluids, be careful of providing too much fluid, especially in the setting of more hemodynamically significant emboli (e.g., significantly increased RV/LV ratio on CT scan). After initial fluid resuscitation, hypotension should be managed mainly with vasopressors in addition to therapy directed towards decreasing clot burden. |
| | ■ Realize that even common medications such as IV fluids (especially in cardiac patients) carry their own risks despite their omnipresence and generally good tolerability. Each therapy should be appraised to the specific applied circumstance. |
| **Antidote** | ■ Stop further IV fluids |
| | ■ Consider gentle diuresis |
| **Common Scenarios** | ■ Not applicable |
| **Note(s)** | ■ Unlike the LV, the RV is perfused during both systole and diastole. This means that the pressure in the RV is important as high pressures may lead to ischemia by decreasing or preventing RCA perfusion during systole. |

## MISTAKE: PHENYLEPHRINE IN HEMODYNAMICALLY SIGNIFICANT PULMONARY EMBOLISM

| | |
|---|---|
| **Case Example** | A 45-year-old male is discovered with a saddle pulmonary embolus with clear evidence of right heart strain on CT imaging (RV/LV ratio of 1.8). The patient receives 2 L of lactated Ringer's but is persistently hypotensive. While administering heparin, you realize that you should not provide too much IV fluids due to ventricular interdependence. Instead, you initiate phenylephrine, which has little effect initially, and quickly uptitrate it to near maximal doses. The patient's hypotension continues to worsen and he eventually codes. |
| **Reasoning Error(s)** | ■ Lack of understanding the pathophysiology of PE |
| | ■ Lack of understanding the physiology of the various vasopressors and inotropes |
| | ■ Using the same first-line vasopressors for hypotension as a reflex without thinking about the individual scenario |

**How to Avoid the Mistake**

- Understand that PE is a form of obstructive shock. This means that the preload and afterload are particularly important in the management of PE. Phenylephrine is a pure α-agonist that raises blood pressure solely through vasoconstriction; in other words, it increases the afterload significantly. In the setting of a significant PE, the increase in afterload makes it even more difficult for the RV to push blood forward, worsening the obstructive physiology.
- The first-line pressor for PE is norepinephrine; in the setting of a dysfunctional RV, inotropes such as dobutamine or dopamine may be considered. Dobutamine is usually preferred as its vasodilatory properties (especially at higher doses) may decrease the afterload.
- Always think about why you are doing what you are doing. Avoid reflexive actions in medicine—though that will be okay most of the times, you may provide inadequate or harmful care in the minority of situations that require critical thinking rather than reliance on reflexes.

**Antidote**

- Stop phenylephrine and switch to an alternate vasopressor or inotrope.

**Common Scenarios**

- Not applicable

**Note(s)**

- In an epidemiologic study of PE by Belohlavek J (*Exp Clin Cardiol* 2013), 9% of patients with acute PE presented with hypotension without shock, 13% in cardiac arrest or shock, 31% without hypotension but with echocardiographic signs of right heart strain, and 47% without hypotension or echocardiographic signs of right heart strain.

## MISTAKE: USING FIBRINOLYTIC THERAPY IN DEEP VEIN THROMBOSIS OR PULMONARY EMBOLISM WITHOUT CAREFULLY CONSIDERING RISK-BENEFIT

**Case Example**

A 70-year-old female with metastatic melanoma to the brain presents with hypotension and acute shortness of breath and is found with a massive saddle pulmonary embolus. You are alone on the night service at the rural hospital without a PE response team and immediately think about how to save the patient's life who is still hypotensive despite gentle IV fluids. You push tPA, and while the patient's hypotension soon improves, the patient suddenly seizes and has new focal deficits consistent with acute hemorrhagic stroke.

**Reasoning Error(s)**

- Quick thinking in a fast and high-pressure environment (acting without deliberately considering the risks of an intervention even in time-sensitive settings)
- Lack of knowledge of contraindications to fibrinolytic therapy
- Not tailoring the decision to each individual patient (including patient-centered decision-making)

**How to Avoid the Mistake**

- Practice medicine carefully and methodically, even in situations that demand quick action. Most massive PEs are not life-threatening to the point of seconds to minutes, and you do have time to carefully assess whether a patient would benefit or not from thrombolysis.
- Common absolute contraindications to thrombolysis include current bleeding, previous intracranial bleeding, known intracranial malignancy, and recent ischemic stroke (within 3 months). Relative contraindications include severe hypertension, vascular malformations, pregnancy, and old age (generally >75 years).

| | |
|---|---|
| **Antidote** | ■ Aminocaproic acid (Amicar) |
| | ■ Tranexamic acid (Lysteda) |
| **Common Scenarios** | ■ Not applicable |
| **Note(s)** | ■ The antidote to thrombolysis is either aminocaproic acid or tranexamic acid, which are both competitive inhibitors of plasminogen activators. This leads to stabilization of the fibrin matrix. |
| | ■ Note that neither aminocaproic acid nor tranexamic acid is a great reversal agents for tPA, but these are the limited agents we can turn toward. |

## MISTAKE: ROUTINE USE OF INFERIOR VENA CAVA FILTERS

| | |
|---|---|
| **Case Example** | A 60-year-old female with no significant past medical history presents with acute shortness of breath and is diagnosed with a submassive PE. The patient is started on anticoagulation with heparin and eventually transitioned to edoxaban. Prior to leaving, the patient exclaims "I never want to experience that again! I'd like to have an IVC filter placed." You agree and refer the patient for an IVC filter but the interventional radiologist declines. |
| **Reasoning Error(s)** | ■ Lack of knowledge regarding the efficacy and risks of IVC filters |
| | ■ Uncertainty about which patients benefit from IVC filters |
| | ■ Well-intentioned and logical but empirically incorrect thinking that IVC filters are beneficial for all patients with PE to prevent further PE |
| **How to Avoid the Mistake** | ■ Understand that overall, IVC filters do not seem to decrease mortality despite preventing future risk of PE. Furthermore, IVC filters may be thrombogenic due to the presence of foreign material and are associated with more DVTs. In the most recent well-conducted meta-analysis of IVC filter clinical outcomes in 2017 by Bikdeli et al, there was notably a significant reduction in PE-related mortality in patients with absolute contraindications to anticoagulation or recurrent events despite therapeutic anticoagulation. |
| | ■ Risks of IVC filters include difficult retrieval, migration to the heart and pulmonary artery (ironically causing a PE), and increased risk of DVT. Furthermore, modern retrievable IVC filters come with risks when kept in too long and unfortunately estimates of filter retrieval estimates sit around 30%. |
| | ■ Consider IVC filters selectively for patients with high bleeding risk that prohibits anticoagulation and those who experience persistent VTE despite anticoagulation. |
| **Antidote** | ■ Continue to assess for IVC filter indication. In a patient who has an IVC filter without a proper indication, consider consultation for its retrieval. |
| **Common Scenarios** | ■ Not applicable |
| **Note(s)** | ■ Most of the larger studies on IVC filter use are old and based on older IVC filter models which were notably very thrombogenic (mostly removed from the market). Furthermore, there is little data related to the newer models which are often retrievable (including data on when it should be retrieved or how long it can safely remain in the IVC). |

**Further Reading**

- An excellent contemporary review on IVC filters: Bikdeli B, et al. Inferior vena cava filters to prevent pulmonary embolism: systematic review and meta-analysis. *JACC.* 2017;70(13):1587–1597.

# Deep Vein Thrombosis

## MISTAKE: REDUCED-DOSE APIXABAN FOR DEEP VEIN THROMBOSIS

**Case Example**

An 81-year-old woman weighing 117 lb (53 kg) is admitted from her nursing home with acute hypoxic respiratory failure. Her legs are asymmetrically edematous, and she is tachycardic on auscultation and recorded vitals. Her creatinine clearance is 53 mL/min, and her creatinine remains stable despite receiving a load of contrast in the emergency department for diagnosis of her PE and deep venous thrombus of the right leg. The patient is admitted and placed on a heparin infusion. Her respiratory failure improves initially, and she is able to transition from high-flow nasal cannula to an ordinary nasal cannula. Her heparin drip is discontinued, and she is switched to apixaban 2.5 mg twice daily. On the second night after switching to apixaban, the patient develops worsening hypoxia and chest pain.

**Reasoning Error(s)**

- Confusion in thinking that apixaban should be dose-reduced for the treatment of venous thromboembolism in the same way that it is for prevention of stroke in atrial fibrillation.
- Forgetting a "loading dose" of apixaban when initiating anticoagulation for VTE because of the lack of a "loading" dose in atrial fibrillation
- Confusing the treatment dose for acute VTE with the sometimes-used lower prophylaxis-dose after extended treatment of VTE.

**How to Avoid the Mistake**

- Clarify the indication for anticoagulation. Remember that there is no adequate evidence thus far suggesting low-dose DAOCs are equally efficacious as full dose. Furthermore, remember that there is a "loading dose," which is in reality a misnomer, for DOAC use in VTE due to risk of propagation of the VTE in the first 1–2 weeks. There is, however, emerging evidence that low-dose DOACs may equally prevent recurrent VTE after 6 months of initial therapy for an unprovoked VTE.
- For treatments shared between multiple indications, consider double checking to ensure the appropriate dosing.

**Antidote**

- Use full-dose dose apixaban with a "loading dose."

**Common Scenarios**

- Venous thromboembolism
- Forgetting a "loading dose" when initiating anticoagulation for VTE

**Note(s)**

- In the acute treatment of deep venous thrombosis and venous thromboembolism, apixaban should be dosed 10 mg twice daily in the first seven days. Following the initial 7 days of treatment, the patient should be dosed 5 mg twice daily. There are no dose-reduction criteria.
- After 6 months of treatment for DVT/PE, the patient can be dosed with apixaban 2.5 mg twice daily.
- For stroke prevention in atrial fibrillation, the dose of apixaban is 5 mg twice daily, unless two of three criteria are met (age ≥80, weight ≤133 lb [60 kg], or serum creatinine ≥1.5 mg/dL), in which case the dose of apixaban should be reduced to 2.5 mg twice daily.

## MISTAKE: USING A LOADING DOSE WHEN RESTARTING CHRONIC DIRECT ORAL ANTICOAGULANT THERAPY FOR VENOUS THROMBOEMBOLIC DISEASE

**Case Example**  A 60-year-old female with a recently diagnosed left peroneal DVT is admitted to the hospital for an elective shoulder replacement. During the hospitalization 3 weeks ago for DVT, the patient was initially started on heparin for 3 days before being transitioned to a higher dose of apixaban for 1 week (10 mg twice daily) followed by the standard dose of 5 mg twice daily. On admission you hold the apixaban per orthopedics. After an uncomplicated shoulder replacement, you restart the patient on apixaban but use a loading dose once again. The patient soon develops a significant hematoma near the shoulder replacement.

**Reasoning Error(s)**
- Lack of understanding the rationale for a "loading period"
- Well-intentioned but incorrect interpretation of the term "loading period" without verifying its true meaning

**How to Avoid the Mistake**
- Understand that acute VTE have a risk of clot propagation in the first 1–2 weeks. This influenced the designs of major DOAC trials for VTE, such as AMPLIFY (apixaban) and EINSTEIN-DVT (rivaroxaban), by mandating a 1- or 3-week higher-dose period. The "loading period" is used when prescribing DOACs for VTE due to this trial design. However, the term is actually a misnomer in that therapeutic levels are achieved without higher dosages, and the reason for the higher doses is the increased risk of clot propagation.
- In chronic DOAC therapy for VTE, the initial period of increased clot propagation has passed. Thus, when restarting or transitioning to a DOAC after the acute period in which the VTE was discovered (generally 1 week of therapeutic anticoagulation with any agent such as heparin is adequate), there is no need to implement another "loading dose."

**Antidote**
- Use the standard DOAC dosage

**Common Scenarios**
- Not applicable

**Note(s)**
- While it is not necessarily incorrect to use a loading dose when restarting or transitioning to DOAC therapy of VTE, the higher doses increase bleeding risk and should be carefully noted.

# Hypertension

Chinelo Lynette Onyilofor

# Diagnosis

## MISTAKE: TRUSTING BLOOD PRESSURE MEASUREMENTS WITHOUT VALIDATING MEASUREMENT TECHNIQUE

**Case Example**

A 75-year-old female is seen in clinic for a recent history of elevated blood pressure (BP). BP readings taken at home were 150/87, 149/83, and 159/86. Given that the average of the three home BP readings was elevated and that home BP is preferred over office BP, alone, to diagnose hypertension (see United States Preventive Services Task Force [USPSTF] 2021 hypertension screening recommendations), you decide to diagnose hypertension and initiate antihypertensive treatment.

**Reasoning Error(s)**

- Taking data at face value without thinking about the possibility of errors in data measurement, especially in nonstandardized settings (e.g., home), though errors in office BP measurement are also very common
- Lack of understanding regarding proper BP measurement technique and the inaccuracies imposed by variations in technique

**How to Avoid the Mistake**

- Understand proper BP measurement technique to be able to counsel patients:
  - Patients should be using a validated home BP device; websites are now available to check whether the home BP device used by your patient is valid (e.g., validateBP.org); for the most part, devices that fit around the upper arm are preferred over wrist devices.
  - Patient should be seated quietly for at least 5 minutes, be relaxed, and have not exercised for the past 30 minutes. Ideally, the patient should also have emptied the bladder.
  - Patient should sit in a chair with both feet on the floor and the back supported.
  - The arm should rest on a flat surface at heart level with the middle of the cuff wrapped on the upper arm.
  - The cuff size is very important; it should wrap comfortably with room for two fingertips at the top of the cuff. If the cuff is too big, the BP may look lower than it truly is.
  - Inflate the cuff and record the systolic and diastolic measurements as well as the pulse.
  - Guidelines recommend that patients check twice in the morning and twice at night for 1 week (28 readings) for diagnosis, but as few as 3 days of home BP readings may be sufficient. Remember to calculate the average of all home BP readings,
- Invite your patient to demonstrate how they measure their BP at home whenever possible so that you can verify that they are using the correct technique; nurses are often available to help with this. There are also excellent patient-oriented materials available online (how-to videos, information sheets) on the American Medical Association and American Heart Association (AHA) websites.
- Remember to trust but verify all critical data whenever possible.

**Antidote**
- Teach proper BP measurement technique during clinic visits.
- Online tools for helping patients understand proper BP measurement technique:
  - AHA Website (https://www.heart.org/en/health-topics/high-blood-pressure/understanding-blood-pressure-readings/monitoring-your-blood-pressure-at-home)

**Common Scenarios**
- Not applicable

**Note(s)**
- White coat hypertension refers to transiently elevated BPs in-office due to a variety of factors such as anxiety. The prevalence of white coat hypertension is at least 10% of the general population and may be as high as a third of patients who have elevated readings in-office. Despite the transient nature, it is important to conduct ambulatory BP monitoring as white coat hypertension is associated with increased cardiovascular events compared to baseline normotensive patients.
- Masked hypertension is the opposite of white coat hypertension where in-office BP is normal and home BP is elevated. It also occurs in approximately 10%–20% of patients. Patients with masked hypertension have similar cardiovascular risk as patients with sustained hypertension.
- Digital BP-measuring devices are always preferred for home measurement.

## MISTAKE: TRUSTING OFFICE BLOOD PRESSURES OVER HOME MEASUREMENTS

**Case Example**

A 50-year-old patient with a history of elevated office BP readings presents for follow-up. Office BPs range from 150/82 to 165/72 on multiple repeats. However, the patient's home BP log shows BP readings from 112/68 to 127/82. You decide to initiate an antihypertensive regimen citing high in-office BP.

**Reasoning Error(s)**
- Lack of understanding the potential variation in BPs between office and home settings.
- Forgetting white coat hypertension
- Not trusting the patient's reported home BPs because you have not witnessed them taking it (including accuracy of technique)
- Not considering alternate methods of obtaining a reliable BP
- Thinking that doctor-performed data are more accurate

**How to Avoid the Mistake**
- Understand that the best BP measurements are obtained in a familiar and comfortable environment (usually the home). A myriad of factors may disturb the BP measurements taken at the office, such as anxiety (white coat hypertension) and measurement soon after walking (incorrect office protocol).
- Teach the patient proper BP measurement technique so home measurements are reliable; evaluate how the patient checks BP at home using their own home BP device so that you are confident in their home BP readings; a nurse may be available to help with this teaching.
- If you continue to lack confidence in the home BP readings, consider referring your patient for 24-hour ambulatory BP monitoring (ABPM), if available.

| | |
|---|---|
| **Antidote** | ■ Compare the average of two or more office BP readings to the average of 1 week of home BP monitoring. |
| | ■ Consider referring to 24-hour ABPM before diagnosing a patient with hypertension if ABPM is available, particularly if you do not trust the capability of patients to correctly follow a home BP monitoring protocol. With ABPM, patients typically have BP measured every 30 minutes such that they get 48 readings in a 24-hour period; BP is averaged separately for awake and asleep periods. |
| **Common Scenarios** | ■ White coat hypertension (i.e., elevated office BP, normal home BP or ambulatory BP) |
| **Note(s)** | ■ For patients with 24-hour AMBM, various societies recommend different BP goals since BPs may vary significantly over the course of the day (e.g., with activity) and especially overnight (usually lower). |
| | ■ According to the most current US-based hypertension guidelines (ACC/AHA 2017), the following are the expert-recommended stages for classifying office BP; prior guidelines used a cutoff of office BP ≥140/90 to diagnose hypertension: |
| | ■ Normal: systolic BP (SBP) <120 mmHg and diastolic BP (DBP) <80 mmHg |
| | ■ Elevated: SBP 120–129 mmHg and DBP <80 mmHg |
| | ■ Stage 1 hypertension: SBP 130–39 mmHg or DBP 80–89 mmHg |
| | ■ Stage 2 hypertension: SBP ≥140 mmHg or DBP ≥90 mmHg |

## MISTAKE: FORGETTING THE BLOOD PRESSURE DIFFERENTIAL BETWEEN UPPER AND LOWER EXTREMITIES

| | |
|---|---|
| **Case Example** | You are called to the bedside for a patient with altered mental status and new-onset hypotension. You recycle the BP and it remains 80s systolic. You move the cuff to the legs and retake the BP. Seeing a reading of 97/70, you reassure everyone that the BP is fine. An hour later, the patient's routine labs are drawn and demonstrate a new transaminitis and acute kidney injury consistent with global hypoperfusion. |
| **Reasoning Error(s)** | ■ Forgetting that BP changes depending on the location of measurement |
| | ■ Selectively relying on a BP measurement that reassures you rather than interpreting a BP in context |
| | ■ Using the same cuff size for measuring the arm and leg BP |
| **How to Avoid the Mistake** | ■ Understand that, on average, BP taken from the lower extremity often has a higher mean BP compared to the forearm (ranging most commonly from 5 to 20 mmHg). |
| | ■ Retake the BP in the opposite side (e.g., right arm if previously on the left arm) for comparison whenever able rather than in the opposite set of extremities (e.g., legs). |
| **Antidote** | ■ Not applicable |
| **Common Scenarios** | ■ Not applicable |
| **Note(s)** | ■ Arm cuffs often do not fit the shape of calves well. Be sure to check whether the cuff fits appropriately if forced to take BP measurements from the lower extremities. |

# MISTAKE: FORGETTING TO WORK UP SECONDARY CAUSES OF HYPERTENSION IN RESISTANT HYPERTENSION

**Case Example**  A patient has been on the maximum dose of hydrochlorothiazide (HCTZ), amlodipine, and lisinopril. However, in-office and home SBP readings show >160 mmHg. You add spironolactone as a fourth-line agent, citing the PATHWAYS-2 trial. The patient returns yet again in 2 weeks with minimal reductions in BP.

**Reasoning Error(s)**
- Limited knowledge on common causes and work up for secondary hypertension
- Misunderstanding the definition of resistant hypertension
- Not considering medication nonadherence

**How to Avoid the Mistake**
- Understand common indications for working up a secondary cause of hypertension:
  - Resistant hypertension is typically defined as taking three BP medications of different classes including a diuretic and BP above goal or taking four BP medications including a diuretic irrespective of BP control status
  - Young age (<30 years)
- Remember common causes of secondary hypertension:
  - Pseudo-resistant hypertension (medication nonadherence)
  - Primary hyperaldosteronism
  - Obstructive sleep apnea
  - Renal artery stenosis
  - Hypo/hyperthyroidism
  - Drug use (e.g., cocaine or amphetamines)
  - Medications (e.g., decongestants, OCPs)
  - Endocrine: pheochromocytoma, Cushing disease

**Antidote**
- Not applicable

**Common Scenarios**
- Not applicable

**Note(s)**
- Pseudo-resistant hypertension refers to BPs that appear to be refractory to treatment when in fact confounding factors (e.g., antagonistic medications, improper antihypertensive dosing, or improper BP measurement) are contributing.
- 5%–10% of resistant hypertension is due to a secondary cause.
- According to the PATHWAYS-2 trial (Lancet 2015), spironolactone is the best fourth-line antihypertensive agent. This is thought to be in part due to a significant proportion of patients with resistant hypertension possessing high aldosterone levels.
- Though it may be tempting to work up all patients for secondary causes of hypertension, it is not feasible in terms of cost and time.

## MISTAKE: FORGETTING TO SCREEN FOR END-ORGAN DAMAGE IN CHRONIC HYPERTENSION

**Case Example**  A patient with long-standing uncontrolled hypertension presents to your clinic to establish care. Office BP is 178/100. The patient is taking only amlodipine 10 intermittently. You prescribe him an additional combination BP pill, losartan-hydrochlorothiazide, and request to see him back in 2 weeks.

**Reasoning Error(s)**
- Not understanding the importance of obtaining insight into the long-term effects of a patient's hypertension
- Lack of knowledge on common end-organ effects of hypertension
- Focusing only on the acute issue at hand

**How to Avoid the Mistake**
- Understand that investigating for end-organ damage due to chronic, often uncontrolled, hypertension serves several purposes: 1) therapies can be initiated for certain complications such as albuminuria, 2) prognostic information, and 3) motivation for increasing patient awareness and adherence to hypertension management.
- Learn the common manifestations of uncontrolled hypertension and how to check for them: chronic kidney disease (creatinine, microalbumin/creatinine ratio), left ventricular hypertrophy (ECG ± echocardiogram), and retinopathy (vision change, fundoscopy).
- Always think about diseases in a systematic way, starting with prevention, immediate management, and long-term goals.

**Antidote**
- Not applicable

**Common Scenarios**
- Not applicable

**Note(s)**
- Chronic uncontrolled hypertension leads to more than just visible signs of end-organ damage. For example, the risk of ischemic stroke increases dramatically; in fact, hypertension is the number one risk factor for ischemic stroke. BP management is often difficult for patients as the condition is asymptomatic and patients do not typically experience any immediate, tangible benefits from treatment.

## MISTAKE: FORGETTING TO MONITOR ELECTROLYTE IMBALANCES WITH ANGIOTENSIN-CONVERTING ENZYME INHIBITORS/ ANGIOTENSIN RECEPTOR BLOCKERS, THIAZIDES, AND MINERALOCORTICOID RECEPTOR ANTAGONISTS

**Case Example**  A patient presents for follow-up after several documented elevated BP readings. You decide to initiate chlorthalidone and schedule a follow-up in 2 weeks. At the follow-up visit, the patient complains of palpitations. You check his electrolytes, which demonstrate a potassium of 3.1.

**Reasoning Error(s)**
- Forgetting that certain antihypertensives may lead to electrolyte derangements
- Lack of knowledge regarding electrolyte disturbances related to common antihypertensives

| | |
|---|---|
| **How to Avoid the Mistake** | ■ Understand which antihypertensives require electrolyte monitoring upon initiation and uptitration:<br>  ■ ACEI/ARB/spironolactone: hyperkalemia<br>  ■ Thiazides: hyponatremia, hypokalemia<br>  ■ No electrolyte derangements: calcium channel blockers (CCBs), α-blockers, clonidine<br>■ Always check a basic metabolic panel (BMP) before initiating antihypertensives (angiotensin-converting enzyme inhibitors/angiotensin receptor blockers [ACEIs/ARBs], thiazides, or mineralocorticoid receptor antagonists [MRAs]) that may cause electrolyte disturbances. Recheck electrolytes as needed, particularly when increasing dosages of the above antihypertensives. |
| **Antidote** | ■ Replete electrolytes as necessary |
| **Common Scenarios** | ■ Not applicable |
| **Note(s)** | ■ Electrolyte derangements need not be an absolute contraindication to usage of essential life-saving medications. Consider workarounds such as potassium-sparing diuretics (Dyazide; HCTZ-triamterene), medications that raise $K^+$ (e.g., ACEIs/ARBs), or if needed, $K^+$ supplements to prevent or treat low $K^+$ in patients prescribed diuretics. Consider loop diuretics, thiazides (especially chlorthalidone), or, if needed, potassium binders to prevent or treat high $K^+$. |

## MISTAKE: FORGETTING TO CONSIDER INVASIVE ARTERIAL BLOOD PRESSURE MEASUREMENTS IN PATIENTS WITH DIFFICULT EXTERNAL BLOOD PRESSURE MEASUREMENTS

| | |
|---|---|
| **Case Example** | A patient is transferred to the intensive care unit for septic shock. BP measurements by the cuff are labile, ranging between 72/49 and 130/89 over the course of 20 minutes. Since the most recent reading was 125/72, team decides to hold off giving additional boluses of fluid. A few minutes later, the patient is found altered and a repeat BP reads 78/60. |
| **Reasoning Error(s)** | ■ Not recognizing the need for closer and more accurate BP monitoring<br>■ Forgetting the possibility of invasive BP measurements<br>■ Self-reassuring selection of BPs with constant recycling of pressures |
| **How to Avoid the Mistake** | ■ Understand the indications for obtaining invasive BP monitoring:<br>  ■ Wide and frequent variations in BP<br>  ■ Severe disease requiring precise BP measurements<br>  ■ Inability to obtain high-fidelity external BP<br>■ Be mindful of convenience bias and obtain accurate BP readings that will help guide optimal medical management. |
| **Antidote** | ■ Not applicable |
| **Common Scenarios** | ■ Not applicable |
| **Note(s)** | ■ The risk of infection with invasive BP monitoring is lower than with a venous puncture given the high velocities associated with arterial blood flow. |

**Further Reading**
- Kaufmann T, et al. Non-invasive oscillometric versus invasive arterial BP measurements in critically ill patients: A post hoc analysis of a prospective observational study. *J Crit Care*. 2020;57:118–123. https://doi.org/10.1016/j.jcrc.2020.02.013.

## MISTAKE: OVERLOOKING ENVIRONMENTAL AND PSYCHOSOCIAL CONTRIBUTORS TO HYPERTENSION

**Case Example**
A 32-year-old female with a history of general anxiety disorder, depression, and hypertension presents for routine follow-up. She has been on amlodipine 10 mg for 6 months, but systolic BPs are frequently in the 160s on late afternoon ambulatory monitoring, though often in the 120s when measured mid-day. You astutely decide to ask the patient about daily stressors, and she notes significant stress when her 6-year-old son with Lesch-Nyhan syndrome returns from preschool.

**Reasoning Error(s)**
- Forgetting that psychosocial factors and social determinants of health can contribute to hypertension and/or antihypertensive medication adherence
- Focusing exclusively on treating hypertension with medications without considering complementary approaches

**How to Avoid the Mistake**
- Obtain a detailed history that includes the patient's psychosocial history or other environmental factors that may contribute to their hypertension.
- Treat patients holistically. For example, patients with significant anxiety may benefit from nonpharmacologic therapy or antianxiety medications though there is yet to be clear data showing anxiolytics improve BP control.
- Explore the factors behind non-adherence. This is much more important than starting more medications!

**Antidote**
- Not applicable

**Common Scenarios**
- Not applicable

**Note(s)**
- Screening for social determinants of health include the following topics: access to health care, education, economic stability, food insecurity, neighborhood/built environment, and social support.

## MISTAKE: FORGETTING TO SCREEN FOR ORTHOSTATIC HYPOTENSION IN ELDERLY HYPERTENSIVE PATIENTS

**Case Example**
A 75-year-old male with hypertension presents to your clinic for an annual visit. Home systolic BPs range in the 130s–140s. In-office BP is 134/61. You decide to increase his losartan from 25 mg to 50 mg daily. At a follow-up visit, the patient notes a few episodes of brief dizziness upon getting out of bed and one mechanical fall.

**Reasoning Error(s)**
- Not understanding the natural history of BP in the elderly
- Forgetting that the elderly are at increased risk for orthostatic hypotension and falls
- Extrapolating the core BP guidelines to beyond the intended population (i.e., lack of individualizing BP goals)

**How to Avoid the Mistake**

- Understand that elderly patients are at increased risk for orthostasis given increased autonomic dysfunction and often decreased oral intake. However, it is important to understand that even with orthostatic hypotension, BP should still be optimized. Tighter treatment does not necessarily worsen orthostasis.
- Understand that guidelines vary across societies and even within societies for elderly patients. Though the SPRINT trial demonstrated the safety of targeting a BP goal <120/80 in patients at increased risk of cardiovascular disease or in the elderly ≥75 years old, the patient population was largely functional and without a history of frequent falls, orthostasis, residing in a nursing home, or with advanced cognitive impairment.
- Use clinical judgment when determining a BP target for patient. This includes factors supporting stricter control, such as increased cardiovascular disease risk, and factors for more lenient control, such as an increased risk of falls.

**Antidote**

- Decrease antihypertensive regimen

**Common Scenarios**

- Not applicable

**Note(s)**

- All elderly adults on antihypertensive therapy should be monitored for orthostatic hypotension, especially in patients with Parkinson disease.
- Interestingly, the SPRINT (and more recently STEP trial from China) did not show increased fall risk with more intensive BP control. These data are reassuring for any higher risk of tight BP control in the elderly.

**Further Reading**

- The landmark SPRINT trial is worth a read! The SPRINT Research Group. A randomized trial of intensive versus standard BP control. *N Engl J Med.* 2015;373:2103–2116.

# Treatment

## MISTAKE: UNDERTREATMENT OF HYPERTENSION

**Case Example**

A 45-year-old female with prior transient ischemic attacks and hypertension (on hydrochlorothiazide) presents for follow-up. Her systolic BPs during the last three visits were 132–139 mmHg; this is corroborated by a home BP log. Given that the patient is fairly close to his target, her antihypertensive regimen is not altered.

**Reasoning Error(s)**

- Forgetting the latest expert recommendations regarding BP targets
- Not realizing that uncontrolled hypertension can lead to serious adverse events such as stroke and cardiovascular disease
- Bias (sometimes patient driven) against strict treatment in the face of an invisible disease that manifests changes only over a long period of time
- Only focusing on pharmacologic therapy in patients resistant to medications
- Attempting drastic changes in medication regimen or lifestyle

| | |
|---|---|
| **How to Avoid the Mistake** | ■ Understand the latest evidence from which new BP goals are based. The SPRINT Trial (*N Engl J Med*, 2015) demonstrated a significant reduction in cardiovascular events and even a mortality benefit in patients at high risk for cardiovascular disease using a more intensive systolic BP target of 120 mmHg. Though slow to be widely accepted, this was a significant driver of the latest major US BP guidelines (2017 ACC/AHA BP guidelines). |
| | ■ Even if the patient has no current complications of hypertension, treating to a goal BP <130/80 is key in prevention. Understand that the manifestations of hypertension are often invisible. |
| | ■ Remember that hypertension treatment includes not only pharmacologic management but also lifestyle modifications (e.g., low-salt diet, exercise, weight loss) and targeting social determinants of health. Do not give up on treating patients who are not as enthusiastic about medications. |
| | ■ Incremental changes are great, especially with lifestyle modifications—listen to the patient and work with them on small steps to optimize control of their hypertension. For BP medication changes, it is reasonable to make fewer but larger adjustments when escalating doses. |
| | ■ Counsel patients on the often invisible nature of the disease. |
| **Antidote** | ■ Not applicable |
| **Common Scenarios** | ■ Not applicable |
| **Note(s)** | ■ First-line antihypertensives include dihydropyridine CCBs, thiazides, and ACEIs or ARBs. Guidelines also recommend combinations of two or more BP medications at low or medium doses for greater reductions in BP with fewer side effects. |
| | ■ Some primary care societies such as AAFP and ACP have not yet adopted the lower BP goal of <130/80. Thus, it is reasonable to involve shared decision-making and tailored BP goals. |
| **Further Reading** | ■ Whelton PK, et al. 2017 ACC/AHA/AAPA/ABC/ACPM/AGS/ AphA/ASH/ASPC/NMA/PCNA guideline for the prevention, detection, evaluation, and management of high blood pressure in adults: a report of the American College of Cardiology/American Heart Association Task Force on Clinical Practice Guidelines. *Hypertension*. 2018;71(6):e13–e115. |

## MISTAKE: OVERAGGRESSIVE BLOOD PRESSURE LOWERING IN HYPERTENSIVE URGENCY OR EMERGENCY

| | |
|---|---|
| **Case Example** | A 43-year-old male presents to the emergency department with a BP of 215/113. Labs are notable for a creatinine of 2.5 (baseline creatinine 0.9). Chest radiograph is notable for pulmonary edema. He is started on nitroglycerin drip. Half an hour later, the BP is 132/85 and the patient complains of blurry vision. |

| | |
|---|---|
| **Reasoning Error(s)** | ■ Primary goal to only improve BP<br>■ Not fully understanding the pathophysiology of hypertensive emergency and the body's short-term response<br>■ Focusing on the maximal recorded pressure instead of average BP readings<br>■ Not differentiating between managing hypertensive urgency versus emergency<br>■ Ineffective choices of medications for managing hypertensive emergency |
| **How to Avoid the Mistake** | ■ Understand the proper management of hypertensive emergency. Given the sustained period of very high BPs that leads to some degree of body acclimatization, it is dangerous to abruptly drop the pressure too much. As such, the usual goal is to lower the BP no more than 25% in the first hour with subsequent reduction within the first 6 hours to no less than 160/110 (if applicable).<br>■ Recognize that there is likely little benefit to abrupt and aggressive lowering of BP in patients with hypertensive emergency, and it still carries the same theoretical risk of underperfusion.<br>■ Always think about the pathophysiology at hand to minimize unintended harm (e.g., overly aggressive BP lowering).<br>■ Understand that the best antihypertensives in hypertensive emergency are those with a fast onset and also offset so that the dosages can be titrated quickly in case of overcorrection or undercorrection. Common choices include labetalol, esmolol, nitroglycerin, and nicardipine. |
| **Antidote** | ■ Decrease antihypertensive therapy if BP is lowered too quickly. |
| **Common Scenarios** | ■ Not applicable |
| **Note(s)** | ■ The 1-year mortality after an episode of hypertensive urgency approaches 10%! Most of the morbidity and mortality in hypertensive urgency actually accrues over months to years; that is, the incidence of adverse events within a week of hypertensive urgency is very low.<br>■ End-organ damage can be evidenced by more than simply lab abnormalities! More severe manifestations include:<br>　■ Vision changes (acute retinopathy)<br>　■ Chest pain (e.g., aortic dissection, myocardial infarction)<br>　■ Shortness of breath (e.g., flash pulmonary edema)<br>　■ Focal neurologic deficits (e.g., intracranial hemorrhage)<br>　■ Anemia (hemolytic anemia) |

## MISTAKE: FORGETTING TO TREAT DIASTOLIC HYPERTENSION

| | |
|---|---|
| **Case Example** | A 43-year-old female presents for her annual wellness visit. Upon her chart review, BP readings from various follow-up appointments within the past year include 128/91, 125/94, and 129/105. Since systolic BP was <130, you decide not to treat. |
| **Reasoning Error(s)** | ■ Not realizing the diagnosis of hypertension includes a systolic BP >130 OR diastolic BP >80<br>■ Lack of understanding of health outcomes associated with elevated diastolic BP<br>■ Lack of a systematic approach to interpreting and treating hypertension |

**How to Avoid the Mistake**

- Develop a habit of paying attention to both systolic and diastolic BPs. If you have a habit of forgetting to consider diastolic pressures, try thinking about management for diastolic BP first prior to interpreting the systolic BP. This can be treated similarly to interpreting ECGs systematically (e.g., not jumping to identify STEMIs).
- Understand the importance of controlling diastolic BP. Per one study (Flint et al, *N Engl J Med*, 2019), diastolic BP was independently linked to a significant increase in cardiovascular events. Notably, systolic hypertension was associated with a greater effect on cardiovascular outcomes.

**Antidote**
- Not applicable

**Common Scenarios**
- Not applicable

**Note(s)**
- Elevated diastolic BP in young patients is associated with future systolic hypertension. It is also more common to find diastolic hypertension in younger patients as opposed to older patients, who often have lower diastolic pressures.

## MISTAKE: FORGETTING LIFESTYLE MODIFICATIONS AND COUNSELING

**Case Example**

A 35-year-old former boxer presents to clinic for hypertension follow-up. He has been on amlodipine for 6 months. Home BPs range between 130s and 140s over 80s. Currently, he smokes 5 cigarettes/day and exercises once every few weeks. You decide to add hydrochlorothiazide 12.5 mg during this visit.

**Reasoning Error(s)**

- Forgetting that nonpharmacologic interventions can be very effective in controlling BP
- Lack of knowledge regarding potential nonpharmacologic interventions and/or their effectiveness
- Receiving bias from patients requesting only medications
- Thinking that patients will be unable to handle the lifestyle modifications
- Considering lifestyle modifications effective only with an all-or-nothing approach

**How to Avoid the Mistake**

- Understand the effect of various lifestyle modifications on BP:
  - Weight loss: up to a 20-mmHg reduction with 20-lb weight loss
  - Dietary Approaches to Stop Hypertension (DASH) Diet: approximately 10 mmHg
  - Physical activity (preferably aerobic): approximately 4–9 mmHg
  - Limiting alcohol: 2–4 mmHg
  - Moderation of salt intake: 2–8 mmHg
  - Overall stress reduction: approximately 5 mmHg
- For all diseases, think about lifestyle modifications as a powerful tool
- Give all patients the benefit of the doubt. Lifestyle modifications may be effective even with partial changes, and small consistent changes should be encouraged over drastic changes. Furthermore, always elicit patient preferences—do not assume patients want to start with medications as this may lead to perceptions that physicians and drug companies are pushing drugs on patients.

**Antidote**            ■ Not applicable

**Common Scenarios**    ■ Not applicable

**Note(s)**             ■ The DASH diet is generally high in potassium and phosphorus and
                          should be avoided in patients who are at risk for hyperkalemia or
                          hyperphosphatemia (e.g., CKD patients).
                        ■ For the typical U.S. diet (~4 g Na/day), the goal is <2 g/day. The
                          typical salt intake is from prepared (e.g., fast food, restaurant) and
                          processed foods as opposed to table salt that is added during seasoning.
                          Thus, education on the source of salt intake is very important.

## MISTAKE: NOT USING FIRST-LINE ANTIHYPERTENSIVES WHEN ABLE

**Case Example**        A patient with a medical history notable only for hypertension is started on
                        metoprolol succinate 25 mg daily. The patient returns in 2 weeks for follow-
                        up, and his metoprolol is uptitrated to 50 mg given inadequate control.

**Reasoning Error(s)**  ■ Forgetting the first-line antihypertensive therapies
                        ■ Lack of understanding the evidence for why calcium channel blockers,
                          ACEIs/ARBs, and thiazides are first line for routine hypertension

**How to Avoid the**    ■ Understand the rationale for using calcium channel blockers, ACEIs/
**Mistake**               ARBs, and thiazides as first-line for hypertension treatment. Large
                          systematic reviews (inclusive of randomized controlled studies such as
                          ALLHAT; *JAMA*, 2002) demonstrated similar efficacy between these
                          three classes in reducing cardiovascular events.
                        ■ When initiating antihypertensive management, use one of the fol-
                          lowing whenever possible: calcium channel blockers (CCBs), ACEIs/
                          ARBs, and thiazides. Notably, in Black patients, ACEIs are not recom-
                          mended as first-line per ACC/AHA guidelines, though ARBs are gen-
                          erally well-tolerated and carry a significantly lower risk of angioedema.

**Antidote**            ■ Not applicable

**Common Scenarios**    ■ Not applicable

**Note(s)**             ■ In patients with stage II hypertension at time of diagnosis, AHA/
                          ACC guidelines recommend initiation of antihypertensive therapy
                          with two first-line agents of different classes at low or medium doses
                          (either as separate or as a fixed-dose combination pill). In practice, it
                          may be worth a more gradual approach including lifestyle changes since
                          most antihypertensive medications will become lifelong medications.
                          However, BPs that are very elevated (e.g., 160/100) or patients with
                          inconsistent follow-up may benefit from more initial aggressive therapy.
                        ■ Patients may be more satisfied with care and may make fewer mistakes
                          following medication regimens when there are fewer medication
                          changes required to achieve goal BPs. Most patients will require at
                          least two BP medications to achieve a BP goal <130/80.
                        ■ Notably, most BP studies have used chlorthalidone, but hydrochlo-
                          rothiazide is more widely prescribed with an assumption that the
                          antihypertensive effects represent a class effect. The most recent 2017
                          ACC/AHA guidelines note a preference for chlorthalidone (though
                          some clinicians believe the electrolyte wasting effects are more potent).

## MISTAKE: FORGETTING TO TAILOR ANTIHYPERTENSIVES BASED ON SECONDARY INDICATIONS

**Case Example**  A patient with HFrEF (EF 25%), atrial fibrillation, and hypertension presents to hypertension clinic. Given inadequate BP control, you decide to treat his hypertension by adding a thiazide diuretic.

**Reasoning Error(s)**
- Forgetting that many antihypertensives possess additional properties beyond simply BP reduction
- Need for additional reasoning regarding ideal antihypertensive regimens based on comorbidities

**How to Avoid the Mistake**
- Think through how to minimize polypharmacy in patients with multiple comorbidities by considering the secondary properties of antihypertensives that can provide additional benefit. For example, ACEIs and ARBs reduce proteinuria in CKD and provide a mortality benefit in HFrEF.
- Realize that patients with certain comorbidities (e.g., HFrEF) may be limited by BP room in the future (e.g., due to GDMT uptitration). Anticipate problems ahead of time when prescribing by setting a goal (e.g., ideal antihypertensive regimen you envision the patient on).

**Antidote**
- Not applicable

**Common Scenarios**
- Chronic kidney disease (especially with albuminuria)
- Heart failure (favor GDMT uptitration)
- Chronic palpitations, anxiety, tremors

**Note(s)**
- The following are additional properties of common antihypertensive classes:
  - ACEIs/ARBs: antiproteinuric, mortality benefit in HFrEF, afterload reduction (e.g., for mitral regurgitation)
  - Dihydropyridine CCBs: smooth muscle relaxation, afterload reduction
  - Thiazides: weak diuretic effect
  - Spironolactone: potassium-sparing, potential mortality benefit in HFpEF
  - β-Blockers: nonselective ones may help control tremors, performance anxiety (but not other types of anxiety such as GAD, panic disorder), and migraine; reduces heart rate and may decrease palpitations; specific β-blockers have mortality benefit in HFrEF
  - α-Blockers: may help with benign prostatic hypertrophy

## MISTAKE: FORGETTING TO CONSIDER CONTRAINDICATIONS TO SPECIFIC ANTIHYPERTENSIVES

**Case Example**  A 37-year-old female with a history of hypertension presents to clinic for an annual follow-up. She is planning to start conceiving. At the conclusion of the visit, you renew lisinopril 10 mg daily. A year later, the patient is devastated to learn that her newborn has renal hypoplasia and growth restriction.

**Reasoning Error(s)**
- Not thinking about contraindications for very common and seemingly well-tolerated medications
- Thinking that first-line therapy for hypertension applies to all populations

| | |
|---|---|
| **How to Avoid the Mistake** | ■ Always elicit a thorough history and think of how to minimize harm with each treatment. Tailor antihypertensive therapy based on individual contraindications. For example, women trying to conceive should be prescribed nifedipine, methyldopa, and/or labetalol during pregnancy. |
| | ■ Seek the aid of pharmacists as needed to help craft optimal and safe medication regimens for patient populations with whom you may have less experience. |
| **Antidote** | ■ Discontinue inappropriate medications immediately. |
| **Common Scenarios** | ■ Pregnancy |
| | ■ Hyperkalemia |
| | ■ Chronic kidney disease |
| | ■ History of angioedema |
| **Note(s)** | ■ In women with hypertension, it is important to have conversations about when they are trying to conceive to transition antihypertensive therapy that will not harm the fetus. The American College of Obstetricians and Gynecologists has a task force report that includes detailed treatment of hypertension in pregnancy. |

## MISTAKE: FORGETTING TO CONSIDER COMBINATION ANTIHYPERTENSIVE PILLS

| | |
|---|---|
| **Case Example** | A patient is on lisinopril 20 mg/hydrochlorothiazide 12.5 mg daily. He explains that he often forgets to take hydrochlorothiazide most days. You continue to encourage him to set reminders every morning, but he continues to forget. |
| **Reasoning Error(s)** | ■ Not realizing that combination antihypertensive pills are available |
| | ■ Not conisidering how to minimize pill burden and/or facilitate improved adherence |
| **How to Avoid the Mistake** | ■ Understand that combination antihypertensive pills exist and are gaining traction around the world. In fact, they are often first-line outside of the United States, such as in many European countries. |
| | ■ Realize that effective treatment is largely dependent on patient adherence, which can be significantly improved by reducing pill burden. For instance, observational studies show a 71%–94% increase in adherence with combination pills. |
| **Antidote** | ■ Not applicable |
| **Common Scenarios** | ■ Not applicable |
| **Note(s)** | ■ Be careful about accidentally combining two medications of the same class when using combination pills (e.g., prescribing both losartan and lisinopril-hydrochlorothiazide). |
| | ■ The majority of patients with hypertension will require more than one BP medication at some point. Based on this, there is increased interest in using combination pills as first-line therapy. |
| **Further Reading** | ■ An excellent review on combination antihypertensives and their potential role as first-line options: Mancia G, et al. Two-drug combinations as first-step antihypertensive treatment. *Circ Res.* 2019;124:1113–1123. |

## MISTAKE: NOT CONSIDERING ALTERNATE ANTIHYPERTENSIVES WITHIN THE SAME CLASS

**Case Example**  A patient with hypertension and long-standing diabetes has been managed on lisinopril 10 mg daily. Home BPs are at goal. However, the patient complains of a new and persistent cough. You decide to discontinue lisinopril and switch to HCTZ on which the patient's hypertension is less adequately controlled.

**Reasoning Error(s)**
- Forgetting alternatives within the same/similar class of medication
- Assuming similar tolerance of medications within the same class

**How to Avoid the Mistake**
- Understand that not all medications within the same class possess the same level of side effects. For example, eplerenone does not cause gynecomastia and breast tenderness, unlike spironolactone.
- Remember that patients may have a strong secondary indication for favoring a particular class of antihypertensive or respond better to one class than another. In these cases, consider trialing a similar medication in the same or similar class. In the case of ACEIs/ARBs, some advocate starting with ARBs since they are now generic (and almost as affordable) and you do not have to monitor for the 10% risk of developing ACEI cough or other allergic symptoms more common with ACEIs.

**Antidote**
- Not applicable

**Common Scenarios**
- Not applicable

**Note(s)**
- Up to 10% of patients on an ACEI experience cough due to the increase in bradykinin. If this is the case, consider switching to an ARB, which does not cause higher bradykinin levels and thus coughing.

## MISTAKE: OVERLOOKING SPIRONOLACTONE AS FOURTH-LINE ANTIHYPERTENSIVE OF CHOICE IN RESISTANT HYPERTENSION

**Case Example**  A 59-year-old female with hypertension is currently on hydrochlorothiazide 25 mg, lisinopril 40 mg, and amlodipine 10 mg daily, yet her BPs remain above goal. You add metoprolol succinate 50 mg daily to her regimen to no effect.

**Reasoning Error(s)**
- Not considering additional data behind other efficacious antihypertensive agents for resistant hypertension

**How to Avoid the Mistake**
- Understand the data for spironolactone use in resistant hypertension. The PATHWAY-2 trial (*Lancet*, 2015) demonstrated a superior reduction in BP with spironolactone compared to other non–first-line agents (α- and β-blockers).
- Many patients with resistant hypertension have a mineralocorticoid excess that may be controlled well with mineralocorticoid receptor antagonists.

**Antidote**
- Not applicable

**Common Scenarios**
- Not applicable

**Note(s)**

- In resistant hypertension, a through history of the patient's lifestyle behavior and medication history should be completed prior to adding more medications. Barriers to adequate control include adherence issues and substances, such as OCPs and stimulants, that oppose the effect of antihypertensives.
- Prior to prescribing spironolactone, it is reasonable to check aldosterone and renin levels. This may provide more evidence that spironolactone is likely to work and may sometimes help with adherence in patients who have been through numerous medications and have medication fatigue.

## MISTAKE: PRESCRIBING NIFEDIPINE TO PATIENTS WITH HEART FAILURE WITH REDUCED EJECTION FRACTION

**Case Example**

A 55-year-old male with HFrEF (EF 20%), CKD III, and HTN presents to establish care at the local primary care office. His BP is noted to be quite elevated and you astutely ask the patient to take home BP measurements. At a follow-up visit 2 weeks later, the patient shows a log of BPs averaging in the 150s systolics. His current heart failure regimen consists of metoprolol succinate 150 mg, Entresto 24–26 mg (maximally tolerated given hyperkalemia), and empagliflozin 10 mg. You decide to add nifedipine 60 mg daily. A week later, the patient is admitted for acute decompensated heart failure.

**Reasoning Error(s)**

- Lack of knowledge regarding differences between CCB generations
- Not knowing empiric outcomes data for nifedipine in HFrEF
- Lack of experience with prescribing nifedipine

**How to Avoid the Mistake**

- Understand that dihydropyridine CCBs come in various generations. Nifedipine is a first-generation agent with more undesirable off-target effects, including negative inotropy. Amlodipine is the long-acting CCB of choice for patients with HFrEF given its higher specificity as a third-generation CCB.
- Note that nifedipine is associated with increased mortality in patients with HFrEF. While the studies reflecting this were conducted using the original (short-acting) form of nifedipine, there will not be equipoise to conduct rigorous studies on the second-generation longer-acting form of nifedipine. Hence, the safest decision for patients is to use a later-generation CCB such as amlodipine.
- CCBs, specifically amlodipine and nifedipine, are commonly prescribed by nephrologists for patients with hypertension and significant CKD/ESRD. Awareness of the increased mortality with nifedipine in patients with HFrEF may be limited, and one should always double check the safety of medications prescribed by consultants. It is a team effort!

**Antidote**

- Stop nifedipine and switch to a later-generation CCB.

**Common Scenarios**

- Nifedipine
- Nicardipine

| Note(s) | ■ First-generation DHP CCBs include nifedipine and nicardipine. They also have a much faster onset of action and shorter half-life, though an extended release formulation of nifedipine exists. Notably, verapamil and diltiazem are also first generation, though they are of the nondihydropyridine type. |
|---|---|
| | ■ Second-generation DHP CCBs include felodipine and long-acting nifedipine. |
| | ■ Third- generation DHP CCBs include amlodipine and nimodipine. |

## MISTAKE: DISCONTINUING ANGIOTENSIN-CONVERTING ENZYME INHIBITORS OR ANGIOTENSIN RECEPTOR BLOCKERS SHORTLY AFTER INITIATION DUE TO RISING CREATININE

| Case Example | A 45-year-old female with hypertension and long-standing diabetes with diabetic nephropathy presents to establish care. For the hypertension, you start lisinopril 10 mg daily. During a follow-up appointment 2 weeks later, her creatinine is 1.2 (baseline 0.7). You discontinue lisinopril and switch to amlodipine. |
|---|---|
| Reasoning Error(s) | ■ Not realizing that a potential rise in creatinine is to be expected when initiating ACEI/ARB therapy |
| | ■ Lack of understanding the mechanism and physiology of RAAS blockade |
| | ■ Jumping to blame a common culprit without ruling out other causes of an elevated creatinine |
| How to Avoid the Mistake | ■ Understand that the creatinine may transiently increase by up to 30% with initiation of ACEIs or ARBs. This is due to constriction of the efferent arteriole transiently until the kidney's autoregulatory mechanism compensates. The glomerular filtration rate is not affected by RAAS blockade despite changes to the renal arterioles. |
| | ■ Recheck the creatinine periodically to assess for a persistent increase in creatinine. Typically, if the creatinine has not normalized within 2 months, consider an alternate medication. |
| | ■ Always rule out other causes of an elevated creatinine (e.g., acute kidney injury or other medications) prior to attributing the increase to RAAS blockade. |
| Antidote | ■ Not applicable |
| Common Scenarios | ■ Not applicable |
| Note(s) | ■ RAAS blockade is an incredible therapy for many patients due to its ability to not only control hypertension but also stabilize the filtration ability of the kidney, help promote positive remodeling of damaged myocardial tissue, and possibly even slow the progression of neuropathy in diabetes. |

## MISTAKE: DISCONTINUING ANGIOTENSIN-CONVERTING ENZYME INHIBITORS OR ANGIOTENSIN RECEPTOR BLOCKERS IN MILD HYPERKALEMIA

**Case Example**

A 45-year-old female with hypertension and long-standing diabetes with diabetic nephropathy presents to establish care. For the hypertension, you start lisinopril 10 mg daily. During a follow up appointment two weeks later, her potassium is 5.0 (baseline 4.4; typical lab range 3.5–5 mEq/L). You discontinue lisinopril and switch to amlodipine.

**Reasoning Error(s)**

- Misunderstanding hyperkalemia as defined by the institution versus levels that cause adverse effects as seen in large trials
- Lack of understanding regarding adverse effects of hyperkalemia

**How to Avoid the Mistake**

- Recognize the difference in how hyperkalemia is defined. In many institutions, hyperkalemia is defined as around 5.0 mmol/L. However, hyperkalemia as an adverse effect is often defined as >5.5 mmol/L in large randomized controlled trials. Most patients who would derive significant benefit from potassium-increasing antihypertensives will tolerate mild hyperkalemia without adverse effects.
- Understand the adverse effects of hyperkalemia. Mild hyperkalemia (5.0–5.5 mmol/L) is most often asymptomatic. Moderate hyperkalemia (5.5–6.5 mmol/L) will have subclinical effects on myocardial conduction (e.g., flattening of P waves and PR prolongation on ECG). Severe hyperkalemia (>6.5 mmol/L) will cause significant conduction abnormalities, leading to QRS widening and even asystole.

**Antidote**

- Not applicable

**Common Scenarios**

- Not applicable

**Note(s)**

- Consider using combinations therapy with diuretics to help offset the hyperkalemia. Though less pleasant for patients and/or expensive, potassium binders may also be considered if necessary to allow for use of important potassium-increasing medications.

## MISTAKE: NOT TRIALING ANGIOTENSIN RECEPTOR BLOCKERS IN PATIENTS WITH ANGIOTENSIN-CONVERTING ENZYME INHIBITOR ANGIOEDEMA

**Case Example**

A 75-year-old female with HFrEF (EF 15%), hypertension, and diabetes is admitted to the hospital for severe angioedema requiring intubation. Her tongue swelling resolves within a week. You work on optimizing her medications and cut RAAS blockade completely from her regimen.

**Reasoning Error(s)**

- Well-intentioned but incorrect thinking that angioedema while on an ACEI equates to a similar risk on an ARB
- Lack of understanding the mechanism behind ACEI-induced angioedema
- Lack of a risk/benefit discussion on ARB use with the patient

**How to Avoid the Mistake**

- Understand that ACEI angioedema is mediated by elevated bradykinin and substance P levels, which lead to vasodilation and plasma extravasation. Since ARBs are not associated with increased bradykinin or substance P levels, this risk is less likely (ranging in studies from 0%–9%). Notably, many other medications that are commonly used, such as NSAIDs, also carry a risk of angioedema.
- Discuss the risks and benefits of trialing an ARB with the patient. This is particularly important in patients who have secondary indications for RAAS blockade beyond simple hypertension. Patients with a history of angioedema with an ACEI can start an ARB 6 weeks after ACEI is discontinued.
- Consider initiating an ARB in the inpatient setting, though angioedema can develop any time after initiation, including months to years out. Provide the patient with ample precautions on what to do if they experience angioedema.

**Antidote**

- Not applicable

**Common Scenarios**

- ACEIs
- Aliskiren (direct renin inhibitor)

**Note(s)**

- The risk of angioedema is similar between ACEIs and Aliskiren. Notably, both medications increase bradykinin and substance P levels.

## MISTAKE: USING THIAZIDES IN SIGNIFICANT RENAL DYSFUNCTION

**Case Example**

A patient with Stage V CKD (not yet on dialysis) and hypertension continues to be above her BP goal of <130/80 despite being on amlodipine 10 mg and lisinopril 20 mg daily. The patient's family verifies good medication adherence. You decide to add hydrochlorothiazide 25 mg to no effect.

**Reasoning Error(s)**

- Forgetting that thiazide efficacy depends on renal function
- Choosing first-line antihypertensives blindly simply based on the fact that they are first line

**How to Avoid the Mistake**

- Understand that thiazides are believed to be dependent on good renal function for their antihypertensive effects. As the GFR decreases, the less effective thiazides become.
- Avoid thiazides for hypertension in significant renal dysfunction if other options are available. If options are limited, consider an empiric trial but pay careful attention to determine if it is working (via other nonrenal mechanisms).
- Always think about appropriateness of medications, including efficacy and side effects, each time you prescribe regardless of whether it is a "first-line" therapy or not. Remember that first line does not necessarily mean best for every patient.

**Antidote**

- Not applicable

**Common Scenarios**

- Not applicable

| | |
|---|---|
| **Note(s)** | ■ Note that new evidence from the CLICK trial suggests that thiazides (particularly chlorthalidone) may retain reasonable antihypertensive efficacy even in advanced renal dysfunction, likely through nondiuretic mechanisms. |
| **Further Reading** | ■ The CLICK trial mentioned above is an interesting read: Agarwal R, et al. Chlorthalidone for hypertension in advanced chronic kidney disease. *N Engl J Med.* 2021;385:2507–2519. |

## MISTAKE: FORGETTING TO OPTIMIZE INTRAVASCULAR VOLUME TO TREAT HYPERTENSION

| | |
|---|---|
| **Case Example** | A 73-year-old female with hypertension and end-stage renal disease presents with hypertensive emergency to 205/114. Nitroglycerin drip is initiated but has little effect. You inquire when her last dialysis session was, and she notes that it was 5 days ago. The patient is urgently initiated on dialysis with aggressive volume removal and her BP soon improves. |
| **Reasoning Error(s)** | ■ Only thinking about antihypertensives as management for hypertension<br>■ Forgetting to assess for the etiology of hypertension |
| **How to Avoid the Mistake** | ■ Always think about the etiology of hypertension. Is the patient volume overloaded? Are they in an adrenergically driven state (e.g., ingestions such as amphetamines or cocaine)?<br>■ Understand that, if volume overloaded, removing volume is an effective means of controlling BP. The excess intravascular volume can lead to significant hypertension! |
| **Antidote** | ■ Offload volume |
| **Common Scenarios** | ■ End stage renal disease or advanced CKD |
| **Note(s)** | ■ Patients who are prone to volume overload (e.g., ESRD) are also unfortunately limited in their use of certain antihypertensives. Commonly used medications in ESRD or significant CKD include hydralazine, long or medium duration nitrates, and CCBs. |

## MISTAKE: NOT SCREENING FOR COMMON MEDICATIONS THAT ANTAGONIZE ANTIHYPERTENSIVES

| | |
|---|---|
| **Case Example** | A 25-year-old patient with a history of attention deficit hyperactivity disorder comes to the ED with BP of 207/120 with headaches. She is treated with an IV nicardipine drip and then discharged two days later on a new oral antihypertensive regimen. She presents to the ED one week later with BP 220/120 and headaches. |
| **Reasoning Error(s)** | ■ Lack of identification of the etiology of hypertension<br>■ Forgetting that common medications can lead to hypertension and/or antagonize the efficacy of antihypertensives<br>■ Not considering common medications that raise BP<br>■ Overlooking clues that argue against primary hypertension (e.g., young age) |

| How to Avoid the Mistake | ■ Understand that common medications may antagonize BP control. These include sympathomimetics (e.g., methylphenidate i.e. Adderall, antihistamines), decongestants (e.g., pseudoephedrine), NSAIDs, oral contraceptives, and recreational drugs (amphetamines, cocaine).<br>■ Always assess for the etiology of hypertension. These include ingestions and medications, adherence patterns, volume status, and family history. Be wary of diagnosing essential hypertension in younger patients without a significant family history. |
|---|---|
| Antidote | ■ Discontinue offending agents as able |
| Common Scenarios | ■ Sympathomimetics<br>■ Decongestants (pseudoephedrine)<br>■ NSAIDs<br>■ Recreational drugs (amphetamines, cocaine)<br>■ Oral contraceptives<br>■ Venlafaxine |
| Note(s) | ■ NSAIDs antagonize antihypertensives by several mechanisms such as decreasing kidney function and thus decreasing the effect of certain antihypertensives such as ACEIs and ARBs. |

## MISTAKE: FORGETTING TO DE-ESCALATE ANTIHYPERTENSIVES AS ABLE

| Case Example | A 48-year-old male is seen in clinic for routine follow-up of his Stage I hypertension. Over the past few months his BP has been under than 120/80 mmHg. He has been on amlodipine 10 mg daily throughout this entire time, has reduced his salt intake, and lost over 20 pounds. You congratulate the patient on all his progress and conclude the visit. |
|---|---|
| Reasoning Error(s) | ■ Forgetting to constantly reassess whether a therapy is needed<br>■ Not realizing that with improved lifestyle, BP may improve<br>■ Fear of trial and error approach to hypertension management |
| How to Avoid the Mistake | ■ Remember that in addition to prescribing medications, stopping medications appropriately is just as important. Assess for changes in the patient that may allow for de-escalation of medications—polypharmacy is a huge issue especially in geriatric patients! On the other hand, younger patients have stronger preferences to be on fewer medications and may often discontinue prematurely.<br>■ Understand that lifestyle modifications are an evidence-based and effective method of reducing BP.<br>■ Understand that the detrimental effects of hypertension result over years and that brief discontinuation of a medication to see if the patient does not need it anymore is worthwhile. In the worst-case scenario, having brief hypertension is unlikely to impact long-term outcomes.<br>■ Encourage patients to be more engaged in their healthcare. Home BP monitoring can be useful for patients to test the benefit of their lifestyle changes and/or medication adherence, but also for helping to bring up the possibility of de-escalating antihypertensive medications. |

| | | |
|---|---|---|
| **Antidote** | ■ | Not applicable |
| **Common Scenarios** | ■ | Not applicable |
| **Note(s)** | ■ | Calculate the ASCVD risk in all adults with Stage I hypertension; if the ASCVD risk <10%, then patients can be managed on nonpharmacologic therapy (e.g., lifestyle modification) and then return to clinic in 3–6 months for BP evaluation. |

## MISTAKE: USING NITROGLYCERIN DRIP IN HYPERTENSIVE URGENCY OR EMERGENCY WITHOUT VOLUME OVERLOAD

| | | |
|---|---|---|
| **Case Example** | | A 63-year-old female with hypertension presents to the ED with a BP 231/125 in the setting of missing her home antihypertensive medications. Labs are notable for a Cr 2.5 (baseline Cr 0.7). Chest imaging shows no evidence of pulmonary edema. You start her on IV nitroglycerin for hypertensive emergency, but her BP hardly improves despite near maximal doses. |
| **Reasoning Error(s)** | ■ | Lack of understanding the mechanism of nitroglycerin in BP control |
| | ■ | Not knowing the etiology of hypertension |
| **How to Avoid the Mistake** | ■ | Understand that nitroglycerin is primarily a venodilator, meaning that it is most effective for reducing BP in patients with volume overload (due to expansion of the venous capacitance). At very high doses, nitroglycerin also has arterial-dilating properties but this pales in comparison to some other common antihypertensives such as nicardipine and nitroprusside. |
| | ■ | Perform a thorough history and physical to ascertain the most likely etiology of hypertension. This will guide you in selecting the most appropriate antihypertensive. |
| **Antidote** | ■ | Switch to another antihypertensive that works well regardless of volume status |
| **Common Scenarios** | ■ | Not applicable |
| **Note(s)** | ■ | A single 0.4-mg nitroglycerin tablet is equivalent to 400 μg (often the max) dose of nitroglycerin drip. Thus, a nitroglycerin tablet can have quite a strong antihypertensive effect in patients who are susceptible, such as those with preload dependence. |

Note: Page numbers followed by '*f*' indicate figures, and '*t*' indicate tables.